Complementary
Therapies in
Maternity Care

by the same author

Aromatherapy in Midwifery Practice
ISBN 978 1 84819 288 1
eISBN 978 0 85701 235 7

Complementary Therapies in Maternity Care

AN EVIDENCE-BASED APPROACH

Denise Tiran

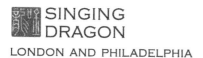

SINGING
DRAGON

LONDON AND PHILADELPHIA

Table 3.3, 7.3, and 8.1 copyright © Expectancy 2014.
Table 4.2 and 7.2 and Box 8.1 copyright © Expectancy 2017.

First published in 2018
by Jessica Kingsley Publishers
73 Collier Street
London N1 9BE, UK
and
400 Market Street, Suite 400
Philadelphia, PA 19106, USA

www.jkp.com

Library of Congress Cataloging in Publication Data
A CIP catalog record for this book is available from the Library of Congress

British Library Cataloguing in Publication Data
A CIP catalogue record for this book is available from the British Library

ISBN 978 1 84819 328 4
eISBN 978 0 85701 284 5

Printed and bound by CPI Group (UK) Ltd, Croydon, CR0 4YY

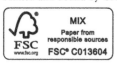

As always, this book is dedicated to my wonderful son, Adam, who is currently working in the African music industry in our beloved South Africa. I miss you. You make it all worthwhile.

Contents

Acknowledgements

I would like to thank, once again, my editor, Claire Wilson, for her help and support with this latest book. It has been particularly difficult to find time to work on the manuscript as my business has grown phenomenally in the past two years and Claire has been very supportive in allowing me the extra time needed to finish the book. Thanks too for all the years we have worked together.

I am immensely grateful to my colleagues and business associates who have offered opportunities to sound out my ideas, who have taken some of my teaching load to enable me to free up some time and who have, on occasion, provided tea and sympathy. You know who you are. Thanks especially to Michelle Weston for reading the manuscript and sharing her experiences of setting up a post-dates pregnancy clinic, and to Cassie Marnoch, who deserves praise for tackling the mammoth task of sorting out the references for me. My Administrator at Expectancy, Anoushka Lucas Howells, has been extremely patient in dealing with matters "back at base" whilst allowing me time to write. Jo Bell and Alex Gwinnell, members of my regular business mentoring group, have offered perceptive thoughts on managing workload and a forum to offload when things got tough. Thanks also to my best friend, Alina Rennie, now living in Glasgow, for hospitality (and wine) when I needed to escape the office in London to crack on with the writing.

Thanks go to all the midwives and students who have attended Expectancy courses, others whom I have met at conferences and other national and international events, as well as to those whom I have not met in person but who have connected with me on social media. Your continuing support and insightful questions and reflections have contributed to the content of the book and enabled me to remain enthused about the subject in difficult times.

Preface

Having only just finished my previous book, *Aromatherapy in Midwifery Practice* (2016a), I somewhat rashly decided to start on this one almost immediately. I have been contributing to the literature on the specialised subject of "complementary therapies in midwifery" since the early 1990s, both through my textbooks and numerous journal papers and via the research projects and conferences in which I have been involved.

I have been very lucky to have been in the right place at the right time, becoming immersed in this clinical field since the early 1980s at a time when complementary medicine was just emerging into the public's consciousness and, over the next two decades, evolving into a specialism in its own right. I was fortunate to have the opportunity to train fully in several therapies, including reflex zone therapy, massage and aromatherapy and to undertake courses specific to midwifery in acupuncture, moxibustion and clinical hypnosis. I have also studied aspects of herbal medicine, homeopathy and Bach flower remedies related to pregnancy and birth. I now have over 35 years' clinical and academic experience in the subject of complementary therapies in midwifery.

Whilst working at the University of Greenwich as a principal lecturer in midwifery in the early 1990s, I was given the opportunity to develop and manage a Bachelor of Science honours degree on complementary medicine. This had evolved from a post-registration module on complementary therapies for midwives and nurses to a Diploma in Higher Education in complementary therapies and finally to a full degree programme, which I managed for 14 years.

As part of this work I established a complementary therapy antenatal teaching clinic at one of the maternity units in southeast London where our student midwives undertook their clinical practice. In order to provide an equitable service the clinic did not offer relaxation treatments; women had to be referred by their own midwives for specific indications such as sickness, backache, breech presentation, post-dates pregnancy and other issues. I treated almost 6000 women over the ten years during which the clinic ran, using an approach in which aspects of several therapies were often combined and women were encouraged to make choices about the therapies they most preferred to receive or self-administer. The clinic had many visitors: midwives, students, even obstetricians, both from around the UK and occasionally from overseas. It gained a reputation as an example of how complementary therapies can be integrated into mainstream healthcare. I was very proud that my work in the clinic was "highly commended" in the Prince of Wales' Awards for Healthcare in London in 2001.

As a university lecturer I was also able to engage in research on my specialist subject, including studies on the self-help strategies used by women for nausea and vomiting in pregnancy (my other specialist interest), a Department of Health-funded project investigating continuing professional development amongst complementary therapists and a study exploring the potential of reflex zone therapy (reflexology) to predict stages of the menstrual cycle. More recently, I have acted as a consultant on a study exploring the use of acupressure for primigravidae with post-dates pregnancy (Gregson et al. 2015). My Masters in Health Research focused on the safety of aromatherapy in pregnancy and childbirth, a subject I have researched, lectured in and written about extensively over the past 25 years.

In 2004 I left the University of Greenwich and set up Expectancy, an education company that provides accredited courses for midwives and student midwives on the safety of complementary therapies in pregnancy and childbirth. Since then I have taught over 2500 midwives, student midwives, doulas, antenatal teachers and therapists on aspects of maternity complementary medicine. I have assisted over 40 maternity units in the UK to establish complementary therapy services, particularly aromatherapy, as well as several units overseas, in Italy, Iceland, Malta, Hong Kong, Japan and elsewhere.

I first started writing on the subject of maternity complementary therapies in 1988 and my first textbook was published in 1993, with a second edition in 2000. This was a multi-contributed book, *Complementary Therapies for Pregnancy and Childbirth* (Tiran and Mack 2000), exploring several different therapies that were popular at the time and applying the principles to pregnancy, birth and postnatal care. *Clinical Aromatherapy for Pregnancy and Childbirth* followed shortly afterwards, with a second edition in 2000 (Tiran 2000). *Reflexology in Pregnancy and Childbirth* (Tiran 2010b) and two editions of *Clinical Reflexology* (with Peter Mackereth) were published in the early 2000s (Tiran and Mackereth 2010), as well as *Nausea and Vomiting in Pregnancy: An Integrated Approach to Care* in 2004 (Tiran 2004). I have also contributed chapters in *Mayes' Midwifery* (Macdonald 2011) and *Myles' Textbook for Midwives* (Fraser 2009). The main focus of the numerous journal papers I have written has always been safety and professional accountability, especially for midwives. Since the late 1990s I have also updated *Bailliere's Midwives' Dictionary* (Elsevier) with my fifth revision published in May 2017 (Tiran 2017).

I am not attempting here to provide readers with my curriculum vitae, nor do I recount my experiences because I want to boast. I only wish to demonstrate how the subject material has developed into a specialist area and I like to think that I have been instrumental in putting the subject of "complementary therapies in midwifery practice" on the map. However, despite the huge increase in interest amongst pregnant and labouring women in the use of complementary therapies and natural remedies, and the corresponding demand from midwives and other maternity caregivers for good quality education on the subject, I have not yet accomplished everything I need to do. The nature of the subject matter means that many people perceive it as being an unimportant side-line or an enjoyable but expensive luxury that the over-stretched maternity services can ill afford to condone. The inference that "natural" equates to "safe" trivialises the inherent power – both in terms of beneficial and possible adverse effects – of the many different complementary disciplines. This is especially noticeable in relation to the use of aromatherapy in pregnancy and labour, with numerous examples of women experiencing problems such as fetal distress, hypertonic uterine action in labour or apparently idiopathic preterm labour from inadvertent misuse of natural remedies including essential oils.

I have campaigned for many years to encourage midwifery lecturers to include the subject in the pre-registration education curriculum for those preparing to become midwives. However, provision remains ad hoc and largely results from the enthusiasm of a few interested individuals who incorporate a session on the subject for small groups of students. So much emphasis is put on safety in conventional maternity care, in terms of managing risk, helping women with complex needs and avoiding litigation, that there is little time to focus on what is seen, at best, as merely a relaxing adjunct to care or, worse, a placebo effect. Conversely, in spite of the possible risks of inappropriate use of complementary therapies and natural remedies, the adverse effects of which are increasingly evident in clinical practice, the Nursing and Midwifery Council still declines to recognise that this is an essential subject that must now be included in the training of midwives.

I do not believe that midwives, at the point of registration, should necessarily be able to practise one or more complementary therapies, apart perhaps from using massage in labour. They require an understanding of the complex issues relating to inappropriate use of complementary therapies, both by expectant mothers and by midwives. The Nursing and Midwifery Council (NMC), in its *Standards for Pre-registration Midwifery Education* (medicines management) (2009), actually requires students to be able to "advise women on over-the-counter natural remedies such as raspberry leaf tea" and to "refer appropriately to a complementary practitioner". Unfortunately, it is rare that students receive appropriate education on the subject because of a lack of midwifery lecturers with the relevant knowledge and clinical experience, meaning that they will be unable to achieve this outcome at the point of registration. As this book goes to press, consultations are underway to revise the *Standards for Pre-registration Midwifery Education*, so it remains to be seen whether or not the NMC will appreciate the need to include the subject of complementary therapies in its new standards.

Yet we know that many women – estimated to be as many as 90 per cent in some areas – are accessing complementary therapies and self-administering natural remedies during their pregnancies and the births of their babies, sometimes with disastrous effects. This alone should alert the midwifery profession to the need to appreciate the benefits and the risks of complementary therapies and natural remedies. Midwives, doulas and antenatal teachers can find themselves in an invidious position when confronted with women using different therapies or requesting information, and their lack of a comprehensive understanding of this vast subject means that women's and babies' lives are being put at risk.

Sceptics, and organisations such as the National Institute for Health and Care Excellence (NICE) and, to a lesser extent, the Cochrane reviews, argue that there is insufficient evidence to support the use of complementary therapies in pregnancy. This is not exactly true, although the research can be difficult to find. In any case, it could be argued that many other initiatives have been introduced into clinical healthcare over the years without first having the research evidence of effectiveness and safety. It seems that political antagonism towards complementary medicine drives this somewhat spurious claim of an inadequate evidence base, but some evidence is there if you know where to look, even though it may be of variable calibre.

It was for this reason that I wanted this latest book to be an examination of some of the research that is available as well as providing a background on the subject for midwives and other maternity workers. I also wanted to demonstrate that, whilst there is evidence, there are problems in applying the results to practice. Perhaps, too, it is not always the primary factor in ensuring that complementary therapies are safe in pregnancy and childbirth. My personal professional philosophy over the whole of my career has focused on safety and professional accountability, and that is what I aim to present in this book.

Unlike *Complementary Therapies for Pregnancy and Childbirth* (Tiran and Mack 2000; first edition 1993), this new book tackles the subject from a woman-focused perspective rather than from a therapy-specific approach. Women do not request complementary therapies from their midwives; they report symptoms and raise issues with midwives for which they are seeking a resolution. Thus, women will not actively request, for example, osteopathy for their backache but will ask the midwife for advice on how to deal with the discomfort they are feeling. Therefore, following a general introduction to the vast number of individual complementary therapies, subsequent chapters cover problems such as sickness, back pain, breech presentation, post-dates pregnancy, intrapartum care and postnatal recovery and explore how complementary therapies and natural remedies can be of use.

I hope that you find this new book interesting and that it may be of some help to you in promoting the safe and effective use of complementary therapies for pregnant and childbearing women.

CHAPTER 1

Introduction to Complementary Therapies in Maternity Care

This chapter introduces the concept of complementary medicine and explores some of the theories that support it. The reasons for the increasing use of complementary therapies and natural remedies in pregnancy and childbirth are explored, together with the growing interest in its use amongst midwives and other maternity professionals. Finally, the main indications for the use of complementary therapies for expectant mothers are summarised in preparation for the detailed debate that follows in subsequent chapters.

The chapter includes:

- introduction to complementary medicine

- the use of complementary therapies and natural remedies in pregnancy and childbirth

- general contraindications and precautions to use of complementary therapies

- conclusion.

Introduction to complementary medicine

Complementary medicine comprises a large number of therapeutic and diagnostic strategies that can be used in isolation or in combination with conventional healthcare. In the 1980s these therapies were considered "alternative", "non-conventional" or "unorthodox" because they were little understood and segregated from conventional healthcare. The term "complementary" became popular in the 1990s as the interest and incidence of use amongst the general public increased and some therapies began to be used alongside medical care. A more contemporary term used by doctors, particularly in the USA, is "integrative medicine", implying that these modalities are integrated within mainstream medicine, although this is still often not the case.

Complementary medicine has previously been marginalised as being primitive, ineffective and, without any real evidence to the contrary, unsafe. In the 1990s a government working party was set up to examine the issues surrounding complementary medicine, concluding that there was a need for greater regulation, more research, better education of practitioners and more integration into the National Health Service (NHS) (British Medical Association 1993). Improved monitoring of conventional healthcare in the 21st century has gone some way towards achieving these aims, although many therapies remain poorly regulated and the amount and calibre of research and preparatory education varies according to the precise discipline. Integration into the NHS care remains sporadic, with the maternity, oncology and learning disability fields being the main specialisms to embrace the benefits, but the NHS generally takes a cautious approach in recommending or advising on complementary medicine (NHS Choices 2017). However, complementary medicine has gradually become more acceptable, with a growing reputation for offering valid, cost-effective options and being worthy of more scientific study to demonstrate efficacy and safety.

There have always been traditional systems of medicine across the world, but the advent of biomedicine relinquished these systems to a place in which they were viewed as inferior to western medicine, the prerogative of tribal cultures, to be derided as being of no value. This disdain for traditional systems, sometimes called "folk medicine", is reinforced by the spiritual beliefs, common in many countries, that evil forces such as witches or malevolent ancestors contribute to illness and disease. There is, however, a necessary distinction to be made between centuries-old practices that have a well-developed body of clinical "wisdom" embedded in the belief system of a particular society, versus practices introduced in recent years by a few well-meaning but unscientific practitioners working in isolation from their peers and without any rigorous testing. The former group includes acupuncture, massage and reflexology, which are thousands of years old, as well as the more recent disciplines of osteopathy and homeopathy, whereas the latter group includes many untested and, frankly, sometimes harmful treatments. This includes numerous therapies claiming (illegally in the UK) to "cure cancer" but which are embraced by desperate people. On the other hand, it is important to be cautious in dismissing those that have not yet been scientifically tested, since this does not mean that they are universally ineffective or harmful.

There is a subtle difference between the terms "complementary medicine" and "complementary therapies". The former is usually applied to modalities used by medical practitioners or by complementary professionals practising more mainstream disciplines such as acupuncture, medical herbalism, homeopathy, nutrition, hypnotherapy or osteopathy. This is politically reinforced by the provision of education on some of these subjects for general practitioners, dentists, anaesthetists and other medical specialists. On the other hand, the word "therapies" implies practices that are more supportive and tends to include those commonly used by midwives, nurses and physiotherapists and by practitioners of therapies that require less rigorous preparation for practice, such as aromatherapy, massage and reflexology. These therapies are often viewed as merely relaxing, without the capability to "cure" disease, although they are extremely popular with the general public.

A further differentiation must be drawn between "complementary therapies" and "natural remedies". The word "therapies" is often used to define manual strategies such as massage, reflexology, shiatsu and other touch techniques such as reiki or the "laying on of hands". However, in the UK, the (non-party) political and medical appreciation of osteopathy and chiropractic, which involve manual manipulation of joints, ligaments and muscles, has elevated these two disciplines above the somewhat dismissive "therapy" group and aligned them with physiotherapy. Statutory regulation, in 1993 and 1994 respectively, has now given osteopathy and chiropractic the status of "professions supplementary to medicine".

The classification of "natural remedies" applies to substances derived from plants and other naturally available elements. Plants have always had an important part to play in human health and wellbeing, providing not only the oxygen we breathe, but also energy from the food we eat and phytomedicines (plant remedies), the value of which is only now being recognised. We can obtain from plants pharmacologically active herbal medicines and essential oils, nutrition and nutritional supplements, as well as energetic medicines such as homeopathy and flower remedies (e.g. Bach or Bush). These remedies are intended for absorption into the body, either through gastrointestinal or respiratory tract administration, dermally or via the mucous membranes such as *per rectum* or *per vaginam*. Other natural elements are also sometimes used in medicines, such as minerals, tissue salts, bacterial cultures and even animal products, particularly in homeopathy.

It is interesting to note the current attention being given by pharmaceutical companies to plants traditionally used by indigenous populations for their apparent therapeutic properties (Drobnik and Drobnik 2016; Rivera *et al.* 2017; Salehi *et al.* 2016; Singh *et al.* 2016). Given that most licensed drugs originate from various plant products, this is perhaps not surprising, but unfortunately, the isolation of identified active constituents when produced synthetically for commercial medicines produces side effects that are not normally apparent in the plants (see Chapter 2, Herbal medicine).

"Whole person" healing: holism and individuality

Complementary therapies and natural remedies are very powerful therapeutic entities which, when used appropriately, have the power to improve health and wellbeing. Although each therapy has its own mechanism of action, all modalities share a common philosophy of treating the "whole person" rather than merely the presenting symptom or condition.

Conventional medicine categorises people, diseases or symptoms, enabling practitioners to apportion a label, using a common language that is understood by the whole medical community. Allopathic (conventional) medicine claims to focus on the bio-psycho-social model, yet the physio-pathological aspects of health and disease predominate in the majority of specialisms. In reality, medical practitioners commonly take a dispassionate, mechanistic and reductionist approach, viewing people essentially as machines in which a single part becomes faulty and requires mending. Resolving the predominating symptoms or condition is seen as "fixing" the person, with little explicit awareness of associated emotional, social or spiritual issues. Causative factors tend to be seen in epidemiological terms rather than considering the reasons *why* a person has developed a particular condition at a particular time. There is a dependence on materialistic interpretation of physical clinical signs with costly, highly technological and invasive methods of treatment (surgery, radiotherapy, etc.). There is little attention to preventative medicine, possibly because health education requires a long-term strategy that is certainly longer than the duration of office of any one political party.

In complementary medicine, each person is seen as a unique individual with her own inner resources. The same symptoms in two different people may have vastly different causes and effects. There is, in fact, no standard by which "normality" can be assessed, nor is there a single treatment for a common set of symptoms. In addition, not relying on diagnostic categorisation leads complementary therapy practitioners to deal with "functional" disorders including pain, nausea, stress or other symptoms conventionally regarded as subjective because they are more difficult to measure, unlike quantitative clinical signs such as blood pressure or urinalysis. Symptoms are regarded by complementary practitioners as precursors to, rather than the results of, disease; treatment is dependent on defining in detail the symptom picture of the individual.

Unfortunately, these methods of diagnosis and treatment are viewed with scepticism because they do not fit with the contemporary biomedical model. The scientific community opines that complementary practitioners lack the training and expertise to diagnose "correctly" – that is, in terms of a medical label – and many doctors believe that this leads to missed or inaccurate diagnoses and, by inference, inappropriate or inadequate treatment. Further, they believe that, whilst complementary therapies may alleviate subjective symptoms, they cannot cure the condition. This is essentially because their views on the manifestation of illness and disease differ from those of holistic practitioners. Doctors are concerned with disease, a relatively passive reaction of the person to invasion with microbes or apparently dangerous external environmental forces. Complementary medicine is concerned with identifying the causes of imbalance *within* the individual, and the therapeutic goal is to return the person to homeostatic equilibrium by whatever method is necessary. Imbalance may occur from invasion by external factors, but these are considered rarely to harm a person who is homeostatically balanced. Complementary healthcare tends to focus on facilitating the self-protective abilities of the individual, regaining, maintaining and strengthening them to prevent future ill health. This, then, is not curing but healing – and healing the whole person.

Prevention of disease is, of course, part of conventional medicine but is achieved through different mechanisms, such as routine immunisation and regular screening. National health policy in all countries aims to work towards the needs of the majority, using drugs, surgery or other strategies to treat only those who are at risk or who have been identified as having a defined medical condition. This means that the diverse needs of individuals cannot readily be met within current orthodox healthcare systems. Their needs and wishes may even be disregarded, particularly when financial factors predominate, as can be seen when new but extremely expensive cancer drugs come on to the market but are offered to only a few in a sort of "postcode lottery". Contemporary adherence to local, national and international guidelines and the use of routine procedures or investigations detracts from the ability of healthcare practitioners to reflect on individuals and may actually increase the chance that the clinical relevance of anomalous features is missed. An example of this is the routine postnatal examination of a mother, which focuses on the completion of "tick charts" in assessing her for pathological complications such as retained products of conception, breast abscesses or perineal infection.

Further, this medicalisation of preventative biomedicine means that the responsibility of individual "patients" is effectively disengaged, tacitly permitting them to engage in risky behaviours, for example smoking, in the unconscious belief that medicine will resolve any adverse effects. Indeed, the use of the word "patient" implies a paternalistic approach to healthcare. Professionals need to redefine their brief for care and treatment, particularly in maternity care, in which a partnership with the individual woman is engaged, and which facilitates an in-depth assessment of the holistic bio-psycho-social aspects of that woman's life. Figure 1.1 provides a model for practice that incorporates the multiple aspects inherent in a holistic approach to care.

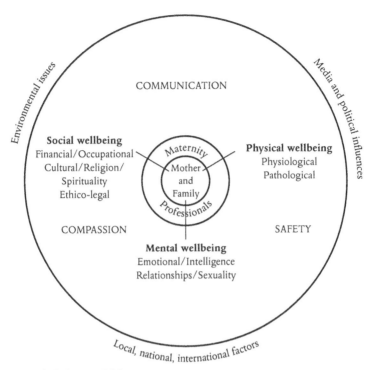

Figure 1.1 The holistic model for practice

Self-healing and the healing reaction

Health is more than the absence of disease or illness. Achieving health may be a means to an end or part of an ongoing process. Wellbeing is more than just psychological equilibrium, and involves an interaction between physical, emotional, social and occupational wellness (Hunter *et al.* 2013). In complementary medicine, achieving wellbeing involves facilitating the inner resources of the individual as an active participant in her own health. Health – or being healthy – is not something magnanimously conferred by professionals but results from the individual's balance of internal resources with the external natural and social environment. Optimum health and wellbeing requires the person to work in partnership with the complementary health professional, who employs gentle methods of alleviating symptoms, usually with fewer side effects than orthodox medicine, and who focuses on prevention rather than the curing of disease. For these reasons alone, complementary therapies fit well with women wanting as natural a pregnancy and birth as possible, without unnecessary intervention, enabling them to remain in control and to have a satisfying psycho-social, physical and spiritual experience.

This concept of the self-healing capacity of the body, with the practitioner merely being a facilitator or acting as a conduit in assisting the client to regain homeostatic balance, is fundamental to the ethos of complementary medicine. The focus is on the person to be healed, rather than on the healer. Clinical assessment involves a consideration not only of *why* the person is unwell but of *how* to facilitate the body to repair itself. There is a complex interaction between the body, mind and spirit in which the individual can influence one part of this trilogy with another. One only has to think of a dying person, who waits for a relative to travel halfway round the world to see them one last time before expiring, to appreciate this dynamic balance. Conversely, over-stimulation of one element can trigger disharmony in the other aspects, such as the impact of emotional stress or distress on the physical body, a feature very common to complementary diagnosis and treatment.

Therapists consider the development of symptoms as a means by which the body attempts to rid itself of toxins in order to return to homeostasis. For example, pyrexia is the body's response to bacterial infection, since heat kills bacteria, sneezing expels cold viruses and vomiting empties the stomach of undesirable substances. Unfortunately, conventional medicine often seeks to suppress these symptoms rather than to determine the underlying aetiology. An example here is that of anti-inflammatory creams that reduce skin irritation (working from the outside) rather than treating the whole person (from the inside) to eliminate the *need* for the skin to react, as it does in response to chronic stress. In this example, identifying the emotional stress warrants treatment with stress-reducing strategies to avoid the manifestation of physical symptoms. A further complication in the conventional treatment of skin conditions is that the application of creams acts not only as a barrier to infection gaining entry to the body but as an obstruction to the release of toxic substances from the body.

Whole person healing occurs in response to one or more strategies facilitated by the complementary practitioner. This may involve physical therapy as with massage or shiatsu, direct psychological treatment such as hypnotherapy or neuro-linguistic programming, or indirect emotional care through the use of relaxation therapies. The process of healing attempts first to rid the body of harmful toxins in order to cleanse the system, which then facilitates a return to homeostasis. Ongoing treatment is designed to maintain homeostatic balance throughout the body, mind and spirit.

However, unlike many of the "quick fixes" of conventional treatment, such as cutting out a diseased organ, healing the whole person takes time. Often the client will experience an exacerbation of the presenting symptoms, or the development of new ones as the body rids itself of the toxins, or even the resurgence of old clinical problems such as pain at a previous surgical or fracture site. This "healing reaction", common to all therapies, is an alien concept to many medical practitioners, who may seek to disparage complementary medicine because it "makes the condition worse". A healing response is a *normal* reaction to the therapy. It should not be confused with the *adverse* reactions which constitute overdose or side effects that may occur from inappropriate use of natural remedies such as aromatherapy oils or herbal medicines. Symptoms of a healing reaction usually occur during the treatment session or within the first 24 to 48 hours afterwards, and are generally worst following the first treatment (Gunnarsdottir and Jonsdottir 2010).

Common reactions that are experienced in response to many therapies include headache, nausea, lethargy, general aches and pains, skin reactions, congestion, mood swings and emotional effects, or worsening of the presenting symptoms. Many pregnant women will report changes in their sleep patterns following treatment, either sleeping better than normally, or experiencing difficulty in getting to sleep, with frequent waking and vivid dreams. Clients should be asked to note any reactions such as these and report them at the next appointment, or beforehand if they have any concerns. It is common – and sensible – practice to advise women to drink plenty of fluids (ideally water) and to avoid stimulants such as caffeine, chocolate, alcohol, cola and other high-sugar soft drinks and to limit excessive activity for a few hours after complementary therapy treatment, to encourage the body to heal itself.

Obviously, in maternity work, it is essential that the practitioner can differentiate between a normal healing reaction, an adverse reaction (side effect) to the therapy through inappropriate or incorrect use, or the onset of a pathological complication of pregnancy. For example, a woman in late pregnancy reporting a headache following treatment could be experiencing a normal healing reaction, a side effect of therapy overdose, a relatively normal stress or tiredness headache, or she could be developing pre-eclampsia. In the event of skin irritation, this could be due to the normal detoxification process of the therapy, a side effect of a natural remedy (such as aromatherapy oils, herbal medicines or energy-based homeopathic or Bach flower remedies), or it could be physiological pruritus or emerging pathological obstetric cholestasis. As a general rule, healing reactions will arise and resolve spontaneously within 24 to 48 hours, whereas side effects may not; untreated pathology will often worsen over a course of hours or days and is, of course, much more serious and requires medical management.

It is worth debating here whether or not women should be warned about a possible healing reaction prior to starting complementary treatment for a specific condition. Some practitioners consider that this could trigger anticipatory symptoms, such as may sometimes be seen in cancer patients: an anticipation of nausea, a common side effect of chemotherapy, may actually induce the nausea. However, this author believes that, in pregnancy, the woman should be informed of the possibility of a healing reaction since lack of knowledge may lead her, in such an event, to report to the maternity unit with symptoms for which no ostensible cause can be found and which may be misinterpreted by colleagues as an obstetric complication. Also, since many pregnant women only seek complementary treatment for specific problems when their symptoms become intolerable, a warning that the presenting problem could potentially become temporarily worse gives her the opportunity to decline treatment if she feels she could not cope. In practice, most women are, by this time, so desperate to feel better that they are prepared to do anything which may help, and the thought of another 24 hours of symptoms somewhat pales into insignificance against the hope that the treatment may improve the condition. Table 1.1 summarises the healing reaction.

Table 1.1 The healing reaction

Common symptoms occurring during treatment	Common symptoms within 24 to 48 hours of treatment (usually worst with first treatment)
Sense of deep relaxation, drowsiness	Tiredness, changes in sleep pattern, vivid dreams
Headache	Headache, usually occipital due to dehydration
Change in body temperature, sweating, clamminess, feeling cold in whole or part of body	Increased perspiration, profuse sweating
Increased thirst	Increased thirst, changes in appetite
Nausea and/or vomiting, retching	Increased urination, changes in bowel habits, flatulence
Increased mucus, saliva, nasal secretions	Increased mucus, saliva, vaginal or nasal secretions, spots and skin irritation

Sneezing, coughing	Cold and influenza-like symptoms
Pain in areas of presenting symptoms or old injuries or surgery	Muscle aches and pains, resurgence of pain in areas of old injuries or surgery
Release of emotions – crying, giggling	Heightened emotions – crying, mood changes, irritability

After-care advice for self-care following treatments: drink plenty of water; avoid stimulants, e.g. alcohol, caffeine, cola; eat lightly; relax to allow body to recover and react to treatment; avoid excessive work, exercise, stress, etc.

The therapeutic relationship and the placebo effect

One of the criticisms often directed towards complementary medicine is that any apparent improvement in the clinical condition is only a placebo effect. Others surmise that, unlike in NHS practice, the facility for the therapist to give each client her time and focused attention in some way makes the client feel better, or even that the fact that the client pays for the service gives her control over her health and contributes to an increased sense of wellbeing. Sceptics also suggest that belief in the therapy has a positive effect on subjective improvement, implying conversely that no relief will occur if the client is unconvinced. In fact, all of these aspects may contribute to the overall positive response – indeed, the placebo response is in itself a powerful entity – but this is not the only mechanism of action.

In medical terms, a *placebo* is generally defined as an inert substance or control method used to evaluate the physio-psychological implications of new treatments or drugs. However, the *placebo response* is somewhat different, being seen by some as unpredictable, unreliable and impacted by non-specific mechanisms that are usually dismissed as immeasurable and irrelevant. It could however be said that every therapeutic intervention, whether conventional or complementary, has a placebo effect, since the recipient is likely to have a degree of faith in its effectiveness, based on her trust in the practitioner. People who seek out complementary therapies tend to have an expectation that their symptoms will be resolved or lessened, but they appear also to be looking actively for practitioners offering a holistic approach that improves their quality of life and facilitates them to be involved in their own care (Richardson 2004). Clients perceive complementary therapists as being "caring" and have high satisfaction levels with their experiences and with the practitioners (Luff and Thomas 2000) with, surprisingly, little difference between consultations in private practice or the NHS (Wye, Shaw and Sharpe 2013).

Subjective improvement in wellbeing can, in fact, assist in overall recovery, activating the individual's coping strategies, not least through the initiation of endorphins and their impact on pain perception. Evidence increasingly demonstrates significant subjective and objective clinical reactions that are unrelated to the placebo effect. Whilst many doctors believe it is unethical actively to encourage a placebo response, the evidence shows that an expectation of recovery can physically and chemically alter the subjective feelings of wellbeing that goes beyond the therapeutic relationship (Price, Finniss and Benedetti 2008). Conversely, research into complementary medicine increasingly demonstrates specific mechanisms of action, including chemical, physiological, energetic and even epigenetic effects that transcend the placebo effect and that cannot be ignored (Kanherkar *et al.* 2017).

The use of complementary therapies and natural remedies in pregnancy and childbirth

The use of complementary therapies before, during and after pregnancy has increased phenomenally in the 35 years since this author started working in this specialist field. In the 1960s and 1970s the medical tragedies of thalidomide and diethylstilboestrol began to turn people away from a dependence on pharmaceutical drugs in pregnancy while, in the 1980s, interest in complementary medicine grew exponentially. At this time, expectant mothers had little idea of how to find reputable, well-trained practitioners, and midwives and obstetricians were largely unaware of the potential benefits – or risks – of these therapies, still seeing them more as the "fringe" ideas of a few mavericks. However, as public awareness grew in the 1990s, pregnant women became possibly the second largest client group (after cancer patients) to embrace the concept of complementary medicine.

Studies of the general population indicate complementary medicine usage up to 71 per cent (Hunt *et al.* 2010), although use by middle-aged women, perhaps seeking relief of menopausal symptoms, may be higher (Lunny and Fraser 2010; Sarris *et al.* 2010). Many people, including those with pre-existing medical conditions requiring medication, such as anti-hypertensives, self-administer natural remedies (Rahmawati and Bajorek 2017), and many patients are willing to pay for complementary (or alternative) treatments (Montross-Thomas *et al.* 2017). Different modalities are used by nurses, dentists, doctors and physiotherapists, as well as by midwives. Research is increasingly being undertaken on ways in which complementary therapies can be incorporated into care of patients with life-limiting or chronic illness such as cancer, HIV/AIDS or Parkinson's disease and peri-operative care (Jaruzel and Kelechi 2016; Lee and Lim 2017; Nlooto and Naidoo 2016). There are also hundreds of papers written on the use of natural remedies around the world, including some of the popular herbs such as St John's wort for mild to moderate depression (see Chapters 2 and 9). Numerous surveys suggest that the primary reasons for turning to complementary medicine are to relieve symptoms, to maintain control over one's own health and for relaxation, and many people would consider using complementary medicine before seeking conventional medical advice (Thomson, Jones *et al.* 2014).

In relation to pregnancy, Broussard *et al.*'s analysis of over 4000 American women (2010) found that around 11 per cent used herbal remedies, most commonly ginger, ephedra, chamomile and herbal teas, whereas an Australian review revealed up to 87 per cent of women accessing massage, aromatherapy and herbal teas (Hall, Griffiths and McKenna 2011). Most surveys suggest that between a quarter and a third of women use complementary therapies (Johnson *et al.* 2016; Jones, Jomeen and Ogbuehi 2013), although Guittier *et al.*'s survey in the USA (2012) found an incidence of almost 70 per cent. Self-administration of natural remedies appears to increase as pregnancy progresses and women prepare for birth, with herbal teas, homeopathic remedies and herbal medicines being the most popular (Bishop *et al.* 2011; Nordeng *et al.* 2011). Kalder *et al.* (2011) largely agree with these findings, adding acupuncture as one of the most frequently accessed modalities. The use of aromatherapy has been formally estimated as being around 15 per cent (Sibbritt *et al.* 2014), but in the UK it is probably considerably higher, due both to self-administration and the increasing use of aromatherapy by midwives (personal communications with women and midwives).

A large study by Kennedy *et al.* (2013) questioned over 9000 women across 23 countries about their use of herbal remedies, indicating an average use of 29 per cent. Women from Russia (69%), Eastern Europe (51.8%) and Australia (43.8%) were twice as likely to use herbal medicines as women from other countries. Women with low risk pregnancies may be more likely to access independent complementary practitioners than those requiring medical care or hospitalisation for a pre-existing or pregnancy-induced complication. Expectant mothers planning home birth tend to be most in tune with the concept of holistic care and are also keen to use any means to facilitate normality so that their babies can be born at home.

It is common for women to seek the use of natural and complementary strategies concurrently with conventional antenatal care, particularly in countries where access to medical or midwifery facilities may be difficult (Dako-Gyeke et al. 2013).

There are, however, some fundamental issues to be taken into account when interpreting these wide-ranging estimations taken from surveys conducted across many countries. It is difficult to draw clear comparisons since the research methodologies vary considerably (Pallivalappila et al. 2013). For example, the formulation of questions may relate only to natural remedies rather than to manual or psychological complementary therapies. Certain strategies to which women may self-refer may not come under the generally understood umbrella of complementary therapies, such as counselling, or may be so obscure that researchers do not include them in the questionnaire options, for example coffee douching. Women may misunderstand the meanings of some questions unless they are very carefully phrased. For instance, researchers studying the use of "ginger for nausea" may intend to determine women's use of ginger tea or capsules taken in therapeutic doses, whereas many women, especially in the UK, may interpret the question to mean the ubiquitous practice of consuming ginger biscuits, which do not contain a therapeutically sufficient amount of ginger (see Chapter 4).

Women who agree to take part in the studies may already be more amenable to the use of complementary therapies; surveys certainly suggest that those who use therapies tend to be slightly older primigravidae, better educated women working in professional roles and non-smokers (Hall and Jolly 2014; Kennedy et al. 2013). Those who have used complementary therapies and/or natural remedies prior to conception are also more likely to continue their use during pregnancy (Frawley, Sibbritt et al. 2016). It may be fair to surmise that women outside these categories could be less inclined to participate in a survey, especially if they know nothing about the subject or are sceptical (Close et al. 2016c). Women may also be questioned, on one occasion or on several separate occasions during pregnancy, or postnatally, during which time the incidence of usage and their views may have changed.

Results and response rates differ according to geographical location. For example in one study, homeopathy was particularly popular, but this survey was undertaken in southwest England, a region which, until recently, had one of the five UK NHS homeopathic hospitals (Bishop et al. 2011). Despite its demise, it is perhaps more likely that appropriately trained doctors in this area would incorporate homeopathy into their practice than those in other areas, especially more deprived areas where other aspects of health and social care take priority. The public may also, perhaps, be more aware of the value of homeopathy, as is seen in other areas of the UK where there have previously been NHS homeopathic hospitals (personal communications).

Attitudes towards complementary therapies also vary between countries and may influence acceptance by medical professionals (Feijen-de Jong *et al.* 2015; Nordeng *et al.* 2011). There may be differences in use between women born in the country and those who have immigrated from elsewhere, as seen in one Swedish study (Robertson and Johansson 2010). Certainly, the use of indigenous herbal medicines by women from developing countries is a growing phenomenon in western maternity units; therefore those units in which the patient demographics include large numbers of women from overseas will see a more prolific, if somewhat covert, use of these remedies.

Acceptance and use of complementary therapies by maternity professionals

The natural desire to want to heal those who are dis-eased, either in body or mind, is fundamental to the role of women. Centuries ago, midwives frequently used herbal concoctions to aid the progress of contractions in labour and manual techniques to encourage the passage of the fetus through the birth canal. In almost all cultures of the world traditional remedies are used to prepare for labour, to ease recovery from birth and to promote lactation. Women often, perhaps subconsciously, view childbirth as the essence of their being, an event which is the ultimate expression of their feminine existence, and at no time more than this are they receptive to ideas that allow them to be in tune with nature.

Since the start of the 21st century, national and international concerns over the huge numbers of interventions in childbirth, such as Caesarean sections and inductions of labour, appear to have given tacit approval to the inclusion of different, perhaps non-conventional strategies in maternity care (King's Fund 2009; NHS Institute for Innovation and Improvement 2009). Most recently, the National Maternity Review (NHS England 2016) has stressed the continuing – and now urgent – need to revert to a focus on birth as a natural bio-psycho-social life process. The philosophy of complementary medicine is very much in harmony with the concept of woman-focused care; using various therapies may contribute to a reduction in medical intervention in childbirth.

Contemporary midwives and doulas appear to be largely accepting of women's use of complementary therapies, but the ways in which they communicate with women on the subject may depend on their personal use and their attitudes to working in partnership with their clients. Most midwives are keen to act as women's advocates by supporting their use of complementary therapies, but are conscious of safety issues. Midwives may also feel threatened by medical scepticism or the possibility of disciplinary action if they work outside defined maternity service guidelines, a fact that may lead some to advise women surreptitiously without recording their discussions (Hall, Griffiths and McKenna 2015).

The experience of this author suggests that midwives and doulas generally fall into five groups in relation to complementary therapies:

- those who are outright sceptics with no knowledge, understanding or interest in the subject, who may use dismissive or even derogatory language to discourage women from using them

- those with an awareness that their knowledge is lacking, who relinquish the responsibility of advising women by stating that they are unable to help them and that women should seek help elsewhere

- those with a little knowledge and a lot of enthusiasm, who overstep the boundaries of their understanding and their midwifery or doula registration because of their desire to help women, but who often provide inaccurate or incomplete information

- those who have undertaken general complementary therapy training, but whose knowledge is not sufficiently comprehensive or applied to the practice of that therapy within midwifery

- those who have been appropriately trained in the use of complementary therapies related specifically to pregnancy and birth, who use or advise accurately and comprehensively on different aspects of therapies or natural remedies within the parameters of their training, local clinical guidelines and their registration (see Chapter 3).

Why do midwives and doulas need to know about complementary medicine?

The increasing use of complementary therapies by pregnant women has fuelled an intense interest amongst midwives and doulas in training in one or more modalities to add to their practice. However, they must be mindful of allowing their enthusiasm for new "tools" to dominate their standard practice. Further, it is worth considering that the desire of women to access complementary therapies in pregnancy is not necessarily a plea for complementary therapies to be incorporated into conventional maternity care. Given the issues around staffing levels in maternity care, trying to implement complementary therapy services within midwifery practice may merely compound the problem unless the introduction of new strategies is tackled carefully.

Not all midwives or doulas need, or wish, to offer complementary therapies as part of their practice, but they must be aware of women's use so that they can advise on safety, particularly in relation to self-administration of natural remedies. Midwives should ask women at booking if they are using any natural remedies or consulting complementary practitioners, and record this in the notes. Failure to disclose self-administration, unless asked directly, is not limited to women in developing countries, nor is it solely the confines of those accessing maternity care. Concern is increasingly expressed by conventional healthcare professionals of all disciplines about the possible adverse effects of complementary therapies and natural remedies, especially when used in conjunction with specialist medical treatments (Henson *et al.* 2017; Kara 2009; O'Connor *et al.* 2011). Conversely, women may be more open about their use of natural remedies in areas where midwives offer one or more therapies as part of the overall care package (personal communications). Sympathetic acceptance by health professionals, coupled with direct questioning in relation to natural remedies when enquiring about medications in general, may offer implied approval sufficient to encourage women to disclose their use of complementary therapies, particularly when they understand the need in the context of potential interactions with drugs or other therapeutic interventions.

General indications for use of complementary therapies in pregnancy, birth and the postnatal period

As with the general population, pregnant women seek complementary therapies for a variety of reasons, including relaxation and relief of stress, to alleviate physiological symptoms, to prepare for birth, facilitate contractions and to aid recovery from birth and the establishment of lactation. The specific therapy may depend on the precise nature and aetiology of the problem, the availability and acceptability of therapies and on client compliance.

Relaxation

The general public's impression of "complementary and alternative therapies" is that they are primarily relaxing, and for many therapies this is a major benefit of the treatment. The aim of all therapies is to facilitate homeostasis by whatever mechanism of action is pertinent to that therapy. The cortisol reduction and rebalancing of other chemicals in the body which occurs with many therapies contributes to improving women's coping abilities when they are faced with the various bio-psycho-social upheavals of pregnancy. A corresponding increase in endorphins and encephalins adds to the overall relaxation effect.

Pregnant women often seek therapies such as massage, aromatherapy, reflexology, shiatsu or reiki specifically for some "me time", for relaxation and to ease tension. The relaxation effect also helps women with fatigue and insomnia, although natural remedies, notably herbs and homeopathy, may have a more direct effect in inducing and improving sleep. Modalities such as acupuncture or osteopathy are not seen as specifically relaxing, but a decrease in stress hormones and an increase in endorphins and encephalins generally occurs irrespective of the primary aim of treatment. Bach flower remedies also provide a means of dealing with emotional problems and can be easily bought and self-administered. On the other hand, where stress has a psychological origin, hypnosis may help and is notably effective for tocophobia, needle phobia and other significant issues (Williamson and Gregory 2015).

Women with specific mental health problems may also find support from accessing complementary practitioners. Although not a maternity-specific study, Hansen and Kristoffersen (2016) found that people with severe anxiety or depression often use complementary therapies in addition to any medical treatment, whereas those with moderate depression tend to access therapies as an alternative option. Ormsby et al.'s Australian study (a 2016 paper was published while recruitment to the study was still in progress) compared acupuncture with mindfulness and with standard antenatal care for women with depression; results are not yet available at the time of writing but it is hoped they may demonstrate possible alternative options for the treatment of mental health issues in pregnancy (see Chapter 9).

Gastrointestinal tract problems

Nausea and vomiting, constipation, diarrhoea and irritable bowel syndrome, heartburn, acid reflux and indigestion, as well as haemorrhoids, respond well to several manual therapies, including reflex zone therapy, massage, osteopathy and chiropractic, pharmacological therapies such as aromatherapy essential oils and herbal medicines, and energy-based therapies, particularly acupuncture, shiatsu and homeopathy. Nutritional therapies are an obvious choice for dealing with some of these complaints which often arise due to food intolerances and allergies (Marchioni, Beery and Birk 2015) (see Chapter 4).

Musculoskeletal problems

Osteopathy and chiropractic are considered the most effective modalities to deal with severe musculoskeletal issues during and after pregnancy, including severe lumbosacral or thoracic backache, neck ache, sciatica, pelvic girdle pain and carpal tunnel syndrome. Post-epidural neck ache and headache also respond well to these treatments and many osteopaths and chiropractors like to see both the mother and the baby at about six weeks postnatal to determine how the mechanics of the birth have affected the maternal pelvis and the baby's skull. Reflex zone therapy and acupuncture also work at a deep level to treat many antenatal musculoskeletal discomforts, whereas massage and shiatsu tend to be more temporarily palliative. Pharmacological therapies may provide a direct analgesic effect but there appears to be a synergistic effect when aromatherapy essential oils are administered via massage. On the other hand, herbal remedies are rarely used for these issues unless a pregnant woman is actively consulting an independent herbal medicine practitioner for some other reason (see Chapter 5).

Malposition or malpresentation of the fetal presenting part

Osteopathy and chiropractic are effective in realigning the maternal pelvis in the event of genetic or traumatic misalignment, thereby facilitating descent of the fetal head (Pistolese 2002). Exercise therapies such as yoga and other methods of encouraging optimal fetal positioning are also popular (Oakley and Evans 2014). Moxibustion, an element of traditional Chinese medicine, is increasingly well known as a means of correcting a breech presentation or occipito-posterior position of the fetus, although acupuncture needling is sometimes also used. Homeopathic remedies may assist in regaining a homeostatic balance between mother and fetus which encourages a normal fetal lie, presentation and position. Hypnosis has also been used to correct malpresentation, with variable success (see Chapter 6).

Preparation for birth

It is well evidenced that women who receive regular complementary therapies in the weeks leading up to the birth, particularly the relaxation therapies, are more likely to commence labour spontaneously within the normal parameters for term, tend to labour well and are more likely to achieve a normal vaginal birth than controls (Fink *et al.* 2012). Yoga, tai chi, pregnancy Pilates and other exercise methods are also popular, both to keep fit and prepare physically for labour and as a means of relaxation (Campbell and Nolan 2016). Many women use strategies to prepare their bodies and minds for the birth, including taking herbs such as raspberry leaf, although not always appropriately. Hypnosis-related preparation has also become very popular as a means of gearing up mentally for the rigours of labour (Finlayson *et al.* 2015; Madden *et al.* 2016) (see Chapter 8).

Natural induction of labour

The desire to end the discomforts of pregnancy and commence labour seems to be a characteristic of expectant mothers around the world. In addition to any physical, emotional or chemical preparation for birth, women seek complementary therapies and natural remedies which can potentially trigger labour onset. This is particularly significant when women, primarily in westernised countries, are advised to have labour induced artificially in order to avoid the purported complications of post-dates pregnancy. Manual therapies such as reflexology, acupuncture, shiatsu and massage are used in various forms, both by professional practitioners and, with some therapies, by self-administration. Aromatherapy oils, herbal and homeopathic, are often used to attempt to induce labour or, in the case of Bach flower remedies, to ease the anxiety about labour that often prevents the natural physiological onset. Therapies such as acupressure or acupuncture may also be effective in accelerating contractions during established labour, if appropriate (Mollart, Adam and Foureur 2015) (see Chapter 7).

Pain relief in labour

Many complementary therapies and natural remedies can be directly pain-relieving. Manual therapies, including massage, aromatherapy, shiatsu, reflexology and acupuncture, have a direct effect on the gate control mechanism of pain relief (Chaillet *et al.* 2014), delaying pain impulses from reaching the brain and positively altering the woman's perception of pain.

Pressure point work with shiatsu/acupressure, reflex zone therapy or even osteopathic/chiropractic techniques can be helpful. Alternatively, the chemicals in many pharmacological remedies, including aromatherapy and herbal medicines, may have a directly analgesic effect. These therapies are especially beneficial during labour, when a combined effect of relaxation and pain relief can redress the cortisol-oxytocin balance and indirectly aid progress towards a normal birth. Homeopathy addresses whole-person issues and determines appropriate remedies based on the bio-psycho-social factors which accompany the mother's pain and discomfort (see Chapter 8).

Wound healing

Some therapies and natural remedies can aid wound healing, especially after the birth, including perineal lacerations, episiotomy and Caesarean section wounds. Some, such as aromatherapy and herbal medicines, have a direct healing effect, combating infection and boosting the immune system, whilst others ease discomfort and aid relaxation, making it easier for the mother to cope. Energy therapies such as homeopathy, Bach flower remedies and acupuncture work at a deeper "whole person" level to facilitate homeostasis (see Chapter 9).

Recovery from the birth

Many therapies and remedies aid in the mother's recovery from labour, providing pain relief and relaxation and facilitating lactation (Nakakita Kenyon 2015). Acupuncture, reflexology and shiatsu can stimulate milk production and ease the pain of breast engorgement or, if necessary, suppression of lactation. Some therapies can contribute to preventing or reducing the severity of postnatal depression, although these tend to require a long-term course of treatment, in which case it could be argued that the continued attendance of a professional practitioner may have some placebo effect (Gong *et al.* 2015) (see Chapter 9).

Table 1.2 summarises the general indications for the use of complementary therapies and natural remedies in pregnancy, labour and the puerperium. Indications for the use of specific therapies or remedies are covered in the sections on each therapy (see Chapter 2).

Table 1.2 General indications for complementary therapies and natural remedies in maternity care

Condition	Acupuncture/pressure	Aromatherapy	BFR	Chiropractic	Herbal med	Homeopathy	Hypnosis	Massage	Osteopathy	Reflexology/RZT	Reiki	Shiatsu
General relaxation Relief of stress, anxiety	*	**	**		*	**	**	**		**	**	**
Mental health issues (depression, anxiety)	**	**	* with caution		**	**	**	**		**	**	**
Tiredness, fatigue, insomnia	**	**	**	*	**	**	**	**	*	**	**	**
Nausea and vomiting in pregnancy/labour	**	*	*	**	**	**	*	*	**	** RZT	*	**
Heartburn, acid reflux, indigestion	**	**	*	**	*	**		*	**	**	*	**
Constipation, diarrhoea, IBS	**	**		**	*	**	*	**	**	**	*	**
Haemorrhoids	**	*	*	**	**	**			**	*	*	**
Varicosities, legs, vulva	**	*	*	**	**	**			**	*	*	**
Oedema	**	**	*	**	**	**		**	**	**	*	**
Backache, sciatica	**	**	*	**	*	**		**	**	**	*	**

Pelvic girdle pain	**	*		**		*		*	**	** RZT	*	**
Carpal tunnel syndrome	**	*		**		*		**	**	**	*	**
Malposition or malpresentation of fetus	** Moxibustion	*		**		*	*	*	**	*		*
Birth preparation	**	**	*	*	*	*	**	**	*	**	**	**
Natural labour induction	**	**	*	*	** NB risks	**	*	**	*	**	*	**
Pain relief in labour	**	**	*		*	**	**	**	*	**	**	**
Acceleration of contractions	**	**			*	**		**		**	*	**
Retained placenta	**	*				**				*		**
Wound healing	*	**	*		**	**		*		*	*	*
Infection	*	**			**	*						
Recovery from birth	**	**	**	**	**	**	**	**	**	**	**	**
Lactation	**	*	*	*	**	**		**	*	**	*	**
Breast engorgement	**	**			*	**		**		**	*	**
Prevent/treat postnatal depression	**	**	**		*	**	**	**		**	**	**

Key: ** directly applicable/appropriate therapy for the condition   * indirect/less dynamic effect   RZT specific reflex zone therapy techniques

General contraindications and precautions to use of complementary therapies

Many complementary therapies, particularly natural remedies, should be avoided or used with caution in the preconception period, during pregnancy, birth and the early postnatal period, or may be contraindicated in women with particular medical or obstetric conditions. Any woman whose pregnancy or labour is not entirely physiologically normal should use complementary therapies and natural remedies with care. Those with major medical conditions, particularly women requiring medication, should be even more cautious, as the effects of some therapies may compromise the maternal or fetal condition or disturb the progress of the pregnancy, whilst the chemicals in some natural remedies, such as aromatherapy oils and herbal medicines, may interact with drugs. Generally, women who require antenatal admission to hospital should avoid receiving or self-administering complementary therapies and natural remedies unless they have been specifically prescribed by an experienced practitioner who is dual qualified in both maternity work and the obstetric use of the specific therapy.

Inappropriate self-administration of natural therapies or the self-use of specific pressure point techniques is a growing problem in western maternity care, particularly as information (and mis-information) is available across all easily accessible media. The misconception that natural therapies are safe means that women keen to avoid medical intervention often resort to complementary and alternative strategies without any knowledge of the contraindications. Whilst a specific therapy in itself may not be contraindicated, inappropriate use can lead to side effects or complications with the pregnancy and women should be advised to take care with all therapies and natural remedies. The message to be highlighted is that "natural" does not always mean "safe".

Table 1.3 lists the general contraindications and precautions to the use of complementary therapies and natural remedies in pregnancy, birth and the puerperium. Therapy-specific issues are covered in the section on each therapy in Chapter 2.

Table 1.3 General contraindications and precautions to complementary therapies in pregnancy

Contraindication/precaution	Justification for caution
Medical conditions	
Anaemia	• Pathological – contraindication, particularly pharmacological therapies – herbal, aromatherapy • Physiological – precaution
Cardiac disease	• Impact of pregnancy on heart exacerbates condition • Significant disease compromises pregnancy progress • Condition may adversely affect fetal growth • Existing major cardiac disease – contraindication • Heart murmur with no previously diagnosed symptoms or effects – precaution
Coagulation disorders, women on anticoagulant medication or other drugs with similar action, e.g. aspirin	• Compromises feto-maternal wellbeing, pregnancy progress • Pharmacological therapies – *serious risk* of interaction with anticoagulant drugs • Herbal medicines – *absolute* contraindication • Acupuncture – contraindication
Diabetes mellitus	• Compromised feto-maternal condition • Insulin-dependent – contraindication to most therapies • Non-insulin-dependent – precaution • Acupuncture – contraindication
Epilepsy	• Medication may be changed to avoid teratogenicity – epilepsy may become more unstable • Relaxation or stimulation effects of some therapies may trigger a fit in susceptible women • Existing epilepsy, drug-controlled – *absolute* contraindication to all therapies • History of previous epilepsy, no recent fits – precaution
Hypertension	• Compromises fetal growth and wellbeing • Exerts additional pressure on maternal cardiovascular system • Fulminating pre-eclampsia or unstable hypertension – contraindication • Mild to moderate hypertension – precaution

Contraindication/precaution	Justification for caution
Medical conditions	
Other medical conditions	• Compromised feto-maternal condition
	• Potential for pharmacological therapies to interact with medication
	• Severe renal disease – compromised kidney function – herbal medicines, aromatherapy contraindicated
	• Liver or gall bladder disease – avoid pharmacological therapies which are metabolised via liver, e.g. aromatherapy, herbal remedies
	• Thyroid disease – caution especially with reflexology
Obstetric conditions	
Vaginal bleeding	• Compromised feto-maternal condition
	• Depends on cause and whether risk of bleeding continues
	• Current bleeding – contraindication
	• Previous bleeding, current pregnancy – precaution
Multiple pregnancy	• Twin pregnancy progressing normally – precaution
	• Twin pregnancy with complications – contraindication
	• Higher multiple pregnancy (triplets +) – contraindication, or may be very strong precaution if in hospital where facilities available to deal with untoward effects
Other obstetric conditions	• Preterm labour treated with drugs – contraindication
	• Late preterm labour committed to delivery – precaution
	• Threatened preterm labour – precaution
	• Reduced fetal movements – contraindication
	• Intrauterine growth retardation – possible contraindication, depends on severity
	• Abnormal fetal lie or presentation – precaution
	• Abnormal liquor volume – precaution
	• Caesarean section – avoid all herbal remedies for at least two weeks prior to elective surgery (risk of bleeding)

Conclusion

The interest in, and use of, complementary therapies and natural remedies by pregnant, labouring and newly birthed mothers has grown considerably in the last 30 years. As more and more women have started to use complementary therapies before, during or after childbirth, midwives have also become ever more enthusiastic about the value of different remedies and techniques, which offer new tools to aid their practice and enhance their care of women. However, it is essential to administer or advise on these modalities with caution. All complementary therapies and natural remedies are powerful entities which can contribute to normality in childbirth when used correctly, but which may cause problems for mothers, babies and midwives when used inappropriately.

It is of paramount importance that midwives and other maternity caregivers using complementary therapies understand the mechanism of action, indications, contraindications and precautions to any therapy they may be incorporating into their practice, and that they can balance their benefits and risks by applying the principles of each therapy to the practice of those therapies within maternity care. Women deserve to receive accurate, comprehensive and, where possible, evidence-based information, advice and treatment with complementary therapies and/or natural remedies in order that their use in pregnancy, labour and the puerperium can be both effective and safe.

CHAPTER 2

Commonly Used Complementary Therapies for Pregnancy and Birth

This chapter provides an overview of the complementary therapies most commonly used in the UK today, including a general description, indications, contraindications and precautions to each therapy, in general and in reproductive health, and some initial debate on the evidence base related to each therapy.

Whilst there are numerous complementary therapies, only about 15 to 20 are commonly in use in the developed world. Some therapies are defined as distinct modalities when, in fact, they derive from other therapies. Some lack any real evidence base and are not generally in common use; others claiming to be clinical therapies fit better into the category of health and wellbeing or even beauty therapy.

In this chapter, 12 therapies appropriate for clinical use in pregnancy, birth and the postnatal period are explored in detail, being those considered to be currently most popular amongst expectant mothers, and of interest to midwives and other maternity workers. Following an introduction to the therapy, the indications, contraindications and precautions and the evidence base are discussed. These therapies are referred to in subsequent chapters, in relation to specific conditions occurring in pregnancy, birth or the postnatal period. Further debate on the research is included in these later chapters.

The following are covered in this chapter:

- introduction
- acupuncture, acupressure and shiatsu
- aromatherapy
- Bach flower remedies
- chiropractic
- herbal medicine
- homeotherapy
- hypnotherapy
- massage
- osteopathy
- reflexology
- reiki
- yoga
- conclusion.

Introduction

Complementary medicine can be classified into several categories. The House of Lords report on complementary medicine (Select Committee on Science and Technology 2000) categorised the main therapies in use in the UK at that time into three main groups. Group 1 included the "top five" modalities, which were the most popular amongst, and sometimes practised by, medical practitioners, namely osteopathy and chiropractic, homeopathy, herbal medicine (relating to herbs indigenous to the UK) and western or "medical" acupuncture. Group 2 listed all the "supportive" therapies, generally thought at the time to be unregulated and lacking an evidence base, although this was challenged vociferously by professionals working in the field. Supportive therapies tend to be those which are not used as discrete systems of medicine in their own right but which enhance other clinical or therapeutic care, both complementary and conventional medicine. This includes massage, aromatherapy, reflexology, hypnosis, hydrotherapy, shiatsu, flower remedies, yoga, stress management, nutrition, reiki, Alexander technique and counselling. Group 3 was sub-divided into traditional systems of (folk) medicine such as Chinese medicine, Indian Ayurveda, Japanese kampo, etc., and alternative diagnostic techniques including kinesiology, radionics and iridology.

There was some controversy regarding these classifications, because the government's reasons for examining complementary medicine in detail were to move towards better education and training, more formal regulation, a greater evidence base and increased integration into mainstream healthcare. However, at the time, some of the therapies included in group 2 were better researched than some of those included in group 1. Sadly, whilst some advances have been made in the last two decades, the aims of the report were never fully achieved. Regulation continues to be a combination of voluntary self-regulation and unregulated therapies, medical science constantly refutes the evidence of research studies that do not fit with the "gold standard" randomised controlled trial methodology, and integration within the NHS remains sporadic. Other challenges focused around specific therapies. For example, acupuncture: western-style (medical) acupuncture as practised by many doctors was, somewhat politically, allocated to group 1 whilst Chinese medicine, including traditional, holistic acupuncture, was relegated to group 3a. The justification for this was that traditional Chinese medicine includes the use of herbal remedies indigenous to Asia and the import and safe use of these remedies in the UK was difficult to monitor.

Today, we could simply consider the differentiation between complementary therapies and natural remedies, as explained in Chapter 1. Alternatively, we could classify the therapies hierarchically from most to least medically accepted or from most to least popular amongst consumers. Therapies can also be categorised according to their mechanism of action, for example pharmacologically active or energy-based modalities, manual techniques or psychological therapies (see also Chapter 1). Several therapies work on more than one level. For example, aromatherapy uses pharmacologically active oils; it is often administered via touch therapy, i.e. massage, and is also thought to work energetically. Erroneously, NICE refers to all therapies as "non-pharmacological" – including aromatherapy. Table 2.1 provides a summary of the various classifications of the main complementary therapies covered in this book and of relevance to maternity care.

Table 2.1 Mechanism of action of commonly used complementary therapies

	Pharmacological	Energetic	Physical	Psychological
Acupuncture		**	**	*
Aromatherapy	**	*	* applied via massage	*
Bach flower remedies		**		**
Chiropractic			**	
Herbal medicine	**			
Homeopathy		**		
Hypnotherapy				**
Massage		*	**	*
Osteopathy			**	
Reflexology		**	**	
Reiki		**	** of the aura	
Shiatsu		**	**	
Yoga		**	*	*

Key: ** primary mechanism of action   * secondary mechanism of action

NB "psychological" refers to the mechanism of action rather than to the effect

Acupuncture, acupressure and shiatsu

Introduction

The term *acupuncture* derives from the Latin, *acus*, for "needle", and *puncture* or "pierce". Acupuncture and acupressure are components of traditional Chinese medicine (TCM), which incorporates other techniques including moxibustion, cupping, Chinese herbs and strong massage called *tui na* (the word meaning "push and grab"). Acupuncture theory is drawn from Chinese texts, thousands of years old, notably *The Yellow Emperor's Classic of Internal Medicine* compiled between 300 and 100BC, which is still regarded as the most authoritative guide to TCM. TCM practitioners would generally use a combination of techniques to treat the person, but a more reductionist way of using acupuncture and/or acupressure alone is used in western medical acupuncture (WMA).

Both systems of acupuncture are based on the principle that the body has energy channels, called meridians, running through it, which link one part of the body to another and help in connecting the whole person. Flowing through the meridians is the individual's life force, a form of energy called *qi* (pronounced "chee"). There are 12 major paired meridians running bilaterally through the body, and two single central meridians, one down the front and one down the back of the body. When the body, mind and spirit are in optimal health, the qi flows through the meridians completely harmoniously (homeostasis), but when one or more aspects of the whole are disrupted, illness or disease occurs and the energy becomes static, deficient or excessively strong. Located at intervals along the meridians are focus points (acupoints) which can be stimulated or sedated according to the requirements of the person's condition. There are over 2000 acupoints, although in modern acupuncture practice only about 200 are commonly used by practitioners.

A further concept in TCM is that of *yin* and *yang*, two opposing but complementary forces which help to balance the person. Imbalance in either yin or yang results in disorder, illness or disease. Yang energy is positive, warm and energetic, whereas yin energy is more negative, cooler and passive. Every aspect of life has a yin and a yang feature, and physiological processes can be viewed in terms of their yin and yang characteristics – see Table 2.2 for a few examples. Each organ is said to have an active, warming function (yang) as well as a cooling, moistening function (yin). An imbalance in the yang energy will also affect the yin qi and vice versa. For example, excessive intestinal energy will increase the qi, causing diarrhoea, whereas increased yin energy causes sluggishness and accumulation of waste, producing constipation. In perimenopausal women, night sweats are a symptom of increased yang energy, which in time depletes the yin energy, causing tiredness and fatigue, because yin and yang are co-dependent.

In TCM, practitioners also consider several other principles, namely the opposing features of excess-deficient energy (qi), heat and cold and what is happening on the interior and exterior of the body. Complex tongue and pulse assessments are used to aid diagnosis. For example, sweating, thirst, a red face and perhaps a predominance of anger in the individual's mood are all yang symptoms and treatment would aim to dispel the excess heat and rebalance the energies by increasing yin energy.

Acupuncture treatment is performed by inserting fine, usually disposable, needles into the relevant acupoints, or by applying thumb or finger pressure (acupressure). A TCM practitioner might also use moxibustion, which involves the application of heat to stimulate points where there is insufficient energy, or cupping, the application of small glass cups over acupuncture points to withdraw excess energy. Moxibustion is increasingly used to turn a breech-presenting fetus to cephalic and is discussed in detail in Chapter 6. Electro-acupuncture, in which leads are attached to the handle of the acupuncture needle, enabling a mild electrical current to pass through the needle to the acupoint, is also widely used by qualified acupuncturists and is similar in principle to transcutaneous electrical nerve stimulation (TENS). Auricular acupuncture, using acupoints on the ears, is also useful for some conditions, particularly when repeated stimulation to certain acupoints need to be carried out manually by the patient over a period of time. Physiological changes which occur during or after acupuncture treatment include changes in blood pressure and cardiac output, blood chemistry, the immune system and peristaltic actions of smooth muscles.

The main difference between TCM acupuncture and western medical acupuncture is that the former uses the full set of opposing principles described above, both to aid diagnosis and to determine the most appropriate treatment. WMA is more focused on anatomical and physio-pathological causes and effects and does not directly consider yin-yang and the concept of qi. The treatment in both styles of acupuncture is similar, using the same acupoints, although WMA practitioners are sometimes said to be practising "dry needling" rather than "acupuncture" per se. However, whilst the more formulaic WMA does not utilise the basic principles of TCM, it is useful for practitioners to have an understanding of them, and in clinical practice, there is often an overlap between the two systems.

It is also necessary here to mention *shiatsu*, which is similar in concept to acupressure but is a completely separate – and more contemporary – discipline. Shiatsu is a Japanese therapy, only developed in the 20th century, although it evolved from the centuries-old Japanese massage called *anma*, adapted from the Chinese *tui na*. The word "shiatsu" means "finger pressure", and treatment involves pressure being applied to the acupoints (called "tsubos" in Japanese) of the whole body, using fingers, thumbs and palms, although some practitioners claim that shiatsu points are unrelated to traditional Chinese meridians. Treatment and diagnosis are undertaken simultaneously, the practitioner working on each set of points to detect abnormalities in the organs and applying different pressures to restore homeostasis. There are several styles of shiatsu, including tsubo shiatsu, meridian shiatsu and Zen shiatsu, which takes a more spiritual approach than other styles. Treatment can be very relaxing and ease stress-related symptoms, and many practitioners use it also to treat specific clinical conditions. Table 2.3 outlines the differences between acupressure and shiatsu.

Table 2.2 Examples of the Yin and Yang characteristics of some physiological processes

Yang	Yin
Stress/hyperactivity	Relaxation/sleep
Testosterone	Oestrogen
Follicular phase of menstrual cycle	Luteal phase of menstrual cycle
Pre-orgasmic stage of sexual response	Post-orgasmic stage
Developing fetus	Pregnancy (mother)
Labour	Post-birth
Oxytocin	Progesterone

Table 2.3 Principal differences between acupressure and shiatsu

Acupressure	Shiatsu
Chinese therapy more than 5000 years old – one element of traditional Chinese medicine	Discrete Japanese therapy; evolved from Chinese medicine over centuries, formally recognised in the mid-20th century
Has its spiritual roots in Chinese Taoism	Has its spiritual roots in Indian Buddhism
Based on rebalancing vital energy within the meridians – qi (pronounced "chee")	Based on rebalancing vital energy within the meridians – ki (also pronounced "chee")
Acupoints are credited with having specific functions – treatment is usually focused on specific points	Tsubos (pressure points) link the whole body – treatment is generally a full-body massage-type treatment
Diagnosis prior to treatment via assessments of energy levels, pulse and tongue assessment and an analysis of the "clues" provided	Diagnosis and treatment undertaken together via palpation of pressure points – practitioners "sense" energy variations during palpation
Pressure applied via the fingers and thumbs	Pressure applied via the fingers, thumbs, palms, elbows, knees
Treatment may also involve use of acupuncture needles, Chinese herbs, *tui na* massage, cupping and moxibustion	Treatment focuses on rebalancing the body's energies by stimulation of the relevant tsubos by leaning into the body, combined with various stretching, holding and manipulative massage techniques
Treatment increases endorphins and encephalins and reduces stress hormones but is not generally given as a relaxation session; reducing stress hormones is a physiological *response* to rebalancing of the qi (homeostasis)	Treatment may be given specifically as a holistic stress-reducing session; it is believed that reducing stress hormones *facilitates* a return to homeostatic balance
Treatment given on a couch in a clinical setting	Treatment often given with the client on a mat on the floor

Indications

Acupuncture is a popular strategy for pregnant women, particularly those who are well educated and keen to take control of their childbearing experience (Soliday and Hapke 2014). During pregnancy, acupuncture may be useful for the relief of musculoskeletal problems including backache, sciatica, pelvic girdle pain and carpal tunnel syndrome. Gastrointestinal conditions respond well to needling of selected acupuncture points, particularly nausea and vomiting, heartburn, constipation and haemorrhoids. Acupuncture and acupressure/shiatsu offer easy, inexpensive and effective treatments for birth preparation, inducing labour in post-dates pregnancy, augmentation of contractions and pain relief in the first stage, as well as helping with intrapartum complications such as retained placenta. Postnatally, stimulation of certain acupoints can aid lactation, ease recovery from birth and balance the psycho-emotional state.

Shiatsu is more traditionally used for relaxation and to ease fatigue, stress, anxiety and related problems such as insomnia, but has also been used to treat gastrointestinal, musculoskeletal, cardiovascular, urinary and neurological conditions.

Contraindications and precautions

Some women should not receive acupuncture. General contraindications include women with coagulation disorders or those taking anticoagulants because there is a risk of bleeding from the insertion of the acupuncture needles, although a systematic review by McCulloch et al. (2015) disputes this. For similar reasons, women who are prone to infection, for example those with diabetes mellitus, should avoid acupuncture as there is a slight risk of infection entering the needle insertion site; practitioners should not needle near open wounds. Women with any major medical or obstetric complication may not be eligible to receive acupuncture, although this will depend on the severity of the condition and on whether the treatment is given in a community-based setting or in the maternity unit where facilities exist for dealing with emergencies. Shiatsu practitioners usually refrain from treating clients with inflammatory disorders, although acupuncturists may view inflammation as a sign of disordered qi. Certain specific acupoints should not be stimulated in pregnancy, either by needling or by pressure, as they may stimulate uterine contractions; these are called the "forbidden points". Shiatsu practitioners generally agree, although they may include more points than acupuncturists.

Evidence base

Conducting randomised double-blind placebo-controlled studies of acupuncture can be difficult. Researchers use different methods in their attempts to reduce bias, often comparing acupuncture to a control group which receives only standard care. A common method is to compare true acupuncture, in which the needles are inserted into the most appropriate acupoints for treatment of the presenting condition, with sham acupuncture. Sham acupuncture may involve the use of specially designed needles in which the needle retracts into the shaft of the handle on insertion, so that the subject experiences the piercing sensation but the acupoint is not stimulated to optimum depth (*deqi*) for a therapeutic response. Less commonly, insertion of a normal needle into parts of the body which do not correspond to specific acupoints may be used. Either method presents difficulties in that, at the very least, there is the possibility of a placebo reaction from the subject as a result of the sensation of the needle puncturing the skin.

Although many of the investigations into acupuncture are naturally published in Chinese language journals, there is an increasing amount of work published in English-language complementary therapy journals and conventional medical, nursing and midwifery journals. There has been a vast amount of research undertaken on the effectiveness of acupuncture for a range of clinical conditions. Whilst there appears to be less evidence to demonstrate safety, acupuncture is generally considered relatively safe, except for the possible risks highlighted by the principles for safe practice (contraindications and precautions). Retrospective systematic reviews of large numbers of cases perhaps offer the most reliable evidence of safety (MacPherson *et al.* 2001; White 2004; White *et al.* 2001; Witt *et al.* 2009).

There is an emerging body of evidence on the mechanism of action of acupuncture. Early work by the North Korean scientist Bong-Han (cited by Soh, Kang and Ryu 2013) appeared to demonstrate the existence of the acupuncture meridians flowing subcutaneously throughout the body, both within and outside blood vessels and lymphatic channels and on the surfaces of organs. More recent work involving injections of radio-opaque dye has shown the structure of the meridians throughout the body, the whole of which has been termed the "primo-vascular system" (Soh *et al.* 2013). It is known that this primo-vascular network is crucial to the cardiovascular system, and is now thought to channel the flow of energy and information around the body, relayed by electromagnetic waves of light (biophotons) and by the DNA. Computerised tomography has also shown the branching tree-like structure of the acupuncture channels (Chen *et al.* 2013), with clear differentiation between the sites of acupoints, corresponding to the original charts of Chinese acupuncture meridians, and non-acupuncture areas. Chinese studies tend to focus on determining the mechanism of action and physiological effects, although much of this work is still evolving (Wang, Chen *et al.* 2016; Wang, Yang *et al.* 2016).

Research on shiatsu is often misrepresented as acupressure, making it difficult to elucidate the specific techniques used. It is for this reason that shiatsu has been included in this section on acupuncture and acupressure, since searching the research databases usually reveals a mixed list of abstracts on both therapies, and in practice the same pressure points are commonly used. An Italian study compared shiatsu with amitryptiline for refractory headaches and found a benefit of manual treatment over the drug (Villani *et al.* 2017), but a prolonged search of several complementary therapy databases indicated that almost all other studies refer to "acupressure" rather than "shiatsu". On the other hand, there are numerous studies on acupressure for a range of conditions, particularly for symptoms such as pain and nausea.

In reproductive health, acupuncture can be helpful for couples experiencing fertility problems (Cochrane *et al.* 2016) and menopausal symptoms (Avis *et al.* 2016). In pregnancy, numerous studies have shown that stimulation of the Pericardium 6 acupoint on the wrists can be an effective treatment for nausea and vomiting, either by needling or acupressure (Can Gürkan and Arslan 2008; Shin, Song and Seo 2007; van den Heuvel *et al.* 2016) (see Chapter 4). Several studies have also been undertaken on the stimulation of acupoints to induce labour (see Chapter 7). Labour pain responds well to acupuncture (Liu *et al.* 2015) and may reduce the duration of labour (Asadi *et al.* 2015) (see Chapter 8).

Aromatherapy

Introduction

Aromatherapy is a scientific therapy in which highly concentrated aromatic essential plant oils are administered in various ways to enhance health and wellbeing. Essential oils are produced naturally and act as a protection for the plant from infection and extremes of temperature. The huge number of chemicals within the essential oils affects the fragrances of each plant so that the appropriate insects are attracted for pollination. These chemicals are also *pharmacologically active*, possessing a range of physical and emotional effects that can be harnessed in clinical practice for therapeutic benefits – but which can also be harmful when used inappropriately.

Essential oils enter the body primarily via respiratory inhalation. This occurs irrespective of the clinical method of administration, but inhalation can be used as a means of administration in its own right. Inhaling the aromas causes the chemicals within the essential oils to disperse around the body via the systemic circulation and also to travel via the olfactory system to the limbic system in the brain, where they impact on the mood. Oils can also be administered via the skin through massage or in water (in the bath or as a compress). Some medical practitioners, notably in France, administer essential oils as drugs via the mucous membranes, rectally as suppositories, or vaginally as pessaries, as well as via the gastrointestinal tract, but these methods are not appropriate in maternity care (and in the UK it is not possible to obtain indemnity insurance cover if oils are prescribed for oral administration). It is a combination of the physiological action of the chemicals, the method of administration and the psychological impact of the aromas which provides a therapeutic treatment according to the client's needs. See Tiran (2016a) for more in-depth information on aromatherapy in pregnancy and birth.

Indications

Aromatherapy treatment is generally relaxing, especially when the oils are administered via massage, the most popular and commonly used method in the UK. Specific essential oils also have pharmacologically relaxing effects, including common lavender oil (*Lavandula angustifolia*) (Sayorwan *et al.* 2012). Conversely, peppermint (*Mentha piperata*), grapefruit (*Citrus paradisi*) and black pepper (*Piper nigrum*) oils are stimulating to specific organs (Butt *et al.* 2013; Nagai *et al.* 2014; Oh, Park and Kim 2014). Lavender and clary sage (*Salvia sclarea*) oils lower the blood pressure (Seol *et al.* 2013), but others, such as rosemary (*Rosmarinus officinale*), will raise it (Fernández, Palomino and Frutos 2014). A predominance of certain chemicals means that some oils are analgesic, for example lemon (*Citrus limon*) (Ikeda, Takasu and Murase 2014) and common lavender (Hadi and Hanid 2011). All essential oils contain chemicals which are anti-bacterial; some are also anti-fungal or anti-viral – thus aromatherapy also offers useful substances to prevent or treat certain infections (Ziółkowska-Klinkosz *et al.* 2016).

It is known that having regular relaxation treatments in later pregnancy provides some much-needed "down time" and may help to prepare women for the birth, facilitating good progress in labour, although this may be due in part to the effects of the massage. In labour, aromatherapy helps the woman's psycho-emotional state and can relieve pain, ease nausea, aid progress and treat retained placenta (Burns *et al.* 2000; Dhany, Mitchell and Foy 2012). Postnatally, the use of lavender or tea tree (*Melaleuca alternifolia*) oils to ease discomfort and aid wound healing following episiotomy is popular.

Contraindications and precautions

Many essential oils should not be used before, during or immediately after pregnancy or may be contraindicated for women with medical or obstetric complications. Women should be advised to avoid self-administering essential oils in the preconception period and during the first trimester, although treatment from an appropriately qualified professional is not, in itself, a contraindication at these times.

Aromatherapy should be used with extreme caution, or avoided altogether, for any woman with a medical condition or obstetric complication. As a general rule, those who are eligible for a home birth or the midwife-led birthing centre can usually receive aromatherapy. Epilepsy is a complete contraindication as the aromas may trigger fits, especially since the woman may have had to change her medication and/or the epilepsy may have become unstable during pregnancy. In addition, some specific oils are known to be neurotoxic, including clary sage and common sage (*Salvia officinale*).

If the woman requires any medication, aromatherapy is usually contraindicated or should be used with caution only under the direction of a dual-qualified practitioner (e.g. midwife-aromatherapist). Drug and essential oil metabolism is similar and there is a risk of interactions or potentiation of either the prescribed medication or the essential oil. Women on anticoagulant therapy or with clotting disorders should avoid essential oils that may have an anticoagulant effect. Those who are admitted to the antenatal in-patient ward are not usually eligible to receive aromatherapy (and if a woman *is* able to receive treatment, care should be taken not to expose other women in the ward to the aroma vapours which may jeopardise their condition). All other women should be assessed carefully to ensure that the oils used are appropriate and safe. These contraindications apply equally to anyone else in contact with the aromas. See Tiran (2016a) for a more in-depth analysis of the contraindications and precautions.

As with any pharmacological therapy, aromatherapy treatment should be determined by the individual's condition, and administered in the correct dosage and by the most appropriate method. Side effects may occur if the oils are used inappropriately, in too high a dose or for a prolonged period of time. Side effects differ from a healing reaction, although the symptoms may be similar. Common symptoms, which are usually dose-dependent, include headaches, nausea, dizziness, lethargy and loss of concentration. Skin sensitivity is a very common adverse reaction, either due to contact with specific chemicals in the oils or to a pre-existing sensitivity to chemicals, including reactions to over-exposure to sunlight's ultraviolet rays.

Respiratory reactions are increasingly common, mainly due to a general over-exposure to chemicals in the environment, our food, toiletries and cleaning products. Severe respiratory effects can be unpredictable, the chemicals in fragrances and aromatic substances such as essential oils causing bronchial and alveolar inflammation resulting in dyspnoea, hyperventilation, air hunger or extreme hayfever-like symptoms. It is for this reason that aromatherapy should never be trivialised by midwives and doulas and the oils should be considered as drugs that need to be prescribed by appropriately trained professionals.

Adverse reactions to essential oils can affect anyone who is exposed to them, including clinicians and any companions of the pregnant woman. Prolonged exposure, for example, when caring for a woman during a long labour, may trigger headaches, nausea, loss of concentration or respiratory reactions in the midwife, doula or birth partner. Use of certain essential oils in labour – notably clary sage (*Salvia sclarea*) – can also cause menorrhagia for attendants who are menstruating. Midwives and others with specific medical conditions may need to decline to use aromatherapy if the oils required are contraindicated. For example, oils to facilitate labour should not be used by midwives who are pregnant, trying to conceive or breastfeeding, and any staff member who has a major medical condition may need to avoid using, or being exposed to women who are using, aromatherapy oils. Table 2.4 summarises the principal contraindications and precautions to the use of aromatherapy in pregnancy, birth and postnatally.

Table 2.4 Contraindications and precautions to the use of aromatherapy in maternity care

Contraindication/ precaution	Justification
Respiratory reactions	• Avoid use of vaporisers, diffusers and burners in institutions such as maternity unit, birth centre – exposure of everyone in the vicinity to the chemicals is unsafe and unethical; burners present a fire risk • Women with history of asthma, hay fever or existing respiratory condition – caution • Women with respiratory reactions to specific oils or perfumes containing these oils – avoid relevant oils, caution with others
Skin reactions	• Avoid oils high in chemicals known to cause skin reactions, e.g. phenols • Avoid specific oils which cause skin reactions in individuals, caution with other oils: common oils include chamomile, tea tree, black pepper • Caution with women with skin conditions, e.g. eczema, psoriasis, or with sensitive skin • Avoid exposure of skin to strong sunlight after administration of citrus oils and others that trigger photosensitivity
Specific oils contraindicated in pregnancy	• Avoid *all* essential oils in pregnancy, birth or postnatal period unless there is reasonable evidence/anecdotal experience of using the oil without major adverse effects
Clary sage oil (*Salvia sclarea*)	• Consider clary sage as "nature's Syntocinon" • Before 37 weeks gestation – contraindication • Labour, contractions well established – contraindication • Mother requiring drugs, e.g. Syntocinon, prostin, Propess, or taking other natural remedies to stimulate contractions – contraindication • Excessive vaginal lochia or retained products of conception in puerperium – contraindication • Attending staff or birth companions who are pregnant or trying to conceive – contraindication • Attending professionals who are menstruating – caution
Medical conditions	• Epilepsy – absolute contraindication • Major cardiac disease – contraindication • Liver disease – contraindication – oils metabolised via liver • Those taking anticoagulants or with coagulation disorder – contraindication • Women on other medication – precaution • Some oils affect blood sugar, causing hyper- or hypo-glycaemia – caution if woman or attendants have diabetes mellitus
Obstetric conditions	• Current vaginal bleeding, placental issues – contraindication • Mild to moderate hypertension – precaution; fulminating pre-eclampsia – contraindication • Twin pregnancy – precaution; triplets or more – contraindication

Contraindication/ precaution	Justification
Neonates/babies under three months of age – *absolute contraindication*	• Baby's skin is sensitive and permeable to essential oils, may cause severe skin irritation • May predispose child to allergies in later life • Baby partially dependent on sense of smell to recognise mother – oil aromas may mask this • Bronchial or sensory hyper-reactivity may occur from inhalation of essential oil vapours – *never* use room vaporisers near babies • Oils are metabolised via liver – neonatal liver is too immature to cope • Newborn immune system is immature: antibacterial properties of all essential oils could compromise immune system, with potential for lifelong difficulties in fighting infection
Homeopathy	• Women using homeopathic remedies should avoid concomitant use of aromatherapy oils by any method of administration because the strong aromas can antidote (inactivate) the chemically fragile homeopathic preparations (see section on homeopathy below)

Evidence base

There is a vast array of evidence to demonstrate the anti-infective properties of essential oils, although many studies involve oils not commonly used in clinical aromatherapy. Tea tree has been shown to be anti-bacterial, anti-viral and anti-fungal. Research on tea tree oil has been ongoing for over 30 years, much of the work being done in Australia (where tea tree grows) (Carson, Hammer and Riley 2006; Hammer, Carson and Riley 1998, 2012). More recent studies by other researchers often replicate or expand on previous studies (Bona *et al.* 2016; Liu *et al.* 2016). One of the largest and most significant studies on the use of aromatherapy for pain relief in labour was conducted by midwives at the John Radcliffe Hospital in Oxford, UK, between 1990 and 1999 (Burns *et al.* 2000) (see Chapter 8). Wound healing with essential oils, notably lavender (*Lavandula angustifolia* and other types), has also been studied. Episiotomy healing is of particular interest, but caution should be taken because the methods of application, types of lavender and doses differ between studies. Whilst it is possible to generalise that aromatherapy, or individual oils, may be effective in aiding wound healing, the specific clinical application should be considered, and the potential for side effects also taken into account with individual women. See Chapter 9 for further debate on aromatherapy for perineal wound healing. Several studies have explored emotional wellbeing, stress, anxiety and pain.

One of the problems with aromatherapy research is that some studies administer essential oils via massage, which presents an interesting confounding variable since the massage in itself may produce positive effects. Whilst some research projects investigate individual oils for their therapeutic properties, other researchers employ a "package" of treatment, often concluding that "aromatherapy" produces a particular effect, almost irrespective of the essential oils used.

Bach flower remedies

Introduction

There are several types of flower remedies, including Bach from the UK, Bush from Australia, orchid essences from Scotland and others from the Far East, but Bach remedies are by far the most well known, particularly in the UK. Bach flower remedies (BFRs) are liquid plant essences thought to have a positive effect on the emotions and on psychological wellbeing. They were devised by Dr Edward Bach (1886–1936), a Welsh microbiologist and pathologist, who became disillusioned with orthodox medicine and its focus on purely physio-pathological aspects of illness. He became interested in the possible impact of the emotions on the human body and the psychology of disease. Whilst working at the London Homeopathic Hospital just after the First World War, he surmised that medicine should treat the whole person, not merely the disease, and that, by working on the emotions through a system of energy-based remedies, this would stimulate the individual's self-healing capacity, a feature of many complementary medical modalities.

Bach (pronounced "batch") developed 37 remedies from different plants, and one from spring water (rock rose), plus Rescue Remedy, which is a combination of five of the original 38 remedies and is a first aid/stress reliever. The remedies are produced by putting freshly picked sun-exposed flowers into spring water. They are said to be similar in principle to homeopathic remedies, although they are prepared quite differently – there is no succussion and dilution, so many homeopaths dispute this claim (see Homeopathy, below). However, as with homeopathy, Bach remedies do not act pharmacologically: they are based on vibrational energy.

Complementary practitioners who use BFRs in their practice are not medically qualified, and although some focus entirely on the remedies as their primary modality, the remedies are mostly used in combination with other therapies such as homeopathy. They are freely available to purchase in health stores and it is relatively simple to self-administer them. The most common method of administration is to use the purchased stock bottle, dilute a few drops in bottled still spring water and then use this as the main remedy source, usually taking two or three drops, perhaps three to four times a day – but this does, of course, depend on the individual's precise symptoms and the reason for using the remedies.

Indications

Rescue Remedy, in liquid form, is used for panic, hysteria and acute anxiety (but is not usually appropriate for prolonged or chronic stress-related conditions). The dose is three to four drops neat on the tongue but it is also available in a spray and a cream for dermal application, as well as lozenges for oral use. However, whilst Rescue Remedy is very effective in acute situations, for example pre-examination nerves, it should not be seen as a panacea for all emotional issues. It is particularly useful for situations in maternity care such as acute anxiety during venepuncture, the transition stage in labour and distress after being given bad news. It is also possible to use a blend of up to seven BFRs to treat more chronic emotional conditions and this would be taken three to four times daily for up to two weeks. Table 2.5 gives some examples of how the full range of 38 BFRs could be of use in pregnancy, labour and the puerperium.

Table 2.5 Examples of situations in maternity care in which Bach flower remedies may be useful

Remedy	General indication	Examples
Agrimony	Mental torment behind a "brave face"	Over-cheerful mother who may be developing postnatal depression
Aspen	Fear of unknown origin	Primigravida frightened of giving birth but unsure why
Beech	Intolerant	Labouring woman who can't stand being touched and becomes irritable
Centaury	Finds it difficult to say "no"	Professional working woman whose pregnancy suffers because she continues to work at her pre-pregnancy pace
Cerrato	Lack of judgement, constantly seeking reassurance	Mother who constantly asks questions, lacks confidence in mothering ability

Cherry plum	Fear of mind giving way, as if she is going to "lose it"	Woman in labour who is becoming "out of control"
Chestnut bud	Keeps repeating the same mistakes, does not learn from experience	Woman who has different relationships with similar, perhaps abusive, men
Chicory	Over-concern for others, controlling	Mother who constantly double-checks the condition of her baby, unable to pass care to others
Clematis	Little interest in what is happening, day-dreaming	Mother who does not attend to her baby, possibly developing postnatal depression
Crab apple	Unable to accept self-image, constantly cleaning	Woman who is overly conscious of the smell of lochia
Elm	Overwhelmed, depressed, too much to do	Woman with several small children, who is overwhelmed by responsibilities
Gentian	Easily discouraged when faced with difficulties	Woman who is discouraged by her slow progress in labour
Gorse	Extreme hopelessness and despair	Labouring woman who feels complete misery, unable to anticipate the birth with joy
Heather	Preoccupied with herself, talkative, demanding attention	Woman after a miscarriage, constantly "de-briefing" her experiences with people
Holly	Feelings of envy, jealousy, suspicion, hatred	Partner who feels jealous of the time that the baby demands from mother, particularly during breastfeeding
Honeysuckle	Over-attachment to past memories, can't let go of the past	Pregnant woman who is constantly worrying about a previous emergency Caesarean
Hornbeam	Mental weariness, "Monday morning" feeling	Midwife at the end of a 13-hour shift
Impatiens	Impatient, easily irritated	Labouring woman who irritably tells the midwife not to touch her
Larch	Lack of self-confidence	Older, highly professional woman, used to being in control, who lacks the confidence to care for her baby
Mimulus	Fear of known things	Woman with needle phobia
Mustard	Depression, deep gloom for no known reason	Postnatal depression
Oak	Exhaustion, burn-out, workaholic, over-achiever	Midwife trying to juggle clinical, academic and personal commitments
Olive	Lack of energy, fatigue	New mother not getting much sleep; midwives on long shifts

Remedy	General indication	Examples
Pine	Guilt, self-reproach, apologetic	Woman feeling guilty about leaving other children at home while she is in hospital
Red chestnut	Worried, over-concern for others	Mother who constantly checks that her baby is breathing
Rock rose	Fear, terror	Woman requiring "crash" Caesarean section for severe fetal distress
Rock water	Self-denial, perfectionist	Mother who is constantly striving to be the perfect parent
Scleranthus	Indecision, usually between two choices	Woman trying to decide whether or not to have external cephalic version
Star of Bethlehem	After effects of trauma, post-traumatic stress	Woman who is completely shocked by an unplanned pregnancy
Sweet chestnut	Extreme despair, hopelessness, anguish	Following loss of baby or birth of baby with abnormalities
Vervain	Over-enthusiastic, hyperactive	Student midwife who does not listen because she is so over-enthusiastic
Vine	Domineering, inflexible, aggressive, bullying	Partner in domestic violence situation
Walnut	Protection from outside influences, adaptation to change	Woman needing to adapt to the role of being a mother
Water violet	Proud, aloof, lonely, anti-social	Woman in parent education class who keeps herself to herself and does not interact
White chestnut	Mind constantly going over problems and worries	Woman unable to sleep because she is constantly worrying that the baby will be all right
Wild oat	Uncertain of correct path, unable to plan and make decisions	Midwife trying to decide on direction of career
Wild rose	Apathy, loss of motivation, resigned to current situation	Midwife suffering "burn out" but without energy to resolve it
Willow	Resentment, self-pity	Woman who resents the interfering help of her mother-in-law

Contraindications and precautions

Although BFRs are generally considered safe to use in pregnancy, the liquid remedies are preserved in aqueous alcohol (brandy), so should be avoided if there is a history of alcohol-related or hepatic disease or if the woman is taking large amounts of medication or herbal remedies that are metabolised via the liver. Occasionally, Rescue Remedy has been reported to cause drowsiness, so women should be advised to try it at home first in order to assess how they respond to it.

Where there are deep underlying psychological issues, care must be taken to assess the woman carefully and observe her closely over a course of treatment. BFRs are said to have an "onion peeling" effect, in which the most dominant emotion is stripped away by the initial administration of combined remedies, often revealing deeper psychological issues hidden below the surface. It is important that practitioners using BFRs also possess good counselling and listening skills and know when to refer to a professional who is more experienced in dealing with women with mental health problems.

Evidence base

There is little robust evidence for the effectiveness of BFRs and, as far as is known, none relating to safety. Rescue Remedy is the most studied of the remedies, mainly focusing on situations such as pre-examination or pre-operative stress (Armstrong and Ernst 2001; Walach, Rilling and Engelke 2001). Ernst (2010) conducted a systematic review of seven flower remedy trials, six of which were placebo-controlled, but none of the studies conclusively demonstrated effectiveness. Similar conclusions were drawn from Thaler *et al.*'s systematic review (2009). One study explored the use of the remedies for children with attention deficit hyperactivity disorder but, again, found no greater benefit of the remedies than with placebo (Pintov *et al.* 2005).

More recently, Rivas-Suárez *et al.* (2015) conducted a small placebo-controlled trial of 43 patients awaiting surgery for carpal tunnel syndrome who used Rescue Remedy cream for 21 days. The results appeared to indicate that it could be helpful in relieving pain, possibly due to a reduction in the emotional perception of pain. Howard (2007) also considered the use of BFRs to relieve pain and surmised that patients' coping abilities were potentially improved through a better mental outlook on the pain, although it is difficult to determine the extent of the placebo effect in this study. Rescue Remedy cream has also apparently been found to control blood glucose and cholesterol levels in rats (Resende *et al.* 2014), possibly providing evidence of physiological effects.

One old obstetric study (von Rühle 1995), a summary of which was found on the Bach Flower Centre's own website, investigated the use of BFRs on primigravidae with a post-dates pregnancy, with three groups receiving individualised flower remedies, additional care and attention or standard care. Although there were no direct effects on the time to onset of labour or mode of birth and results were not statistically significant, the researchers found that women in the flower remedy group appeared to have a perception of less labour pain and nausea and possibly required less intervention than women in the other two groups. It would, however, be difficult to replicate this study since the remedies were individualised to each subject within the original study, a factor that detracts from the robustness of randomised controlled trials.

The general conclusion in most studies is that there is a placebo effect, a factor which is increasingly recognised as a powerful therapeutic response in itself (Ernst 2010). BFRs are very popular amongst certain sections of the public. However, taking into account the lack of any real investigative support, there is little direct cross-referencing to BFRs in the condition-specific chapters in this book as they seek to examine the evidence base for the use of complementary therapies for each condition.

Chiropractic

Introduction

Chiropractic was founded in the 1890s by the Canadian Daniel David Palmer, a magnetic healer. Since 1994 it has been a statutorily regulated profession in the UK in the same way as medicine, nursing and midwifery. Chiropractic deals with the diagnosis, treatment and prevention of mechanical disorders of the musculoskeletal system and the effects of those disorders on neurological functioning and on general health and wellbeing. Treatment normally involves manual manipulation and/or adjustment to rebalance the whole and to help the person regain and maintain homeostasis. It is similar in principle to osteopathy but has some differences in philosophy and the management of conditions. See Table 2.6 for a summary of the similarities and differences between chiropractic and osteopathy. See also Osteopathy, below.

Table 2.6 Similarities and differences between chiropractic and osteopathy

Similarities
• They share a common history and philosophy
• Both work on the musculoskeletal system, including bones, joints, ligaments and tendons
• Both work on the neurological system and blood supply to influence other bodily systems
• Both use observation and touch as part of the diagnostic process

Differences	
Osteopathy	**Chiropractic**
Osteopathy was founded 21 years earlier than chiropractic	Chiropractic was developed from the principles of osteopathy by a group of osteopaths with opinions that differed from their colleagues
Takes a more holistic approach, considers the body as a whole, aims to improve function by correcting the overall structure of the body	Focuses mainly on realignment of the spine to treat pain, preventing neurological system compromise
Treats a wide range of functional conditions including circulatory and digestive system disorders	Treats primarily musculoskeletal issues
Diagnosis is by history-taking and physical examination, referral for other diagnostic tests as necessary	Diagnosis may include X-rays, MRI scans, urinary analysis and blood tests as well as history-taking and clinical examination
Treatment involves a wide variety of techniques including muscle and soft tissue work, such as massage, joint articulation and manipulation	Treatment involves more manipulative techniques to aid adjustment of the vertebrae and facilitate optimal nerve transition
Treatments may be over a prolonged period to allow for holistic assessment and therapy, with appointments being spaced out to facilitate recovery	Treatments are often short but frequent

The primary concept of chiropractic is that joint subluxation (dislocation) is the cause of disorders within the body and that spinal manipulation assists in correcting the relationship of the joints, ligaments and tendons in order to treat the consequent illness. Spinal manipulation involves high-velocity, low-amplitude manual thrusts applied to spinal joints, which cause extension of the joints beyond the physiological range of motion. This is different from the spinal mobilisation used in physiotherapy in which manual force is applied to the joints without thrusting movements and within the normal passive range of motion.

Indications

Chiropractic is used to treat a wide range of illnesses, including stress, respiratory conditions such as asthma, to irritable bowel syndrome, cardiovascular problems and, of course, musculoskeletal issues. In pregnancy, backache, particularly lumbosacral pain, sciatica, pelvic girdle pain and carpal tunnel syndrome appear to respond well, but chiropractic can also be used to treat soft tissue conditions including nausea, constipation, heartburn, oedema and even pelvic floor problems (Bernard and Tuchin 2016; Haavik, Murphy and Kruger 2016; Henry 2015; Tuchin 1998).

Contraindications and precautions

Women with coagulation disorders or taking anticoagulants should not receive chiropractic, especially the high-velocity manipulations which can occasionally induce internal tissue tearing. Chiropractic is also contraindicated in those with osteoporosis, malignant or inflammatory disease, fractures or spondylolisthesis. It is important that expectant mothers seeking treatment inform the chiropractor of their pregnancy because X-rays are often used to aid diagnosis. It does, however, seem to be safe during pregnancy and for the treatment of neonates (Todd *et al.* 2015).

Evidence base

Research into chiropractic commonly revolves around treatment of backache and other major spinal disorders. A systematic review by Blanchette *et al.* (2016) found that chiropractic appears to be at least as effective as physiotherapy for the treatment of low back pain (in non-pregnant patients) and that it is relatively safe. Unfortunately, many of the papers involve small studies or comprise single case reporting (Howell 2012). Conversely, studies on pregnant women with back pain show good results (Murphy, Hurwitz and McGovern 2009; Peterson, Mühlemann and Humphreys 2014). A systematic review by Close *et al.* (2014) indicated similar results for both chiropractic and osteopathy, although methodology was considered to be of variable quality and it was suggested there was an element of bias in the studies reviewed. An additional problem is that many studies have been undertaken in Canada, the "spiritual home" of chiropractic, implying that there may be an expectation by clients of its potential success (Sadr, Pourkiani-Allah-Abad and Stuber 2012). See Chapter 5 for further discussion on back pain in pregnancy.

Herbal medicine

Introduction

Herbal medicine (phytotherapy) is the therapeutic use of plants and plant substances. Plants contain numerous chemicals which, when administered correctly, work synergistically to facilitate homeostasis. Although still not accepted by the medical professions, there is a great deal of research ongoing by pharmaceutical companies keen to harness the therapeutic properties of individual constituents so that they can be isolated and produced synthetically as drugs. Commonly used drugs which have been derived from plants include aspirin (from willow bark and meadow sweet), digoxin (from foxglove), cannabis (from opium) and quinine (from the bark of the cinchona tree), used for malaria. Plants have been used as medicines for centuries all around the world, particularly for childbirth problems.

Indications

Women frequently use herbal remedies, including herbal teas, to treat physiological disorders such as nausea and vomiting, constipation and other gastrointestinal discomforts in pregnancy. Use in pregnancy is often unrelated to previous use (Nyeko, Tumwesigye and Halage 2016), with older, better educated primigravidae being the most likely to use herbal remedies (Forster *et al.* 2006). Antenatal use is also common in developing countries, especially in rural areas with little access to conventional healthcare (Yemele *et al.* 2015). Women may also attempt to treat what they perceive as "minor" complaints with herbal medicines, including the rather worrying use of cranberry for urinary tract infection or St John's wort for clinical depression (Frawley *et al.* 2015; Izzo *et al.* 2016).

Expectant mothers' use of herbal remedies increases as they approach term, with many using herbal medicines specifically to prepare for and initiate labour (see also Chapter 7). Self-administration tends to decline during the early postnatal period, although some women take substances such as fennel or fenugreek to stimulate milk production. Traditional Chinese medicine is of particular concern in the UK because it can be difficult to elicit precisely what remedies have been prescribed; a survey of 54 Chinese medicine shops in London (Teng, Shaw and Barnes 2015) indicated potentially misleading information and unsubstantiated advertising claims that could lead to inappropriate consumer choices. Of more concern is the sometimes injudicious use of herbal teas to calm babies, especially, but not exclusively, in developing countries (Abdulrazzaq, Al Kendi and Nagelkerke 2009; Savino *et al.* 2005; Sim *et al.* 2013).

Contraindications and precautions

The most important factor which conventional healthcare professionals need to take into account is that *all* herbal remedies, including herbal teas and essential oils, act pharmacologically, their metabolism being the same as for other medication, whether prescribed or recreational. The risk of adverse effects is probably greater than with any other complementary or alternative therapy (Langhammer and Nilsen 2014). Women perceive herbal remedies as being safer than drugs and do not consider any potential risk to fetal development when taking natural remedies, although ironically their approach to prescribed medication is more cautious (Petersen *et al.* 2015).

One of the major problems of inappropriate use is the potential for overdose, side effects and interactions with other herbs or with prescribed or recreational drugs. As with drug medication, it is imperative that herbal remedies are taken for the correct purpose, in the correct dosage and frequency. Many side effects occur because of the public's widespread misconception that plant remedies are safe because they are natural.

Concern has been expressed by numerous authorities about the use of herbal medicines in the preconceptional period and during pregnancy, childbirth and lactation (Boltman-Binkowski 2016; Budzynska *et al.* 2013; Johnson *et al.* 2009; Sim *et al.* 2013; Teoh *et al.* 2013). In pregnancy, the main issues centre on the impact of harmful chemicals on the mother and fetus and on the progress of pregnancy. Some plants are genuinely known to cause side effects, but others will only cause problems if taken to excess, and the difficulty in differentiating these two aspects further confuses the picture. The evidence for safety in pregnancy can be scarce simply because the individual herb has not been studied, or because there is no evidence of risks such as miscarriage or fetal anomalies in relation to the remedy. However, this does not mean that phytomedicine is safe in pregnancy – an absence of evidence of risk is not the same as proof of safety (Tiran 2012).

Research undertaken to elicit therapeutic effects in order that active constituents can be isolated and extracted for the development of drug manufacture can also be applied. For example, if a study finds that a herb has a hypertensive effect, it is obvious that caution should be taken in pregnancy even if there is no evidence of direct reproductive toxicity. In addition, there is a need to apply knowledge of the mechanism of action of the relevant herb to the physiology of pregnancy; for example, juniper berry may decrease blood sugar (Orhan *et al.* 2011), cause urinary tract irritation and even epileptiform fits if taken in excess and may significantly interfere with drug metabolism (Tam *et al.* 2014).

Medical practitioners rightly take a cautious approach to the use of herbal remedies in pregnancy, although this is mainly through lack of any in-depth knowledge. The general public takes the opposite approach, believing that herbal remedies must be safe (or safer than drugs) because they are natural. Conflicting information and evidence on individual herbal remedies abounds, even in relation to those which are very popular such as ginger, echinacea, chamomile and St John's wort (Cuzzolin *et al.* 2010). Although the proportion of harmful chemicals tends to be less than in commercially prepared herbal remedies, excessive consumption of herbal teas can also lead to complications such as hepatotoxicity, as reported in a (non-pregnant) case related to rooibos (red bush) tea (Reddy *et al.* 2016), or airborne allergic reactions to chamomile tea (Anzai, Vázquez Herrera and Tosti 2015; Benito *et al.* 2014).

It is safest to advise women that herbal medicines should be avoided completely in pregnancy unless they have been prescribed by a qualified practitioner. This commonsense approach extends to the preconception period as many herbal remedies may interfere with fertility or early embryonic organogenesis. This applies across most cultures and in almost every country in the world. Women should avoid any plant remedies which are not essential during the first three months of the pregnancy, since many are known, even anecdotally, to trigger miscarriage; this rule is even more essential if there is a history of difficulty in conceiving or recurrent miscarriages. Certain remedies are, however, very commonly used in later pregnancy, not least those which are thought to prepare the woman's body for labour.

Numerous plant remedies have strong anticoagulant effects and should be avoided by anyone, pregnant or otherwise, with haemorrhagic or coagulation disorders, or who is taking warfarin, aspirin or other drugs or herbs with anticoagulant effects (McEwen 2015). There are numerous published papers expressing concern about the effects of herbs on blood clotting, sufficient to prompt some anaesthetists to advise discontinuation of all herbal remedies at least two weeks prior to elective surgery (Leite, Martins and Castilho 2016). This practice should extend to women due to have an elective Caesarean section, to reduce the risk of haemorrhage during or after surgery.

From a maternity professional's point of view it is paramount that women are asked about their use of herbal remedies before and during pregnancy, in preparation for the birth and when breastfeeding. Some herbal medicines can be used effectively to treat specific conditions during the childbearing year, but it is far more common for maternity professionals to be faced with untoward adverse effects of inappropriate use, often without their knowledge.

There are several hundred herbal remedies used by qualified medical herbalists. Table 2.7 highlights some of the common herbs considered unsafe, in therapeutic doses, to use during the childbearing period as they may cause birth defects and are systemically toxic or utero-tonic (NB this list is not exhaustive). The key points are that herbal medicines act pharmacologically and can interact with prescribed medications, with each individual remedy having its own indications, contraindications and precautions in the same way as pharmaceuticals. Women should be advised to be extremely cautious in using herbal remedies, including excessive consumption of herbal teas or individual culinary herbs, during the preconception, antenatal, labour and postnatal periods.

Table 2.7 Herbal medicines considered unsafe to use before and during pregnancy, labour and breastfeeding

Plant	Reason	Reference
Aloe vera (oral)	May cause birth defects, miscarriage and have strong purgative effect on bowel	Ulbricht *et al.* 2007
	May cross to breast milk	
Basil	May cause miscarriage, preterm labour	Mohammed *et al.* 2016
	May affect blood glucose; avoid with diabetic medication	
	Small amounts suitable for culinary use	
Black cohosh	May cause miscarriage, preterm labour	Blitz, Smith-Levitin and Rochelson 2016
	Avoid in hepatic conditions, or with antidepressants or sedatives	
	Possibly acceptable in labour (see Chapter 8)	
Blue cohosh	May cause miscarriage, preterm labour; developmental abnormalities in fetus	Dugoua *et al.* 2008
	Major vascular problems in neonate	
	NOT to be used for natural induction of labour	
	Avoid completely in pregnancy and labour (see Chapter 8)	

Clary sage	Strong uterine stimulant, may cause preterm labour, hypertonic uterine action in labour, postpartum haemorrhage Avoid with oxytocics, antidepressants, alcohol (see Chapter 8)	Anecdotal evidence – personal experience and communications with midwives (see Tiran 2016a)
Comfrey	May cause miscarriage, preterm labour Hepatotoxic	Stickel and Seitz 2000
Dong quai (angelica)	May cause miscarriage, preterm labour, diarrhoea, sensitivity to sunlight Avoid with bleeding, coagulation disorders, anticoagulants	Chuang et al. 2006
Fennel	May cause miscarriage, preterm labour, dermal irritation May inhibit strong antibiotics	Trabace et al. 2015
Fenugreek	Large amounts may cause miscarriage, preterm labour Consumption immediately prior to delivery may cause baby to have unusual body odour similar to that with maple syrup urine disease Avoid with anti-diabetic medication, bleeding, coagulation disorders, anticoagulants	Ouzir, El Bairi and Amzazi 2016
Feverfew	May cause miscarriage, preterm labour May cause nausea, diarrhoea, constipation, headache, abdominal pain, bloating Avoid with bleeding, coagulation disorders, anticoagulants	Yao, Ritchie and Brown-Woodman 2006
Ginger	Use in small amounts for no longer than three weeks Anticoagulant effects – avoid with bleeding, coagulation disorders, anticoagulants	McEwen 2015 See Chapter 4
Ginseng, Asian	May cause fetal abnormalities Avoid with bleeding, coagulation disorder, anticoagulants, anti-diabetic medication, immunosuppressants, alcohol, caffeine	Seely et al. 2008
Juniper berry	Toxic to kidneys, may cause difficulties with conception, miscarriage Avoid with anticoagulants, renal complications	Butani et al. 2003
Motherwort	May cause miscarriage, preterm labour Avoid with antihistamines, drugs with sedative action	Ernst 2002
Mugwort	May cause miscarriage, preterm labour; may contain lead traces NB mugwort sticks for moxibustion are safe as not used orally; see Chapter 6	Aziz et al. 2016

Plant	Reason	Reference
Nutmeg	May cause miscarriage, preterm labour, thrombosis, hallucinations, changes in consciousness Avoid with pethidine or similar-acting drugs	Ernst 2002
Parsley	May cause miscarriage, preterm labour, birth defects Avoid with anticoagulants, aspirin, anti-diuretics Culinary use acceptable in small amounts	Ciganda and Laborde 2003
Passiflora (Also known as passion flower)	May cause miscarriage, preterm labour Avoid with sedatives	Boeira *et al.* 2010
Pennyroyal	Toxic to liver, kidneys May cause dizziness, bloody vomiting, delirium, fits, raised blood pressure, blood clotting disorders May cause miscarriage or preterm labour	Jalili *et al.* 2013
Sage	May cause miscarriage, preterm labour, postpartum haemorrhage May affect milk supply postnatally Avoid with anticonvulsants, anti-diabetic medication	Ernst 2002
Senna	Long-term frequent use may cause laxative dependence, liver toxicity Purgative effects may cause miscarriage, preterm labour, abdominal pain, cramps, nausea, diarrhoea Avoid with other laxatives, anticoagulants	Vanderperren *et al.* 2005
Squaw vine (also known as partridge-berry)	May cause miscarriage, preterm labour; use only under supervision of medical herbalist	Chevalier 2016
St John's wort	Mechanism of action similar to antidepressants and may cause same side effects Not a replacement for antidepressants	Moretti *et al.* 2009
Thuja (also known as arbor vitae)	May cause miscarriage, preterm labour Can cause epileptiform fits; avoid with anticonvulsants, antibiotics, antidepressants	Naser *et al.* 2005

Evidence base

There is a phenomenal amount of good quality research evidence to support the benefits and risks of herbal medicine. Many studies have been undertaken by pharmaceutical companies wanting to isolate active ingredients in order to develop and patent drugs. Whilst this gives us some relevant information about the mechanism of action of specific herbal remedies, it is the isolation of active constituents and the production of a synthetic form to be patented which is likely to lead to the appearance of side effects in patients taking the drugs. However, there is no clear evidence as to the safety of specific herbal medicines in pregnancy since it is impossible to conduct appropriately designed research studies on pregnant humans. Much of that available focuses on the risks to embryonic/fetal development and is usually performed on animals or in the laboratory. Other evidence is anecdotal and arises from reports of adverse effects, often from poisoning through inadvertent misuse.

Homeopathy

Introduction

Homeopathy is a gentle system of healing developed in the 18th century by Dr Samuel Hahnemann who became disillusioned with the medical practices of the day, for example blood-letting, purging or using toxic substances, which often caused severe side effects. Hahnemann discovered that, rather than treating people with opposites (such as treating constipation with laxatives), the principle of "treating like with like" was gentler and more effective. He challenged the popular belief that quinine from cinchona bark cured malaria due to its diuretic properties: after self-administering quinine he discovered that it *produced* malaria-like symptoms, which led him to the theory that "like cures like". He later experimented with ever-smaller doses and realised that an infinitesimal dose worked even more effectively, especially when it was shaken vigorously – a process called succussion. Essentially, he discovered that when the person's individual symptom picture is matched to a remedy (this is termed a proving), that same remedy, in extremely diluted form, will actually treat the same symptoms. Examples include a remedy derived from coffee (coffea) that may treat insomnia, or one from arsenic (arsenicum) that may ease profuse vomiting. The remedy resonates with the body's vital force (internal harmonising capacity) to raise its energetic vibration, facilitating healing. This concept of the vital force is similar in principle to that of qi, as harnessed in traditional Chinese medicine.

Sceptics argue that because homeopathic remedies are so dilute, their action is purely a placebo effect. However, homeopathy does not work pharmacologically (i.e. chemically) but through a process of quantum physics in which the vibratory (dynamic) structure of a substance can be altered by violent shaking (succussion). For most physiological conditions in pregnancy and postnatally, a single tablet, taken three to four times daily for no more than four days, should be sufficient to resolve or lessen the symptoms. Taking an inappropriate remedy for longer than this can cause a "reverse proving", in which symptoms intended to be treated by the remedy develop in addition to existing symptoms. For labour, a more acute phase, one tablet of 200C may be effective or, for more prolonged symptoms, one 30C tablet every one to two hours. It is the *frequency* of administration which affects the dose, *not* the number of tablets taken at each administration. If the correct remedy has been selected, the mother may initially feel worse (an anticipated healing aggravation) but her condition should then improve within a few days.

Indications

The essential method of diagnosis employed in homeopathy aims to determine ways to treat the whole person. Every aspect of the individual's symptom picture is vital to choosing the most appropriate remedy. Different women with the same condition – for example, nausea and vomiting in pregnancy – may be prescribed different remedies because their overall symptom picture may differ. Conversely, the same remedy may be used to treat several different conditions because the underlying characteristics of the remedy match the symptom pictures. Women who are familiar with the principles of homeopathic remedy selection will often choose to self-administer remedies for the various physiological conditions of pregnancy and the postnatal period, including nausea, constipation, oedema and lactation issues. In labour, homeopathy can be useful for pain relief and to stimulate contractions, to help women overcome anxiety, fear and the various emotional changes occurring as labour progresses; it can also be effective for critical problems such as retained placenta. However, given the acute nature and possible dangers of a mismanaged third stage of labour, this would need to be prescribed by an experienced homeopath and should not be attempted by novices, particularly when midwives have access to other, proven, pharmacological and surgical treatments. Whilst the use of homeopathic remedies can be helpful, labour is a dynamic, constantly changing event and it can take some skill to identify the most appropriate remedy for each woman.

Contraindications and precautions

Homeopathic medicines are chemically very fragile, and although they will not interact with drugs, some medicines, such as antacids and certain strong antibiotics, can inactivate the remedies. Remedies must be stored carefully to avoid being inactivated by other chemicals or the environment, including exposure to bright light, radiation such as microwaves, televisions and mobile telephone energies, mint and other strong flavours and aromas (including aromatherapy essential oils), coffee, eucalyptus and embrocations for muscle pain such as Deep Heat™.

A healing reaction is a very common effect of treatment when the correct remedy has been selected. This is not the same as an adverse (side) effect of a pharmacological therapy such as herbal medicine or aromatherapy. In homeopathic medicine, the presentation of symptoms following administration of a remedy is more commonly known as a homeopathic *aggravation* and needs to be distinguished from adverse effects arising from inappropriate administration, such as taking the wrong remedy, or taking the right remedy too frequently or for too long. For example, a reverse proving can occur if a woman takes arnica tablets excessively frequently after delivery, causing her to develop severe systemic bruising.

Parents familiar with homeopathy often use remedies to treat their children, believing that it is gentler than pharmaceutical drugs. However, in the USA, over 400 reports of adverse reactions of infants given homeopathic teething granules or gels have been received by the Federal Drug Administration (FDA) since 2011 (Abbassi 2017). The reports included infants suffering convulsions, dyspnoea, drowsiness, coma and gastrointestinal complaints, and ten deaths. The FDA has advised parents not to use the products, several companies have voluntarily withdrawn stock from sale and one company issued a recall on a homeopathic teething product found to contain inconsistent amounts of belladonna; analysis by FDA laboratories found excessive levels of belladonna in another product. The FDA investigation continues at the time of going to press but this is likely to be another setback for the acceptance of homeopathy. However, as with any therapy, there is a correct method of administration and a correct dose to which people should adhere. It is probable that many of these children either suffered severe reverse provings or that some had underlying medical conditions which would make the use of the specific remedies inappropriate at that time. Unfortunately, as with herbal remedy adverse effects, problems with homeopathy most likely occur with inappropriate use due to lack of knowledge and understanding. Box 2.1 outlines the criteria for effective and appropriate use of homeopathic remedies.

BOX 2.1

Criteria for effective use of homeopathic remedies

- Avoid food, drink, toothpaste or cigarettes in the mouth for 15 minutes before or after taking the remedy.

- Avoid substances which antidote remedies: aromatherapy essential oils, coffee, strongly spiced foods, peppermint, mint-flavoured toothpaste or chewing gum, eucalyptus, decongestants, Olbas™ oil, mobile telephones, metal spoons, X-rays, microwaves.

- Avoid with drugs which block homeopathic action: analgesics, antacids, antibiotics, aspirin, steroids, laxatives, decongestants, cough lozenges.

- Remedies should not be taken prophylactically – await the occurrence of the condition.

NB It is particularly important prior to an elective Caesarean to avoid taking remedies such as arnica in advance of surgery as prolonged administration will cause a reverse proving.

Evidence base

Despite the current attempts to discredit homeopathy, a systematic review of the use of homeopathy by people in 11 countries (UK, USA, Germany, Australia, Canada, Switzerland, Norway, Japan, Israel, South Korea and Singapore) showed that up to 4 per cent regularly use homeopathic medicines, either bought over the counter for self-administration or by consulting qualified practitioners (Relton *et al.* 2017). However, the evidence for the effectiveness and safety of homeopathy is, as with several other therapies, relatively scant, inconclusive and fraught with the risk of criticism about methodology. Unfortunately, as this book went to press, the NHS, in an apparent cost-saving exercise, has produced new guidelines stating that homeopathic remedies, together with some herbal and nutritional supplements, will no longer be available on NHS prescription (Davis and Campbell 2017).

The greatest difficulty for those researching homeopathy is that every single subject with a particular condition may present with a different symptom picture, each requiring a different remedy. It is therefore extremely difficult to conduct randomised controlled trials in which a group of subjects with the same condition (in conventional terms) receives the same test remedy. Criticism is levied at the use of substances which apparently contain little, if any, active molecular ingredients – the dilution and succussion of the original substance means that the final product contains none of the original chemicals. Studies appearing to demonstrate the efficacy of homeopathy are often dismissed as placebo effects or spontaneous healing. A few studies attempt to compare a homeopathic remedy with a conventional drug but, again, the need for individualisation of the prescription often produces results which appear at best inconclusive and, more often, negative (Zafar *et al.* 2016). Conversely, criticism has been levelled at scientists who conduct systematic reviews without adequate understanding of homeopathic concepts, which leads them to conclude that very few studies meet the inclusion criteria for meta-analysis (Vithoulkas 2017).

An additional complication when searching for papers is that the remedies often have the same name as substances studied in herbal medicine. It is essential to differentiate between trials on homeopathic and on herbal preparations, which have a different mechanism of action; for example, *Hypericum perforatum* (St John's wort) is both a herbal and a homeopathic remedy. However, unfortunately, there are also occasions when even the researchers (usually conventional medical or nursing practitioners) fail to appreciate the difference between homeopathic and herbal medicine (Boltman-Binkowski 2016). However, this modality is one in which veterinary medicine studies can be useful as of course there is no placebo effect, in terms of expectation of effectiveness, in animals.

One of the most common homeopathic remedies studied is *Arnica Montana*, a remedy for the treatment of shock and trauma. Many women use homeopathic arnica cream or tablets immediately after the birth to ease the pain of perineal lacerations or episiotomy. Most arnica research is inconclusive, perhaps because there are other remedies which may be more effective, depending on the cause of the trauma. Arnica research is further complicated by the practice in some countries, such as Germany, of using combination remedies, whereas in the UK it is more common to administer single remedies and await a reaction (Paris *et al.* 2008). See Chapter 9 for more discussion on arnica for perineal healing.

Hypnotherapy

Introduction

Hypnotherapy involves the induction of a trance-like state to facilitate relaxation and make use of enhanced suggestibility to treat psychological conditions and effect behavioural changes. The first therapeutic use of the hypnotic state is attributed to the Austrian physician Franz Anton Mesmer in 1778, from whom the word "mesmerism" is derived. In the UK, the physician James Braid is credited with making the therapeutic modality of hypnosis respectable to the medical community, and in the 1950s the British and American Medical Associations recognised hypnosis as a legitimate medical procedure.

The aim of hypnotherapy is to facilitate the person to regain control over her behaviour, such as stopping smoking, losing weight, resolving emotional issues (for example, needle phobia) or habitual or stress-related physiological processes, including nocturnal enuresis in children. This is achieved by the induction, under professional supervision, of the altered state of consciousness or hypnotic trance so that the person focuses her attention inwards, thereby allowing easier access to the non-critical unconscious mind which is more susceptible to suggestion. The client remains under her own control and not that of the practitioner, implying that this altered state of consciousness is, in fact, self-hypnosis with the practitioner as a facilitator.

Hypnosis is physiologically similar to meditation or guided imagery, sometimes referred to as visualisation. However, Facco (2017) argues that the hypnotic state is usually induced by a practitioner with specific therapeutic aims, whereas meditation is self-induced with full awareness and is often more a way of life with greater philosophical implications. There are several commonalities: induction of the subconscious state is based on focused attention, and the conscious-unconscious processes in both modalities can lead to behavioural change. Unfortunately, hypnotherapy has received negative coverage in the press on occasions, largely due to stage hypnosis, although encouraging audience participation for entertainment purposes is very far from clinical hypnotherapy.

It is also necessary here to mention "hypnobirthing", which is a very popular contemporary trend. "Hypnobirthing" is *not* hypnosis, nor should it be classified as a complementary therapy. It is essentially a form of guided deep relaxation, meditation and visualisation based on the early teachings of the obstetrician Grantly Dick-Read who first wrote about "childbirth without fear" in the 1930s. It is a technique to be commenced during pregnancy and practised at home, rather than simply being applied in labour. "Hypnobirthing" is specific to preparation for childbirth and differs from hypnotherapy in that it taps into certain features of inducing the hypnotic state but is not generally individualised. It is often combined with antenatal education to inform prospective parents about the birthing process, specifically explaining the fear-tension-pain cycle and its effects on the progress of labour. See Chapter 8 for more on hypnobirthing. Table 2.8 explains the differences between hypnotherapy and "hypnobirthing".

Table 2.8 Differences between clinical hypnotherapy and "hypnobirthing"

Hypnotherapy	"Hypnobirthing"
Clinical modality, regulated as a complementary therapy	A tool used within maternity care, unregulated, not classified as a complementary therapy
A form of clinical psychotherapy, used to treat a range of psychological and behavioural issues	Pregnancy-specific relaxation techniques taught to couples to prepare them for childbirth
Derived from the 18th-century work of Anton Mesmer	Derived from the 1960s work on preparation for childbirth by Grantly Dick-Read
Individually prescribed and delivered	Usually conducted in group settings
Practitioner acts as a facilitator to induce the hypnotic state and provides suggestions to effect required therapeutic changes	Teacher provides information to aid expectant parents' understanding of labour, plus deep relaxation and visualisation to practise at home and to use in labour
May include additional self-hypnosis to aid treatment	Encourages a subconscious state of deep relaxation similar to self-hypnosis
Generally used as a discrete clinical modality, or may be combined with other psychological therapies such as neurolinguistic programming or biofeedback	Classes may incorporate other aspects to prepare women for labour, e.g. massage

Indications

Common indications for clinical hypnotherapy include addictions such as smoking, weight loss and eating disorders. It is also useful for patients with phobias, such as fear of dentistry, needles or spiders. Clinical hypnotherapy is often used to treat anxiety, pain relief, post-traumatic stress disorder and various psychosomatic conditions. It has been used to enhance fertility (James 2009) and may improve the chances of success when used during in vitro fertilisation (Levitas *et al.* 2006).

Women are considered to be more hypnotisable during pregnancy – thus the structured use of clinical hypnotherapy may be particularly effective (Alexander, Turnbull and Cyna 2009), especially for women with extreme tocophobia or anxieties based on previous childbirth experiences. Other factors that may influence hypnotisability include age and educational level, as well as individual motivation to achieve the planned outcomes of treatment. For example, although hypnosis can be very effective in changing behaviour such as stopping smoking or losing weight, the impact of treatment will be greater in those truly committed to the objective.

Contraindications and precautions

Generally, hypnotherapy is relatively safe, and any problems tend to arise from the use of unintended suggestions or failure to identify physical health issues. However, hypnotherapy, and "hypnobirthing", should not be used for women with epilepsy, major mental health problems or significant emotional issues such as a recent bereavement. It is also contraindicated in women with a history of alcohol or drug dependence.

Side effects in response to clinical hypnotherapy can include tiredness, insomnia, dizziness, nausea, headaches and unexpected thoughts or feelings such as irritability, fear, anxiety and occasionally the creation of false memories. These effects are usually transient, although reactions under hypnosis can be stronger than anticipated. In some women, especially those receiving a long course of treatment, panic attacks may occur, and in more serious situations, delusions, identity crisis, personality changes, psychotic episodes and even suicidal tendencies can ensue.

Another effect of hypnosis is *abreaction*, an emotional or physical reaction caused by re-living highly emotional thoughts and feelings associated with the memory of an earlier traumatic event. Abreaction may occur because the subconscious mind is accessed during the hypnotherapy session and given "permission" to bring past thoughts and feelings to the fore. Abreactions may occur while working through a trauma, such as a woman who has had a previous traumatic birth experience.

Worryingly, some courses preparing maternity professionals to teach "hypnobirthing" do not adequately explore the possible complications that can occur within the hypnotic state, nor how to help a woman who experiences a negative effect such as not emerging from a deep trance. The trend of offering group sessions, in which several women and their partners undergo the "hypnobirthing" experience together, is usually done without any history-taking to determine individuals' psycho-emotional wellbeing, nor does it enable the facilitator to observe all participants for abreactions. Further, since people respond to different hypnotherapeutic cues (e.g. visual, auditory, kinaesthetic), a "one size fits all" approach is neither appropriate nor safe for everyone in a group setting. This does not mean that "hypnobirthing" is without merit, since it offers options for birth preparation, relaxation and social interaction with other expectant parents which are increasingly absent from the conventional maternity services. See Chapter 8 for more discussion on "hypnobirthing" to prepare for labour.

Evidence base

There is some good calibre research on hypnotherapy, and the results of non-maternity trials can often be applied to pregnancy and birth. Several studies, particularly those on people with dental phobia, show positive results and attempt to explain the mechanism of action of clinical hypnotherapy, in terms of neurological functions (Facco, Zanette and Casiglia 2014; Halsband and Wolf 2015; Meyerson and Uziel 2014). Hypnotherapy has been shown to be more effective than nicotine replacement to help people stop smoking (Hasan *et al.* 2014); other studies explore the changing perceptions of peri-operative pain (Del Casale *et al.* 2015; Wolf *et al.* 2016). Contemporary research aims to determine the neuro-physiological effects of hypnosis and the factors that affect susceptibility to hypnosis induction (de Pascalis, Varriale and Cacace 2015; Jiang *et al.* 2016). Electroencephalogram and magnetic resonance imaging of the brain have shown definitive changes in cortical and sub-cortical activity during hypnosis, with a marked difference in particularly susceptible subjects (Del Casale *et al.* 2015; Jensen, Adachi and Hakimian 2015).

In maternity care, early hypnosis studies demonstrated decreased use of intrapartum analgesia and duration of first and second stages (Freeman *et al.* 1986; Guthrie, Taylor and Defriend 1984; Harmon, Hynan and Tyre 1990; Jenkins and Pritchard 1993; Rock, Shipley and Campbell 1969). Mehl-Madrona (2004) also showed potential effectiveness for women using self-hypnosis in preparation for birth, with better psychological and birth outcomes, as did Abbasi *et al.* (2009). Conversely, the reduction in duration of first stage labour was not supported by later work (Werner *et al.* 2013). There is also some suggestion that clinical hypnotherapy can help women with a breech presentation, either using it as a relaxation strategy prior to external cephalic version or facilitating muscle relaxation to encourage spontaneous version (Mehl 1994; Reinhard, Heinrich *et al.* 2012).

Unfortunately, most of the more recent studies exploring hypnosis for labour do not differentiate between self-hypnosis, "hypnobirthing" and clinical hypnotherapy, so it is often difficult to extrapolate the findings to establish a common theme in the results. It is interesting to note that the early maternity-related studies applied true clinical hypnosis principles whereas more recent studies appear to confuse hypnosis/hypnotherapy with "hypnobirthing". Sado *et al.* (2012) investigated the use of clinical hypnosis for the prevention of postnatal depression but found no evidence to support their hypothesis. There are also several case studies in the literature, including the use of clinical hypnotherapy for antenatal post-traumatic stress (Slater 2015) and excessive salivation associated with hyperemesis gravidarum (Beevi, Low and Hassan 2015). However, this latter case involved a prolonged course of treatment from 16 to 36 weeks gestation, suggesting that there could have been a spontaneous resolution of the hypersalivation that was unrelated to the clinical intervention or possibly that, if the problem was exacerbated by stress, the client-therapist interaction over a 20-week period contributed to reducing the symptoms.

Massage

Introduction

Massage is the applied use of touch in which the practitioner uses various stroking, kneading, rolling and pressure movements of the hands, arms and elbows to manipulate the soft tissues of the client's body. Other techniques, such as traction, may also be used. Massage is one of the oldest forms of medical treatment and has been used by midwives for centuries. Modern massage development is attributed to the Swede Per Henrik Ling, who developed an integrated system of massage with passive exercises performed by the practitioner: this was later termed "Swedish massage". There are, however, many other types of massage, each using different pressures and techniques.

A base oil is usually used to prevent the friction of skin-to-skin contact, and essential oils are sometimes added, as in aromatherapy. Most traditional forms of medicine include some massage techniques, including *tui na* in Chinese medicine, Ayurveda and Indian head massage. Deep tissue massage targets the deeper layers of muscles and internal tissues, and incorporates slow strokes and friction techniques which are beneficial for chronically tight sore muscles and repetitive strain injury and is generally not appropriate for pregnant clients. Rolfing involves intense deep manipulation of the fascia of the muscles and internal organs in order to relieve both physical and emotional tension. Hot stones may be placed over chakra points on the body and used in addition to the base oil to warm the muscles, or sticks may be used to stimulate specific points.

Other modalities incorporate manual techniques which are sometimes misrepresented as simply "massage", including reflexology, acupressure, shiatsu and craniosacral therapy, but the mechanism of action in these modalities is somewhat different from that of basic massage. For the purposes of this book, these latter techniques are identified as specifically different therapies in their own right and are dealt with elsewhere in this chapter.

Indications

Massage can be used for a variety of physical and emotional indications. It is traditionally employed as a general relaxation technique, easing stress and tension. It is often revitalising, even though it may initially relax the client and aid sleep. In pregnancy, massage is popular to help the woman mentally prepare for the birth. Touch is a means of communication and can enhance the relationship between the expectant mother and father, or between the woman and her professional caregivers. It can also aid emotional release, through the healing reaction experienced by many who receive massage. Physically, massage is useful for relieving pain, oedema, aiding excretion and lymphatic drainage. It stimulates the circulatory and cardiovascular systems, reducing blood pressure and regulating the heartbeat. In labour, massage can ease pain and tension, aid progress and contribute to achieving a normal birth and reducing intervention. Postnatally, it can aid the recovery of the mother from childbirth.

Perineal massage, performed before or during labour, may reduce the need for episiotomy or the risk of severe lacerations (Beckman and Stock 2013; Demirel and Golbasi 2015), although a meta-analysis by Bulchandani *et al.* (2015) suggested that current evidence for the effectiveness of perineal massage is inconclusive and maternal awareness of the practice is low (Ismail and Emery 2013) (see also Chapter 9).

Contraindications and precautions

Little evidence could be found on the risks of massage beyond those aspects normally considered to be contraindications to treatment. Massage should be avoided if there is a current deep vein thrombosis or if the woman is pyrexial and should not be performed directly over areas of phlebitis, burns/scalds or skin issues such as infection or eczema. Cancer was traditionally considered a contraindication to massage but is more of a precaution, especially in pregnancy – for example, a pregnant woman with breast cancer may enjoy a short relaxing hand or foot massage but, of course, direct work over the breast area should be avoided.

Care should be taken to ensure that women are emotionally comfortable with the concept of massage and close physical contact, particularly if it involves the removal of clothing. Many women will experience a normal healing reaction, either physical and/or emotional, but adverse effects are extremely rare when massage is performed appropriately. The practitioner should ensure that a comprehensive history has been taken, including the possibility of allergic reactions to the base oil used, for example nut oils. Some concern has been expressed about certain base oils used in massage (and aromatherapy). An Italian study (Facchinetti *et al.* 2012) suggested that regular dermal applications of sweet almond oil in pregnancy could precipitate preterm labour. Indeed, it is known that approximately 1 per cent of the population is allergic specifically to certain chemicals in sweet almond oil and therefore women should be assessed for potential allergy to almonds prior to using the oil for massage. It is essential to differentiate between sweet almond (*Prunus amygdalus var. dulcis*) and bitter almond (*Prunus amygdalus var. amara*), the latter containing toxic elements, although this generally applies more to oral than to dermal use.

The safety of olive oil has also been challenged, particularly when used for baby massage, as it is thought that the oleic acid content may adversely affect skin integrity (Darmstadt *et al.* 2002), although Kiechl-Kohlendorfer, Berger and Inzinger (2008) dispute this and suggest that olive oil-based creams can actually reduce the risk of dermatitis in preterm neonates. Similarly, a review by Carpenter and Richards (2011) found no definitive evidence on the risks of olive oil to newborns. However, delayed-onset dermatitis has been reported following prolonged use of olive oil by a massage therapist (Isaksson and Bruze 1999), and maternity professionals would be wise to be cautious in their own use of carrier oils.

Evidence base

Different types of massage have variously been found to reduce blood pressure, cortisol and perceived stress (Bennett *et al.* 2016). Muscular relaxation is thought to be aided by the increased blood flow and raised skin temperature which occurs during massage (Plakornkul *et al.* 2016). It is known that touch impulses reach the brain quicker than pain impulses via the gate control mechanism; thus massage can be an effective analgesic, possibly through sensory responses and the action of chemical mediators such as substance P and various inflammatory processes (Sejari *et al.* 2016). Massage can also increase mobility and movement range associated with musculoskeletal disorders (Field *et al.* 2014, 2015), especially when moderate pressure is used, which stimulates the relevant skin receptors (Field, Diego and Hernandez-Reif 2010a).

Tiffany Field and her team have researched all aspects of massage and touch therapies at the Touch Research Institute in Miami, USA, and have found it useful for antenatal and postnatal depression, stress, hypertension and pain (Field 2016a; Field, Diego and Hernandez-Reif 2010b). Antenatal massage may reduce the incidence of prematurity and low birth weight in the babies of depressed mothers (Field *et al.* 2009) and impact positively on the duration of breastfeeding (Adams *et al.* 2015). It may offer a useful tool for women with post-Caesarean section pain (Saatsaz *et al.* 2016) and has been found to reduce pain in labour (McNabb *et al.* 2006) and post-operatively (Boitor *et al.* 2015).

The effect of massage on delayed-onset muscle action in athletes (Han *et al.* 2014; Visconti *et al.* 2015) may partly account for its physical, as well as emotional, benefits in preparing women for labour. In combination with antenatal education and, perhaps, other aspects of complementary therapy, it may contribute to women's greater understanding of the process of birth and contribute to an increase in normal births (Levett *et al.* 2016a). Research by Bolbol-Haghighi, Masoumi and Kazemi (2016) also showed a positive impact on labour, with a significant decrease in the duration of both first and second stage labour and an increase in neonatal Apgar scores. A Cochrane review on the effect of relaxation techniques on preterm labour suggests that massage could, theoretically, be helpful (Khianman *et al.* 2012). However, midwives and other maternity professionals should employ restraint in using massage for women in preterm labour, ensuring that techniques used will not exacerbate the situation.

Osteopathy

Introduction

Osteopathy is a form of manual diagnosis and treatment involving manipulation of soft tissues and mobilisation of peripheral and spinal joints and ligaments. Osteopathy was founded in the USA by Andrew Taylor Still in 1874 but the therapy has had a turbulent history since then. It is now well accepted and was statutorily regulated in the UK in 1993, becoming a profession supplementary to medicine rather than a complementary therapy. Practitioners are regulated by the General Osteopathic Council.

Osteopathic philosophy is based on the premise that the practitioner facilitates the client's body to heal itself and that the structure and function of the body are closely related. The musculoskeletal system is considered to act as the body's main supporting framework, and any misalignment, caused by genetics, injury or disease, exerts tension on the soft tissues contained within the framework. Re-alignment corrects imbalances in the systems and eliminates obstructions in lymphatic or blood flow to maximise health and function. Several techniques are used in the process of re-alignment, including direct high-velocity, low-amplitude thrusts, techniques to encourage muscle energy and articulation of joints, indirect counter-strain and balancing techniques, myofascial release, trigger point and neuromuscular release movements and others to encourage lymphatic drainage. For a comparison between osteopathy and chiropractic, see Chiropractic, above.

Cranial osteopathy, or craniosacral therapy, is an off-shoot of osteopathy, developed by Dr William Garner Sutherland (1873–1954), who adhered to more gentle touch techniques. Sutherland believed that the bones of the cranium (skull) are not rigid, even in adult life, and that they move in a cranial rhythm. Craniosacral therapy addresses the delicate balance between the cranium, spine and sacrum, connected by a continuous membrane of connective tissue, the dura mater, and enclosing the brain and central nervous system. Sutherland recognised that the cerebrospinal fluid rises and falls within the compartment of the dura mater, a movement he termed the "primary respiratory impulse", now known as the cranial wave. Practitioners employ a highly refined sense of touch around the skull and sacrum to detect subtle changes in the tension and tissues of the body. This enables them to diagnose dysfunctional areas, often those that have been affected by past trauma. Although the body naturally compensates for past injuries or disease, the individual may be unaware that current symptoms could be relevant to these old traumas. Treatment aims to harmonise the natural rhythm of the central nervous system to help the client regain homeostasis.

Indications

Conditions typically treated by osteopaths include back, neck, shoulder, pelvic, knee and other musculoskeletal problems, particularly when affected by posture, strain or pregnancy. Many soft tissue problems can also respond well to treatment, including duodenal ulcer and other digestive tract symptoms, neuralgia and circulatory issues. In pregnancy, osteopathy is one of the best treatment modalities for lower and upper backache, neck and shoulder pain, carpal tunnel syndrome, pelvic girdle pain, sciatica and problems resulting from the impact of increased weight on the abducted knees. It can also be useful for heartburn, nausea and vomiting, and constipation. Postnatally, it can assist in returning the mother's body to full alignment.

When a new mother attends for treatment she is usually invited to bring her baby with her and to discuss the birth, so that if necessary the baby can receive some gentle treatment to correct structural issues caused by labour and transit through the birth canal (McGlone et al. 2016). Craniosacral therapy is ideally suited to the treatment of babies and children because it is so gentle. It is often used for babies born prematurely, fractious babies with colic, and for older children with attention deficit hyperactivity disorder, temporo-mandibular dysfunction or autism. It has also been used to discourage thumb-sucking in infants and for the treatment of certain birth defects.

Contraindications and precautions

Osteopathy is contraindicated if there is osteoporosis, or any coagulation or bleeding disorder. Treatment is usually postponed in the event of an existing infection or pyrexia. Very few adverse effects occur with osteopathy which employs gentler techniques than chiropractic, although tiredness and a healing reaction are common. Cranial osteopathy should be avoided if there is acute systemic infection, recent skull fracture or intracranial haemorrhage or aneurysm.

Evidence base

The body of evidence for osteopathic manipulation is still emerging. There is a reasonable amount of research on its use for back pain in the general population (Licciardone, Gatchel and Aryal 2016; Tamer, Öz and Ülger 2016), and some recent investigation of its value in treating other conditions such as gait disturbance in Parkinson's disease (Di Francisco-Donoghue et al. 2017).

A recent trial of the use of osteopathy in pregnancy – the Pregnancy Research on Osteopathic Manipulation Optimizing Treatment Effects (PROMOTE) study (Hensel, Buchanan et al. 2015; Hensel, Carnes and Stoll 2016) – compared 400 women with back pain who were randomised to receive third trimester osteopathy or usual care plus ultrasound placebo treatment or usual care only. It was found that osteopathic treatment during pregnancy reduced the incidence of operative and instrumental birth, episiotomy and perineal tearing and of fetal distress. Interestingly, it was found to increase the duration of labour compared to women in the other two groups. Osteopathy has been shown to be safe, with no unanticipated adverse effects (Hensel, Roane et al. 2016), and appears to be acceptable to women.

Ruffini et al. (2016) conducted a systematic review of osteopathy trials in pregnancy but found only limited evidence to support its use for back pain. Hall, Cramer et al.'s systematic review (2016) similarly found the body of evidence lacking but indicated that women commonly seek osteopathy for back pain. Martingano (2016) suggests that osteopathy may also be useful for women wanting a successful vaginal birth after a previous Caesarean section, particularly where the Caesarean may have been attributed to musculoskeletal misalignment preventing adequate descent of the fetal presenting part.

On the other hand, general studies of craniosacral therapy demonstrate effective treatment of back and neck pain and headache, and may have a possible role in treating post-traumatic stress disorder (Arnadottir and Sigurdardottir 2013; Castro-Sánchez et al. 2016; Davis, Hanson and Gilliam 2016; Haller et al. 2016). A single-blind, randomised controlled trial of pregnant women with pelvic girdle pain found that morning symptoms improved with craniosacral therapy but treatment had little overall effect on pain experienced in the evenings or on the amount of sickness absence from work taken as a result of the pain (Elden et al. 2013). Cranial osteopathy appears to be a safe option in the treatment of preterm babies

(Raith *et al.* 2016) and may facilitate feeding to enable earlier discharge from the neonatal unit (Quraishy 2016).

Reflexology

Introduction

Reflexology is a generic term for a range of therapies based on the principle that one small area of the body represents a "map" or chart of the whole. In general, the two feet are used for this microcosmic map, although the hands, tongue, back, ear, face or head can also be used in some types of treatment. The concept of reflexology is derived from ancient Chinese, Indian and Egyptian techniques. Modern reflexology evolved in the late 19th and early 20th centuries when the American ear, nose and throat surgeon William Fitzgerald noticed that patients would often subconsciously apply pressure to their hands in an attempt to suppress surgical pain. He discovered that indigenous American Indians also applied pressure to points on the feet and hands for relaxation and to ease pain, and he defined the "maps" of reflex zones on the feet and hands. Further work in the USA by the masseuse Eunice Ingham produced the first modern foot charts and use of the word "reflexology". In 1950s Germany, Hanne Marquardt, a midwife, further refined the reflex zone concept and coined the term "reflex zone therapy" or "reflexotherapy". Reflex zone therapy is a clinical modality that has been used extensively in European midwifery practice, notably in Germany and Switzerland.

However, reflexology is not simply foot massage. Application of pressure to specific points on the feet aims to stimulate or sedate reflex zones that link to organs and other parts of the body via a network of channels or transmitters, in order to rebalance and maintain homeostasis. Some believe it is simply through the placebo effect or via touch receptors, which aid endorphin and encephalin release, reduce cortisol and adrenaline and aid relief of pain, perhaps along the lines of the "gate control" theory of pain relief originally discovered by Melzack and Wall (1965). Nevertheless, reflexology appears to act more deeply than basic touch and massage, working as a somatic therapy (working from inside-outwards), whereas massage generally facilitates topical relief of muscular and joint pain (working from outside-inwards). Different sensory nerve receptors in the skin make the feet sensitive to pressure and movement, pressure or touch causing the cells to emit an electrical current (an "action potential"), which is carried to the brain via sensory nerves, then to local muscles for a response. The various different styles of reflexology have varying mechanisms of action; some are based on Chinese meridians as with acupuncture, some are more akin to massage. The German style of reflex zone therapy focuses on a thorough understanding of anatomy and physiology and is more of a clinical modality than simply a relaxation tool.

Indications

Reflexology aims to stimulate the body's self-healing capacity, working with, rather than against, altered homeostasis. It is generally relaxing and de-stressing, but this is not necessarily the primary aim of clinical treatment. Reflexology also relieves pain and inflammation, aids circulation and excretory processes, may indirectly promote muscle tone and appears to have a neurological effect (Tiran 2010b). In maternity care, reflexology can be used as a means of alleviating stress, tension and anxiety, and women who receive regular treatments experience an accumulative effect. The Marquardt system of reflex zone therapy can also significantly relieve a range of symptoms in pregnancy, labour and the puerperium, including physiological disorders and psycho-emotional issues, and prevent or reduce the impact of pathological complications.

Contraindications and precautions

In addition to the general medical and obstetric contraindications, reflexology/reflex zone therapy should not be performed on women with foot- and leg-related problems such as deep vein thrombosis, phlebitis or fractures, and care should be taken if there are varicosities, verrucae, athlete's foot or other skin disorders, although these should be noted as they may be clinically relevant depending on the precise location on the feet. If a woman is pyrexial, the warming effects of reflexology preclude her from having treatment. Some authorities cite the post-operative period as a contraindication, although Tiran (2010b) disputes this in relation to post-Caesarean section treatment.

Healing reactions during and after treatment are common, indeed desirable, as they indicate a systemic response to the reflexology. However, pregnant women can have excessively strong and quite rapid reactions during treatment and a prolonged effect afterwards. In pregnancy, hands-on work should not exceed 35 minutes (a traditional treatment is usually about 50 to 60 minutes' duration) (Tiran 2010b), and application of pressure to the relaxation point (coeliac plexus reflex zone on the sole) should be *extremely* light to avoid rapid and dynamic adverse effects. Women requiring prescribed medication should be treated by experienced practitioners since over-stimulation of the reflex zone for the liver can potentiate the metabolism of drugs.

Evidence base

One of the most significant difficulties when searching for reflexology research is that there is considerable confusion between foot reflexology and foot massage. Reflexology used in a clinical setting (as opposed to salon reflexology) is *not* massage, although relaxing massage techniques may be incorporated into the overall treatment. Further, there are several styles of reflexology, and many variations on the location of specific reflex points on the maps or charts used by different schools of thought; for example, the heart reflex zone may differ with different styles. Also, as with aromatherapy research, some papers explore the *concept* of reflexology, concluding that reflexology treats a specific condition, but there is very little work on the precise stimulation or sedation of specific points related to the individual's condition. This perpetuates the notion that the primary effect of reflexology is one of relaxation and not specific to the treatment of conditions other than those which are stress-related.

Criticism is often levelled at reflexology studies, claiming that any positive results are due to a placebo effect, an issue compounded by the fact that many reflexologists are unable to debate at an academic and scientific level, and some are even unable to justify or challenge elements of treatment that they have been trained to do. Unfortunately, the calibre of reflexology studies cannot always be assessed by reviewers examining papers for possible publication because the reviewers themselves may be unaware of the variations in styles (even those who are qualified in reflexology). Thus there is a plethora of research studies appearing to show success in using reflexology for various situations, yet which are of poor quality, both in terms of research methodology and reflexology knowledge.

Some studies combine "foot reflexology" with other modalities such as foot, hand or back massage, which makes interpretation of the results difficult. A variety of control treatments is used, including foot massage or foot baths, but rarely are there any studies comparing true reflexology with sham reflexology points, a strategy used in some acupuncture research.

The duration of single treatments varies, as does the number of treatments provided for different client groups. Authors almost universally fail to specify the style of reflexology or to identify the specific points used and their location, describing merely "reflexology treatment", which often also incorporates considerable massage. A few studies describe techniques which are unsafe, for example direct stimulation of the reflex zones for the uterus to ease pain relief in labour (Valiani *et al.* 2010). Some studies, such as one on women with sub-fertility, fail to acknowledge the related complex patho-physiology, in this case describing a generalised treatment without any apparent understanding of the multifactorial aetiology of fertility issues which would often require different, individually prescribed reflexology treatments (Holt *et al.* 2009). Others appear to confuse reflexology with acupressure (Khorsand *et al.* 2015).

Several non-pregnancy reflexology studies show reduced pain and anxiety, or improved relaxation and quality of life (Aydin, Aslan and Yalcin 2016; Nazari *et al.* 2016; Valizadeh *et al.* 2015). There is some evidence to support the use of reflexology in pregnancy and labour, albeit with small numbers, not always robust methodology and occasionally some sweeping conclusions. Moghimi-Hanjani, Mehdizadeh-Tourzani and Shoghi (2015) compared reflexology with a standard-care control group and demonstrated a perceived reduction in labour pain and anxiety. Li *et al.* (2011) appeared to show that regular evening reflexology for five consecutive days improved sleep quality in postnatal women. Mollart (2003) undertook a single-blinded study in which women with leg oedema were randomised to receive either general reflexology or reflexology incorporating specific lymphatic drainage techniques or to a control group (rest only). Although there were no real statistically significant effects on the reduction in oedema, women perceived the lymphatic reflexology to be most likely to relieve some of their symptoms.

Reiki

Introduction

Reiki is a Japanese therapy, the name deriving from two Japanese words, *Rei*, meaning "God's wisdom", and *Ki* (pronounced "chee"), which refers to the universal energy within us, the same as in acupuncture (qi). It is sometimes referred to as spiritual or faith healing, and is similar to the Therapeutic Touch® (TT) system devised by American nursing professor

Dolores Krieger in the 1970s. However, unlike TT which developed from a sound scientific background, reiki has only recently become recognised as a credible therapeutic technique.

Practitioners of reiki are prepared for practice through a process of "attunement" in which the ability to sense clients' energies is passed on by an experienced reiki practitioner or "Master", enabling the student to tune in to the energies in and around people and to harness them for healing purposes. Treatments do not always involve touch of the client's physical body, but focus on massaging the energetic aura surrounding the person. Practitioners use a process often called the "laying on of hands" in which they become aware of the energy surrounding the client and can use their own energy to facilitate a return to homeostasis. The client may feel a tingling or warm sensation during the treatment and is usually relaxed at the end of it. A few practitioners claim to be able to perform "distant healing" without having a face-to-face consultation with the client.

Indications

Reiki is relaxing and can be used to treat stress-related conditions. It is not usually employed to treat specific medical conditions but aims to relieve the symptoms associated with stress such as headaches, backache and psycho-emotional disturbance. Reiki, or TT, has been used in several clinical settings including palliative care and appears to ease pain (Tabatabaee et al. 2016). The relaxation effect may also relieve pain.

An abstract was found of a recent international study exploring the energetic concept, in which experienced practitioners were asked to focus on the vibrational state of water molecules (Matos et al. 2017). This study found interesting, though not significant, changes in electrical conductivity and magnetic field of both the water and the magnetic field and radiation close to the experimental area, suggesting that brain waves of the practitioners may have an impact on external energy.

Contraindications and precautions

Some sources of information, notably several reiki websites, claim that there are no contraindications, whereas others suggest that reiki should not be used during surgery as it may decrease the effects of anaesthesia. It is also claimed that reiki may, in people with fractures, accelerate bone sealing before the fracture has been professionally re-set. Whilst these apparent contraindications are somewhat spurious, anyone suffering from psychiatric illness should avoid having treatment which may produce strong healing reactions. The spiritual nature of the therapy may be difficult for some women to accept, so it would be important to explain the concepts of reiki prior to use. Many practitioners claim that it is almost impossible to "switch off" the channelling of reiki energy and that they use it, perhaps unintentionally, raising an ethical issue about using it without having first gained informed consent from the client.

Evidence base

Searching databases for research abstracts on reiki is difficult. Using words such as "therapeutic touch" often produces studies on massage or reflexology, rather than those specifically on reiki or the American style of Therapeutic Touch®. It is also necessary to use search terms such as "spiritual healing" or "faith healing", but these tend to reveal papers on prayer or on the spiritual aspects of nursing care. However, there is a growing body of evidence on the benefits of reiki and similar energetic practices, although some literature is merely individual case reports.

Reiki appears to be helpful in stress-related conditions, aiding sleep and reducing agitation (Bukowski and Berardi 2014; Kumarappah and Senderovich 2016), although as with other therapy research, the technique is sometimes combined with strategies such as massage which may skew the results (Kurebayashi *et al.* 2016). A randomised controlled pilot study on knee surgery patients indicated that reiki can aid in relieving post-operative pain, modulate blood pressure and respiration and alleviate anxiety (Baldwin *et al.* 2017). A Brazilian study on patients with cardiovascular patients also found that spiritual healing eased pain, muscle tension and anxiety and improved oxyhaemoglobin saturation levels (Carneiro *et al.* 2017). Reiki is purported to aid wound healing, although a review by O'Mathúna (2016) found variable results from a small number of studies and concluded that there is insufficient evidence of good calibre to support its use in wound management.

One obstetric study, a randomised, controlled, single-blinded trial, found that reiki reduced post-operative pain when applied to the wound incision area 24 and 48 hours after Caesarean section and decreased the need for pharmacological analgesia (Sagkal Midilli and Ciray Gunduzoglu 2016), although distant reiki has not been found to be effective (Vandervaart *et al.* 2011). A systematic review by Ferraz *et al.* (2017) comparing reiki, prayer and drugs for perioperative pain relief in women having Caesarean sections found slight, but insignificant, evidence that both reiki and prayer meditation may have an indirect analgesic effect. One Canadian study suggested that Therapeutic Touch® reduced anxiety in pregnant women with drug dependency (Larden, Palmer and Janssen 2004). However, the use of reiki within UK maternity care, particularly by midwives, remains limited.

Yoga

Introduction

Yoga is a mind-body intervention that involves the practice of gentle stretching exercises, movement, breath control and meditation. The word "yoga" is derived from the Sanskrit word *yuj*, which means "to yoke" or to join the body and the mind in harmonious relaxation. It is thought to have been around for over 3000 years as part of Ayurvedic medicine. Yoga is believed to increase the body's stores of *prana* or vital energy (similar to Chinese qi in acupuncture or the "vital force" in homeopathy) and to facilitate the energy flow by improved posture and movement. Devotees practise regularly and achieve a deep sense of relaxation and peace from it, as well as increased muscular strength and suppleness.

The style most widely used in the west is hatha yoga, involving postures (*asanas*), breathing (*pranayama*) and meditation, which aim to achieve a state of stillness and heightened awareness. This is the safest method for pregnant women. *Iyengar* yoga is more physical and involves the use of props such as blocks or straps. Other styles, such as *ashtanga* yoga, involve more movement or holding poses for longer and can be very physically challenging. For pregnancy, the techniques and postures are usually adapted and focus on muscular strength and wellbeing.

Yoga is generally taught in group classes for relaxation with continued practice at home or, increasingly, on a one-to-one basis for specific therapeutic purposes (Ross *et al.* 2016). Women who only practise at home on their own perceive yoga as a means of preparing them for birth and promoting a healthy approach, whereas those who also attend classes appear to view yoga as a preventative measure and one which can be effective in reducing symptoms such as nausea and vomiting or backache (Cramer *et al.* 2015).

Indications

Yoga has become very popular as a therapeutic intervention for certain groups, including peri-menopausal women, for whom it may ease stress, resolve sleep disturbances or regulate blood sugar levels (Buchanan *et al.* 2016; Chaturvedi *et al.* 2016; Jorge *et al.* 2016). Mental benefits appear to include deep relaxation, feelings of wellbeing and reduction in stress levels, not least because of the effect of the breathing exercises on the increased respiration which is a feature of the stress response, and on increased expansion of the lungs from the movements used in practice. Other stress-related conditions such as headache, irritable bowel syndrome, premenstrual syndrome and back pain may also respond to yoga. In pregnancy, it is increasingly popular as a means of preparing for the birth, and the availability of pregnancy yoga classes has grown in the last few years.

Contraindications and precautions

There are no specific contraindications but extreme or prolonged postures should be avoided in pregnancy. Women should be advised to notify their instructor of their pregnancies so they can be helped to reduce the intensity of their movements and breathing. Physical damage can be precipitated by excessive posturing, especially given the action of progesterone and relaxin on the musculoskeletal system in pregnancy. Poses that accentuate muscular and ligamental stretching should be avoided, and women should be advised to ensure that the instructor is experienced in working with pregnant clients. The meditation can cause some women to feel a sense of distancing from reality and therefore yoga should not be practised by anyone with a severe mental health issue, notably psychosis, nor by those with a personality disorder.

There do not appear to be any untoward adverse effects, although some people can feel drowsy after practising yoga and should be advised to rest before driving. Yoga is thought to reduce blood pressure, although recent studies have found no statistically significant difference between yoga and control groups (Cohen *et al.* 2016; Wolff *et al.* 2016). It is possible, however, that the endorphin effects of yoga may be addictive and accumulative, with a corresponding impact on blood pressure, suggesting that women taking anti-hypertensive medication should refrain from or limit their practice of yoga to avoid severe hypotensive effects. On the whole, however, practising yoga appears to be safe during pregnancy with no adverse fetal effects or excessive maternal energy consumption (Babbar *et al.* 2016; Peters and Schlaff 2016; Polis, Gussman and Kuo 2015).

Evidence base

Several studies have been conducted on the practice of yoga in pregnancy. Kusaka *et al.*'s randomised controlled study (2016) demonstrated a reduction in salivary cortisol and improvement in mood, depression and anxiety scores. Similar findings relating to depression were obtained by Kinser and Masho (2016) and Uebelacker *et al.* (2016). A Japanese observational study suggests that regular, sustained yoga practice in pregnancy may reduce the incidence of preterm labour and the need for ritodrine hydrochloride (Kawanishi *et al.* 2016). In her review of meta-analyses and empirical studies, Field (2016b) argues that there is good evidence to demonstrate the benefits of yoga, without any real evidence of adverse effects; she goes so far as to suggest that it is now ethically questionable to assign subjects to a non-participation control group.

Conclusion

There are several hundred different complementary and alternative clinical modalities, although this chapter has discussed only those therapies most commonly used in the UK. These are popular with the general public, but not all are accepted by the medical professions or the scientific community. The amount and calibre of evidence on both effectiveness and safety of these therapies is variable, and it is interesting to note that some of the less well regarded therapies may have more research available than medically acknowledged disciplines. For example, there is a plethora of studies on aromatherapy and essential oils, whereas osteopathy has not, until recently, been particularly well researched.

Many therapies have an application to maternity care and are frequently accessed by pregnant women, and increasingly used or recommended by maternity care professionals. The fundamental premise of using complementary therapies in pregnancy and childbirth must be safety, effectiveness and evidence-based care. Professionals must be able to apply the theory of the therapy to its use within standard maternity care, with particular reference to the health and wellbeing of the individual woman, her growing baby and the progress of the pregnancy. Further chapters in this book examine this application and the benefits and risks of a variety of complementary therapies and natural remedies for specific conditions experienced by women during pregnancy, labour and after the birth.

CHAPTER 3

Professional Issues

This chapter explores some of the professional issues affecting midwives and doulas in relation to the use of complementary therapies in pregnancy and childbirth. Maternity professionals have specific responsibilities towards their clients according to whether women wish to self-administer natural remedies or consult independent practitioners. Different matters arise if the midwife or doula refers to a therapist, or when complementary therapies are incorporated into mainstream maternity care. Further obligations apply when midwives choose to offer complementary therapies in private practice. The chapter concludes with a suggested professional code of practice for safe use of complementary therapies in pregnancy and birth.

This chapter includes discussion on:

- introduction

- autonomy, advocacy and equity

- safe, effective and compassionate use of
  complementary therapies in maternity care

- education and training in maternity complementary therapies

- regulation and indemnity insurance

- responsibilities of midwives in relation to
  complementary therapies and natural remedies

- midwives implementing complementary therapy
  services in conventional maternity care

- midwives working in private practice
  offering complementary therapies

- professional code of practice for maternity complementary therapies

- conclusion.

Introduction

The fundamental tenet of healthcare is that all clinical care, whether provided by conventional health professionals or those working outside mainstream services, either publicly funded or private, must be safe, effective, compassionate and preferably cost effective for both users and providers of the services.

Statutorily regulated healthcare professionals complete accredited theoretical and practical educational programmes and are registered with a national member organisation which has a code of professional conduct/practice and a mechanism for dealing with members who do not adhere to specified parameters. For midwives, the NMC provides guidelines and directives for its registrants, but the principles for good practice are essentially similar for all other conventional healthcare professionals and for complementary therapy practitioners. For the purpose of debate in this chapter, the professional criteria for midwives set out by the NMC are addressed, but doulas, antenatal teachers and complementary therapists working with expectant mothers will appreciate the application of these principles to their own areas of practice.

All professionals providing complementary therapies for pregnant and childbearing women must treat clients as individuals, uphold their dignity, work in partnership with them and act in their best interests, respecting their right to privacy and confidentiality (NMC 2015: 1, 2, 4, 5). They have a duty to work effectively, preserve safety and promote professionalism and trust. The use of complementary therapies should be based on a thorough working knowledge and understanding of the therapy in relation to pregnancy and birth and, where possible, supported by currently available contemporary evidence (NMC 2015: 6).

All practitioners must maintain comprehensive contemporaneous records of any treatments and/or advice given to women (NMC 2015: 10). It is, however, concerning that many apparently informal conversations which midwives have with women on the subject of complementary therapies and natural remedies go unrecorded (Hall, Griffiths and McKenna 2013, 2015; personal communications with UK midwives). An example of this is the issue of raspberry leaf tea (see Chapter 8), a common question often asked casually by the woman at the end of a clinic visit. However, rarely do midwives adequately assess the woman for contraindications and precautions before advising her whether or not it is appropriate to take the remedy. Complementary practitioners should also record any conversations they have with clients relating to their pregnancies and avoid offering well-intentioned but sometimes misguided information outside the parameters of their therapy training. For example, it would be inappropriate for a hypnotherapist or acupuncturist to answer questions from clients on foods to be avoided in pregnancy unless the practitioner is qualified in nutrition and/or is up to date with current government recommendations on diet in pregnancy.

All caregivers should reduce as far as possible any potential for harm associated with their use of complementary therapies and should ensure that the therapies/remedies used are compatible with other care, treatment or medication that the woman may be receiving (NMC 2015: 18 and 19). This can be difficult if the midwife is unfamiliar with the mechanism of action of different therapies and remedies, in which case, expert advice should be sought.

Autonomy, advocacy and equity

Women have a right to use complementary therapies or self-administer natural remedies (NMC 2010). Midwives, doulas and others should support women's choices and act as their advocates, but be prepared also to advise those whose conditions warrant discontinuation of the therapies/remedies (see Chapter 1, General contraindications and precautions to use of complementary therapies). Expectant mothers should be empowered to be autonomous in their decision-making but may need professional help to do so with regards to safety. However, this can sometimes cause conflict for midwives with little or no knowledge of the vast subject area of complementary therapies. Expectant mothers' own lack of awareness can result in clinical situations in which either the materno-fetal condition or the safety of staff or other pregnant women may be at risk. Examples of this include the concomitant use of herbal remedies which have an anticoagulant effect by a woman who is taking warfarin or aspirin, or the use of uterotonic aromatherapy oils such as clary sage in an area where women (and midwives) in early pregnancy are also present (see Chapters 1 and 2; Tiran 2016a).

There has been a change in emphasis in healthcare generally since the 1990s, when national interest in integrating complementary therapies into conventional healthcare was at its highest and the process of implementing new strategies into mainstream healthcare was relatively lenient. However, in the 21st century, increasingly stringent clinical governance, the litigious nature of society and health service policy and funding have become central to the provision of maternity care, particularly in the UK. Whilst midwifery has always purported to be an autonomous profession, decades of conflict with other professionals over the "ownership" of birth, compounded by the current state of the maternity services, has diminished that autonomy to a level where midwives could admit to feeling unsure of their role. Incorporating complementary therapies into maternity care enables self-motivated midwives to extend their therapeutic repertoire and suggests that they may be able to regain some of their lost autonomy, although this is often not the case (Cant, Watts and Ruston 2011). The "alternative" genre of complementary therapies remains a barrier to complete integration, both in practice and in education. It is necessary first to convince sceptics of the value of introducing aspects of complementary therapy into mainstream care, and to justify that their benefits can exceed merely a relaxation or placebo effect, whilst being able to rationalise the use of modalities which often lack robust evidence and for which the scientific underpinning may be difficult to elucidate.

Conversely, it is vital that midwives can truly substantiate that their desire to include complementary therapies in their care of women is altruistic and not purely an unconscious means of regaining power and redefining their professional identity (Adams 2006). Even within the profession, there are examples of insidious battles for control, with the suggestion that those midwives who use complementary therapies somehow have supremacy over those who do not. This extends beyond the grass-roots clinical staff to managerial and operational levels, in which the belief that providing services not available in other local maternity units in some way raises the profile of those units offering complementary therapies. However, the principle of beneficence dictates that women's wellbeing should be at the forefront of care provision and should guide clinical decision-making which, in turn, should be justifiable to the women.

Further, any demand for additional, extraneous services such as complementary therapies should be balanced with the priorities for existing service provision. The use of complementary therapies must be for the benefit of the women and their babies, and not for the egotism of midwives or other care providers. Where maternity managers wish to introduce complementary therapies into the maternity unit, a sound rationale must be identified based on how it can improve current services. Rather than enthusiastically and randomly attempting to "implement (one or more) complementary therapies" midwives would be wise to explore the issues facing the contemporary maternity services, such as unacceptably high levels of Caesarean sections and inductions of labour, or poor maternal satisfaction scores. Attempting to redress these issues through the use of complementary therapies provides a more sound rationale for implementation and can be more robustly audited and more easily compared to current conventional strategies in order to demonstrate their value to the overall service. Incorporating complementary therapies into care in this way can also provide a vehicle for research studies to underpin practice.

It is also easy to misinterpret the statistics on the increasing use of complementary therapies by pregnant women to assume that they are demanding that complementary therapies be provided within mainstream maternity care. It is well known that conventional maternity services in the UK and elsewhere are over-stretched, with excessive workloads, poor staffing levels, disillusioned midwives and a large percentage of the midwifery workforce approaching retirement age. Women often feel dissatisfied with their maternity care provision and may choose to consult independent practitioners to supplement what they perceive to be missing in the maternity services. Many women continue to work until term and are often physically and emotionally stressed, so they value the opportunity for some relaxation when visiting a complementary practitioner. Also, reductions in NHS services such as physiotherapy mean lengthy delays awaiting treatment for excessive physical discomforts such as backache, so women opt for alternative treatments – in this example, perhaps acupuncture or osteopathy.

It is not appropriate for a maternity unit to train just a few midwives in several different therapies in an attempt to be able to offer a range of services. This will result in an inequitable service, fragmentation of treatment and a hierarchical system in which only a few select midwives are able to provide the therapies. A limited service which only enables a small proportion of the women to access it is morally indefensible, not cost effective and less likely to be allowed to continue in the long term. In today's large maternity units in which there may be over 6000 births, it is logistically impossible to provide an equitable "relaxation service" with complementary therapies. It is preferable that several, if not most, of the midwives in a unit are able to incorporate into general care a range of complementary strategies for specific purposes. For example, aromatherapy or massage can be specifically applied and taught to all community and birth centre midwives so that it can be offered to women in normal labour, or groups of midwives could learn specific acupressure techniques known to initiate labour for women with post-dates pregnancy. Alternatively, providing services for specific groups of women also facilitates the identification of need, rather than simply a desire; for example, hypnotherapy services could be provided for women with a previous poor obstetric history, needle phobia or tocophobia; massage services for teenagers may improve antenatal clinic attendance and compliance. It may also be appropriate to train a limited number of midwives in a very specific aspect of complementary therapy which can be delivered in a cost effective way. An example of this would be providing moxibustion as part of a specialist clinic for women with breech presentation, which perhaps also includes facilities for external cephalic version, discussion of the option of vaginal breech birth and pre-operative planning for women needing or desiring Caesarean section (see Chapter 6).

Within conventional maternity care, the use of complementary therapies offers a mechanism to enhance care for women, by giving midwives some new tools, but enthusiasm can occasionally cloud the judgement of individuals (personal communications with midwives). Implementation must be coordinated within and between maternity units in a single health board or trust so that all midwives practise according to defined criteria and all women, except perhaps those with high-risk pregnancies, can be assured that they may have the opportunity to receive therapy as appropriate and that the quality is consistent. Offering strategies which are relaxing and which may contribute to a more normal birth is exciting, pleasurable and satisfying, but midwives need to be mindful of working within boundaries set by the NMC, by guidelines and protocols laid down at national level or by local maternity service employers, and by the extent of their complementary therapy training.

Safe, effective and compassionate use of complementary therapies in maternity care

Martin Bromiley, an airline pilot, founded the Clinical Human Factors Group[1] after the death of his wife from minor surgery, which was later found to be due to "human factors", including poor communication between individuals and departments. He reasons that a good safety record is seen as an essential feature when prospective passengers are choosing an airline with which they wish to fly. If we apply this principle to healthcare, patients should be able to choose those hospitals or practitioners with the best safety record.

Bromiley asserts that safety is integral to compassionate care and cannot be separated from it. Given that obstetrics has the highest expenditure on compensation for negligence than any other clinical field, it stands to reason that safety is fundamental to good maternity care. Safe practice involves everyone working in, and receiving, healthcare services. It is ongoing, with adjustments and adaptations being made, either directly as a result of safety incidents or indirectly, in response to efficiency drives and client and staff feedback. Safety is not achieved simply through the use of guidelines, policies or standardised processes; indeed the ease with which staff can adhere to these means that they risk doing so in an unthinking manner. Further, safe practice should not be based on a punitive measure of accountability in which it becomes an obligation for more personal reasons (such as avoiding disciplinary action) than for the overall wellbeing of those receiving care.

Safe practice requires commitment from every member of the team, with careful forethought and ongoing reflection. *Every* aspect of the healthcare experience must be safe, from the environment to the equipment and technology, and from the procedures, work schedules and staffing levels to the actual treatment and care provided. Communication is vital to this process, as are good team leadership, peer support and, importantly, a change from the current blame culture to one of mutual respect and learning. A safety culture, in which everyone shares the same values, beliefs and attitudes, is essential to compassionate care. A report from the Clinical Human Factors Group (Illingworth 2015) advocates that:

> the pursuit of safety depends on volunteerism…and…is more about what people *choose* to do than about what they are required to do.

---

1   See www.chfg.org

Safety cannot, in any meaningful sense, be required of a workforce or, for that matter, of those they serve. (this author's italics)

Barratt (2017) argues that the ability to provide compassionate care cannot be learned and that it is incumbent on the individual practitioner first to develop self-compassion and mindfulness. Unfortunately, cultural mores may inhibit the ability of individuals to become self-compassionate, which then impacts adversely on the degree of compassion exhibited in healthcare provision (Campion and Glover 2016). Beaumont *et al.* (2016) further explore the concept of self-compassion as a means of responding to the self-critical element that is inherent in health services where the risk of litigation is implicitly used as a "sword of Damocles" to threaten individuals and to police standards of care. Without an internal self-appreciation of what constitutes compassionate care, it is impossible to deliver it to others. This seems to be particularly entrenched in the maternity services.

If maternity care is unsafe then it cannot claim to be compassionate. This applies equally to the use of complementary therapies in pregnancy and birth. Midwives justify their use of complementary therapies as enabling them to return to being "with woman", offering relaxing and pleasant strategies to help women through pregnancy, birth and new motherhood. They defend their practice by alleging that complementary therapies combat the negative, often unwanted and unwarranted interventions which are so prevalent in maternity care today. They use the misconception that complementary therapies are "safe" because they are "natural" as an argument to support their introduction into maternity care. However, this unthinking and incorrect declaration is, in itself, unsafe, adherence to which risks the wellbeing of mothers and babies, and of staff.

Where midwives have long-standing complementary therapy services in place, there is a risk of complacency which could threaten the safety – and thus the compassionate delivery – of the strategies provided. Midwives cannot assume that they can continue to practise any element of care continuously for several years without constantly reviewing and reflecting on it. All aspects of midwifery practice evolve and develop as a result of experience and the availability of new evidence. Services adapt in response to client and staff feedback, including formal audit processes and informal evaluation. This should apply equally to the incorporation of complementary therapies within maternity care, especially since these "alternatives" are often required to justify themselves twice over in order to convince the sceptics that they are safe, effective, satisfying and cost effective. Several maternity units are known to this author where, it could be argued, midwives no longer provide compassionate – or safe – complementary therapies to pregnant and childbearing women because there has been little, if any, ongoing updating, evaluation or development. Further, midwives often lose sight of the fact that their use of complementary therapies must be within the parameters laid down by their initial registration, namely by the NMC, and by the parameters of the culture in which they work.

Leading on from this, the NMC (2015: 16) requires midwives to act on any concerns they may have in relation to client or public safety. For this author, this particular clause has elicited much soul-searching, because there are numerous safety incidents relating to the use of complementary therapies by midwives, or by women being cared for by midwives, including some which have caused serious adverse maternal or fetal effects. The inadvertent misuse of complementary therapies and natural remedies is usually due to lack of knowledge and a misunderstanding of the power of these substances and techniques. This applies equally to mothers and to midwives and doulas. Caregivers' lack of knowledge and absence of any real appreciation of safety also contributes to serious professional issues, for example relating to drug administration when aromatherapy essential oils are used or herbal remedies are advised (Tiran 2016b).

Enthusiasm to use new, ostensibly pleasant and relaxing therapies can often override midwives' adherence to NMC directives, putting them in a situation which, at the extreme, could jeopardise their registration. For example, in 2016, three midwives were brought before an NMC professional conduct hearing for failing to transfer a woman with fetal distress from her home to a main obstetric unit – because the labouring woman was apparently due to receive an aromatherapy treatment from one of the midwives. On eventual transfer to hospital an emergency Caesarean section was performed but the baby suffered brain damage and multiple organ failure; a claim for compensation was pursued in the courts. Interestingly, despite the NMC's Code (2015) requiring midwives to prioritise care needs and to act in the woman's best interests, the midwives were judged by the NMC *not* to have practised unsafely, particularly as it was not possible to establish if the delay in transfer, or the use of aromatherapy, contributed to the baby's condition (Butterworth 2016). The lack of any punitive action by the NMC means that the case is not recorded on their website and information on this case has been found only in local newspapers. The fact that the midwives appeared to favour aromatherapy over transfer to hospital suggests misplaced obligations and a conflict between advocacy and accountability. However, it is, of course, impossible to judge without being in possession of the full facts and it is probable that other factors, perhaps involving the mother's or family's demands, may have contributed to the situation. In another case in 2009, a midwife in Wales was removed from the NMC register for inappropriate administration of aromatherapy oils to a labouring woman. Despite the maternity unit not having clinical guidelines for aromatherapy, the midwife used some of her own essential oils for a woman in labour. Unfortunately, she failed to give adequate information, resulting in the woman mistaking the blend for medicine, which she proceeded to drink. This case raised issues around drug administration and record keeping (Tozer 2009).

Education and training in maternity complementary therapies

It must be acknowledged that each complementary therapy is a clinical profession in its own right, some of which require many years of training in order to qualify and practise safely. Training for most disciplines involves both theory and practice. Safe practice necessitates an understanding of the therapy's specific mechanism of action, indications and benefits, contraindications and precautions, side effects and possible complications. This always includes an in-depth study of the relevant anatomy and physiology and may, depending on the therapy, involve learning chemistry, physics, pharmacology and pharmacokinetics, psychology, sociology and other disciplines. Training also includes legal, ethical and professional issues and, since most complementary therapy practitioners work in private practice, business management.

Nevertheless, some complementary therapy training courses are relatively short in terms of the required number of pre-qualifying hours and may be taught at a fairly basic academic level, particularly the supportive therapies. Worryingly, it is actually possible to find online distance learning courses in some therapies for a nominal fee, and it is still legally permissible under common law in England and Wales for "graduates" to start offering their services to the paying public (unless the therapy is statutorily regulated as in the case of osteopathy and chiropractic). On the other hand, since all health practitioners are now required to have professional indemnity insurance applicable to the specialism in which they work, those who have not completed an accredited course will find it difficult to obtain insurance cover (see NMC 2015: 12.1). This is especially relevant to the use of complementary therapies in pregnancy and even more so when it comes to caring for women in labour.

For midwives and doulas seeking complementary therapy training, clarifying the calibre and appropriateness of the numerous, widely available courses is complicated by the fact that many supportive therapies are not nationally regulated and there may be several regulatory organisations covering the same therapy, for example reflexology, of which there are several different styles (see Chapter 2). However, whilst most accredited training courses for supportive therapies, such as aromatherapy, massage and hypnosis, are part time, they often last 12 months or more, with considerable practice and case study work undertaken between taught sessions. Other therapies, notably those which are statutorily regulated (osteopathy, chiropractic) or voluntarily self-regulated at a national level, such as acupuncture and medical herbalism, may be full-time university degree programmes completed over several years.

The NMC permits midwives to use complementary therapies in their practice but specifies that they must be adequately and appropriately trained to do so and must practise in accordance with set parameters (NMC 2010: 23; 2015: 6.2). The issue of what constitutes "appropriate" education is contentious and very much open to debate and clarification. The NMC puts the onus of responsibility on the individual midwife to ascertain whether or not her training is appropriate, but this can be difficult if the midwife (or manager) is unaware of the requirements of the therapy and the issues related to using that therapy in relation to NMC registration and other directives and guidelines. Midwives wishing to learn specific therapies must ensure that the training is *midwifery* focused and not merely a generic qualification or a maternity-related course intended for therapists with no knowledge of pregnancy and birth. Indeed, it can sometimes be difficult for midwives with qualifications in particular therapies to apply the principles of those therapies to their use within midwifery practice.

Those who have fully qualified in one or more therapies may require some further learning, perhaps in the form of an "adaptation" course, as well as a comprehensive understanding of the NMC regulations and how these relate to the use of complementary therapies within midwifery practice. These same midwives also need to be up to date in the practice and theory of the specific therapy and should not assume that a complementary therapy qualification which they gained several years ago is still valid today, especially if they have not practised regularly since their initial training. In any case, many pre-registration therapy courses exclude maternity work as they view it as a post-qualifying area for continuing professional development (CPD). Even those CPD courses for therapists which claim to prepare them to specialise in working with pregnant clients are often taught by tutors with an enthusiastic interest in the subject but with little or no real clinical experience or in-depth knowledge. Personal experience of this author in teaching several hundred therapists from different disciplines indicates a concerning lack of understanding of basic issues, particularly the justification for specific practices. A very basic example is that many therapists who claim to have attended maternity CPD courses still lack adequate knowledge of anatomy and physiology to explain why a heavily pregnant woman should not lie flat on her back. It is also known that some therapists treat pregnant women without any training, maintain no records, never communicate with midwives or doctors and even, in the case of one reflexology clinic in London, arrogantly claim to be able to help a woman start labour without ever taking a history, referring to the woman's handheld maternity notes or liaising with the woman's midwife or doctor (personal communications).

Conversely, numerous complementary therapy regulatory and training organisations have expressed grave concerns about conventional healthcare professionals, including midwives, presuming to practise therapies without adequate education, not least from a safety perspective (personal communications at a national level). There is also the issue of professional identity which causes some disquiet. Midwives have a responsibility to provide *midwifery* care under their NMC registration. This does not currently include the practice of different complementary therapies, and midwives must be careful to examine their motivation, competence and justification for incorporating aspects of complementary therapies into their care of women.

Furthermore, some midwives have an increasingly self-important attitude to the inclusion of complementary therapies in their practice. This has resulted in midwives who complete introductory courses preparing them to use very limited aspects of a therapy who then presume to be competent and knowledgeable enough to teach other midwives (numerous personal communications with midwives and managers around the UK). This level of "cascade training" of complementary therapies is inappropriate, unsafe, unprofessional and unethical. Any midwife using aspects of complementary therapy in her own practice must not only be a "knowledgeable doer" (Cant 2011) but must also *understand* what she is doing, based on extensive clinical experience, before attempting to teach others. Clinical practice incorporating the therapy into midwifery care is essential to gain sufficient experience of the positive and negative effects of the therapy in pregnancy, birth or the postnatal period. Also, since students only retain a proportion of what they learn in the classroom, there is a natural dilution of content with each successive "cascade". This egotism is misplaced, particularly since midwives would not condone therapists undertaking a short course on midwifery and then attempting to teach others.

Similarly, doulas, maternity support workers and antenatal teachers should also be mindful that the courses they attend are sufficiently applied to their area of work and enable them to acknowledge their boundaries. For example, it is not fitting for a doula to perform moxibustion to turn a breech presentation to cephalic or acupressure to trigger contractions for a woman with a post-dates pregnancy without a thorough understanding of the individual woman's underlying pregnancy physiology, the potential complications of inappropriate use of the therapy and a comprehensive understanding of the intricacies of the therapy they wish to use. Unfortunately, it is known that many doulas use complementary therapies and prescribe natural remedies for women yet may have either received only nominal training or have acquired "knowledge" from colleagues in a "Chinese whispers" fashion (Tiran 2010a). Antenatal teachers should also ensure that information given on aspects of self-help strategies or natural remedies is based on comprehensive knowledge of the indications, contraindications and precautions and be able to refer women to more authoritative sources of information and advice if necessary.

Given the number of women now using complementary therapies, it is also imperative that student midwives are provided with an overview of the whole subject area, with specific reference to pregnancy and birth. It is, in fact, the ill-informed and injudicious use of complementary therapies, especially natural remedies, that predisposes women to iatrogenic complications, such as intrapartum uterine hypertonia and fetal distress. Despite the NMC's *Standards for Pre-registration Midwifery Education* (NMC 2009) requiring midwives, at the point of registration, to be able to advise women on over the-counter remedies, this subject remains an area which is given scant coverage in midwifery training. Enjoyable "taster" sessions on massage and aromatherapy do *not*, in any way, equip student midwives to advise women knowledgeably and comprehensively on the safety of different therapies and remedies, nor can they adequately address the relevant professional accountability issues. Furthermore, these sessions perpetuate the trivialisation of complementary therapies as merely relaxation strategies, a factor which detracts from their therapeutic power when used appropriately and their potentially serious risks with inadvertent misuse or abuse. Complementary therapies education for students and midwives should provide sessions that help midwives to comply with NMC requirements and, once qualified, are suitable for NMC revalidation. Midwives with a particular interest in one or more therapies applied to pregnancy and birth should have the opportunity to study them as post-registration activities when they can consider the scientific basis of the therapy, its application to midwifery practice and the process of change management required to implement it in the workplace.

Continuing professional development is also essential for all those using complementary therapies with pregnant and childbearing women. Midwives, doulas and antenatal teachers should ensure that they update regularly, both in terms of the therapy and its application to maternity care. Therapists wanting to specialise in working with pregnant clients require further study and supervised experience of treating expectant mothers. They should acquire a good working knowledge of reproductive anatomy and physiology, and appreciate the conventional maternity services and any contemporary developments, as well as their roles and responsibilities when caring for maternity clients. Table 3.1 outlines the minimum requirements for education and training by midwives and doulas in any individual complementary therapy.

Table 3.1 Education and training requirements for maternity complementary therapies practice

Maternity-related content	Complementary therapy-related content
• understanding of anatomy and physiology of pregnancy, labour, puerperium • ability to determine possible pathology, recognition and actions to be taken • professional responsibilities, limitations of role when using complementary therapies in maternity practice • the context in which maternity complementary therapies are set, i.e. NHS • practice of complementary therapies based on safety, professional accountability and evidence-based practice	• philosophy of complementary medicine and its place within contemporary healthcare provision • mechanism of action of the specific therapy including related pharmacology, pharmacokinetics, chemistry, physics, anatomy and physiology as appropriate • indications, contraindications and precautions to use of the therapy, in general and specifically in pregnancy, labour and postnatal period • the healing reaction, side effects, complications of the therapy and how to deal with them

Adapted from Tiran (2016a)

Regulation and indemnity insurance

Within the complementary medicine arena, early attempts at regulation commenced with the results from two government working parties which produced reports into "alternative" medicine (BMA 1986) and "non-conventional" medicine (BMA 1993). During the 1990s there was a demand from the government, complementary therapy organisations and conventional healthcare practitioners for better regulation, improved education and training, more evidence-based practice and greater integration of complementary therapies into mainstream healthcare. In addition, major health-related controversies, such as the case of Dr Harold Shipman in the late 1990s and the maternity-related deaths at Morecambe Bay Hospital in the early part of the 21st century, have led successive governments to impose ever-tighter controls on health and social care provision, organisations and individuals working in the services with the aim of improved protection for the public.

A regulatory body (for example, the NMC) is accountable to, and acts in the best interests of, the public and is independent of individual professional organisations. It sets criteria for safe practice, education, continuing professional development, codes of conduct and practice and disciplinary and complaints procedures. It provides information to the public about each modality (in this case, each therapy) and what a prospective client or patient can expect when consulting a practitioner. The regulatory body also liaises with governmental and other organisations as required. Conversely a professional organisation or association acts in the interests of the profession and its members and is independent of the regulatory establishment. In complementary medicine it acts as a membership organisation for practitioners of specific therapies and upholds education and practice standards to which members are expected to adhere. A professional association ensures that any member training organisations provide courses that meet specified core curricula. Some organisations are linked to individual colleges, whilst others maintain lists of approved training schools. Professional associations may have opportunities to liaise with governmental, national or international bodies but are not the official "voice" of the discipline. In midwifery, an example of a professional organisation would be the Royal College of Midwives.

However, in midwifery and other statutorily regulated health professions, the situation is much clearer than for many complementary therapies. Many of the principal complementary therapies have evolved a system of voluntary self-regulation, although both osteopathy and chiropractic were regulated by statute in 1993 and 1994 respectively. However, there remains a confusing plethora of organisations claiming to be the "lead body" for a particular therapy, and this can be confusing for the public and for conventional healthcare professionals. There are some overarching bodies with member organisations from various complementary disciplines, as well as associations related to just one therapy or a series of therapies with similar principles, for example massage therapies. Some therapies have more than one body, sometimes differentiating between "medical" or "western" reductionist therapy and holistic, "classical" or "traditional" practice, as with both acupuncture and homeopathy. Table 3.2 provides a summary of the main complementary therapy organisations in the UK.

Table 3.2 Regulatory organisations for commonly used complementary therapies in the UK

General organisations covering a range of therapies	Complementary and Natural Health Care Council (CNHC) www.cnhc.org.uk	Principal UK voluntary regulator, accredited by Professional Standards Authority for healthcare (NHS compliant); accredits training and member organisations from different therapies (not individual practitioners)
	General Regulatory Council for Complementary Therapies (GRCCT) www.grcct.org	Claims to be the UK federal regulator for complementary therapies but now superseded by CNHC
Acupuncture	British Acupuncture Council (BAcC) www.acupuncture.org.uk	Largest UK self-regulatory organisation for acupuncturists practising traditional acupuncture
	British Medical Acupuncture Society (BMAS) www.medical-acupuncture.co.uk	Voluntary self-regulation for those trained in western medical acupuncture (doctors, nurses, midwives, etc.)
Aromatherapy	The Aromatherapy Council www.aromatherapycouncil.org.uk	Lead voluntary self-regulatory body
	International Federation of Aromatherapists (IFA) www.ifaroma.org	Regulates and accredits standards for both training courses and practitioners
	Aromatherapy Trade Council (ATC) www.a-t-c.org.uk	Self-regulatory trade organisation for manufacturers and suppliers of essential oils

Bach flower remedies	Confederation of Registered Essence Practitioners (COREP) www.corep.net	Voluntary self-regulation of all practitioners using flower essences of any kind
Chiropractic	General Chiropractic Council (GCC) www.gcc-uk.org	Statutory regulation for chiropractors in UK
Herbal medicine	National Institute of Medical Herbalists (NIMH) www.nimh.org.uk	Main self-regulatory body for herbal medicine practitioners
Homeopathy	British Homeopathic Association (BHA) www.britishhomeopathic.org	Voluntary self-regulation for medical homeopaths – doctors, nurses, midwives, dentists, osteopaths, chiropractors, podiatrists, pharmacists, veterinarians
	Society of Homeopaths www.homeopathy-soh.org	Largest organisation for non-medical homeopaths (classical homeopathy), registered with Professional Standards Authority for healthcare
Hypnotherapy	General Hypnotherapy Standards Council (GHSC) www.general-hypnotherapy-register.com and General Hypnotherapy Register (GHR) www.general-hypnotherapy-register.com	Largest professional body and register of clinical hypnotherapists in the UK
Massage	Complementary and Natural Health Care Council (CNHC) www.cnhc.org.uk or General Regulatory Council for Complementary Therapies (GRCCT) www.grcct.org	There are several regulatory bodies for different types of massage but CNHC or GRCCT register massage therapists who comply with specified general criteria
Osteopathy	General Osteopathic Council (GOC) www.osteopathy.org.uk	Statutory regulation for osteopaths in the UK

Reflexology	Association of Reflexologists (AOR) www.aor.org.uk or British Reflexology Association (BRA) www.britreflex.co.uk	Leading self-regulatory organisation for all styles of reflexology; member of CNHC
Reiki	UK Reiki Federation www.reikifed.co.uk	Voluntary self-regulation body accredited with CNHC
Shiatsu	Shiatsu Society www.shiatsusociety.org	Accredited with CNHC
Yoga	British Council for Yoga Therapy (BCYT) www.bcyt.co.uk	Self-appointed regulatory body for all styles of yoga; members can join CNHC

Responsibilities of midwives in relation to complementary therapies and natural remedies

Women have the right to self-administer natural remedies and should be facilitated in their wishes where possible (NMC 2010). If the midwife is unsure whether the remedy is safe or appropriate, she should discuss this with the woman and consult a midwife or doctor who specialises in this field, or a therapy organisation. Women should be asked periodically throughout the pregnancy about their use of complementary therapies and natural remedies, for example at the booking visit, early in the third trimester in preparation for the birth and at the start of labour. Importantly, if the midwife feels unable to advise the woman, this must be recorded in the maternity notes, together with any advice about where to obtain appropriate information. Any informal advice given to the woman must also be recorded.

Frequently women self-administer natural remedies without informing their midwife, but this can lead to complications, which may be considered idiopathic by uninitiated staff, but which are, in fact, iatrogenic. For example, if a woman is admitted in preterm labour, or with complications for which no medical cause can be determined, it is wise to enquire of the woman if she has used any natural remedies, including herbal medicines or herbal teas, homeopathic remedies or aromatherapy essential oils, as these may have contributed to the onset of contractions. Also, many women from overseas use traditional remedies which are often strongly embedded in their own cultures, particularly plant remedies in preparation for birth and during labour.

The midwife should, if she is aware of the fact, record contemporaneously in the woman's notes (and on the partogram and cardiotocograph printout, if in use) when the woman administers a remedy to herself, even if the midwife is not familiar with its actions. The midwife also needs to be aware of the risk of interactions between pharmacologically active natural remedies and any prescribed drugs, as many have similar mechanisms of action. Some remedies may also interfere with the results of investigations; for example, therapeutic doses of ginger tea or capsules for nausea (see Chapter 4) may reduce platelet aggregation, potentially increasing measures of bleeding time (Chen *et al.* 2011). If complications arise the midwife may need to advise the woman against continuing her use of natural remedies (see Chapter 2) and record in the notes whether the woman agrees to this.

If an independent therapist or doula accompanying a woman in labour administers complementary therapies or natural remedies, she is responsible for her own practice, but the midwife is ultimately responsible for the care of the woman during labour. Midwives should try to encourage women wishing to be accompanied in labour by a practitioner who intends to use complementary therapies to discuss this in advance, perhaps by including a question in their discussions on preparation for the birth. This may help to avoid any conflict when the woman is in labour. Doulas and other birth companions attending in a professional capacity should ensure that they inform the midwife of any natural remedies they administer or any complementary manual treatments they give to the woman.

Some maternity units require therapists and doulas to confirm in writing that they are in possession of professional indemnity insurance and that they understand they cannot rely on the hospital's vicarious liability insurance to protect them in the event of complications leading to a compensation claim. It may also be wise to clarify professional boundaries and to ask the practitioner to acknowledge in writing that the midwife and/or doctor remains responsible for the mother's and baby's care and that, in the event of an emergency, the therapist/birth supporter agrees to step aside if asked to do so and/or to discontinue the complementary therapy. The midwife should record in the woman's notes when therapy is in progress or remedies are given. A note here that therapists using aromatherapy should be forbidden to use any form of diffuser, vaporiser or burner whilst in the maternity unit or birth centre, and with caution in the woman's own home, because of the risk to the mother, baby and other people (see Chapter 2, Aromatherapy).

The field of complementary medicine is a minefield, not least because there are so many different therapies, many of which lack a robust theoretical underpinning or evidence base. Unlike midwifery, nursing, medicine and related professions such as physiotherapy, there is little compulsion to "professionalise" many of the therapies and the majority remain largely unregulated. It can, however, be difficult for midwives, doctors and birth workers to identify how or to whom they should refer women seeking complementary therapy services outside the maternity care system. There is certainly a need for greater collaboration and communication between conventional maternity care providers and complementary practitioners, as well as an increased ability to discuss the subject of complementary therapies with pregnant clients (Adams *et al.* 2011). The NMC requires midwives to work cooperatively with colleagues, respecting their skills and expertise, and referring to others when necessary (NMC 2015: 2.1, 8.2).

It is interesting to note that the NMC also requires midwives to be able, at the point of registration, to "refer appropriately" to complementary therapists (NMC 2009). However, referral to the most appropriate practitioner is a very refined clinical skill which midwives studying limited components of one or two therapies are highly unlikely to be able to do. At the very least, it requires a good working knowledge of *each* of the numerous individual therapies. Additionally, unless they have personal clinical experience of combining several complementary therapies, they are unlikely to be able to appreciate the potential interactions that can occur when therapies are mixed with one another or with aspects of conventional maternity care. Without adequate understanding of the specific therapy, midwifery referral of a woman to a particular therapy may be inappropriate or, occasionally, unsafe.

Sometimes, midwives with no knowledge of complementary medicine may be sceptical and dismissive or, conversely, may view a therapy as purely for relaxation, with no appreciation of the potential risks associated with inappropriate referral. This is often seen when women seek complementary therapies at term to initiate contractions in order to avoid medical induction of labour. The therapist may request the client to check with her midwife as to whether she can receive the therapy; the midwife, with no understanding, perceives that anything that may help the woman to relax has some benefit and tacitly gives "permission" to the woman, who then returns to her therapist with the notion that the midwife has agreed that it is safe to go ahead. At no point has there been any specific professional, clinical debate and yet both practitioners believe that their indirect communication has sufficed.

It is also important to advise the woman not to engage in "therapy shopping" in which she seeks one therapy (or therapist) after another, nor that she combines several therapies at the same time, unless a combination strategy is advocated by a single therapist. Any therapy takes time to take effect, especially if the clinical picture of the woman's condition is complex. There is often a healing reaction (see Chapter 1), and the practitioner needs to differentiate these from potential adverse effects of the therapy or, indeed, from an unrelated complication of the pregnancy. This particularly applies to therapies such as homeopathy, which treats the "whole person" but which can take time to resolve the symptoms fully, first producing the normal homeopathic aggravations which can be misconstrued by the uninitiated as side effects or complications of the treatment (Stub, Alraek and Salamonsen 2012).

Complementary practitioners also need to consider when and to whom referrals of their pregnant clients become necessary. Their role in maternity care is to supplement the care provided by members of the conventional maternity services, either midwives or doctors; they are not, by law in the UK, permitted to take on the sole provision of care during pregnancy and birth. Practitioners should be aware of the reasons not to treat potential clients (often referred to as "red flags"; see Chapter 1), or to discontinue or suspend treatment of current clients. If there is any cause for concern, the therapist should either advise the woman to contact her midwife or doctor, or make the initial contact themselves, by telephone or email, depending on the severity of the situation. In an acute emergency, the therapist should call an ambulance.

Midwives implementing complementary therapy services in conventional maternity care

The increased use of complementary therapies by pregnant and childbearing women has resulted in midwives wishing to introduce aspects of complementary therapy into their own practice, and many maternity units now offer aromatherapy, acupuncture, "hypnobirthing" or moxibustion. However, it is paramount that midwives implement complementary therapies within the framework of the NHS and their NMC registration, taking into account national directives and recommendations such as NICE, local limitations and even international law. There needs to be adequate rationalisation and justification for the introduction of a therapy, based on clinical need, patient demand and satisfaction and financial and practical considerations. The first priority is to the safety of women and babies, and the justification for any new initiatives must be based around this in order to offer complementary therapies in a safe and compassionate way.

The production of a business plan enables those wishing to introduce an element of complementary therapies to justify their proposal. This should include all costs, notably initial and ongoing training, equipment or products required and the time taken to implement, provide, maintain, audit and review the service. The implementation of a new service is about managing change and this can be difficult for many midwives, particularly those at "grass roots" who have the enthusiasm but who may not possess the skills to take the initiative forward.

It is essential to develop clinical guidelines to support those midwives who will be providing the service and to protect mothers and babies. These may also need to be cross-referenced to other clinical guidelines, in order to alert other caregivers to their use. For example, a guideline on moxibustion should be cross-referenced to the one on management of breech presentation; an aromatherapy guideline should be linked to those on intrapartum care, epidural anaesthesia and Caesarean section. Where a unit provides more than one complementary therapy, it is wise to develop just a single clinical guideline. For example, if aromatherapy, massage and reflexology are provided, it would be preferable to have one guideline with general issues such as training, indications, contraindications and precautions, followed by specific points for each therapy. This avoids repetition and prevents the inappropriate predominance of clinical guidelines on complementary therapies, possibly at the expense of others. Box 3.1 provides a summary of points to include in a clinical guideline for complementary therapies and gives guidance on the issues to be considered when implementing one or more complementary therapies into conventional midwifery practice.

BOX 3.1

Development of clinical guidelines on complementary therapies

- policy statement or Statement of Intent
- definition of the complementary therapy (or therapies) to be implemented
- rationale for implementation – in terms that are valid to the organisation, for example to reduce interventions, to normalise birth, for pain relief in labour
- benefits of the therapy supported by contemporary evidence where possible
- training and continuing professional development requirements of those providing the service (NMC 2015)
- a statement relating to the need for midwives to justify their use of complementary therapy and that this must be in the best interests of the woman/baby and not at the expense of other clinical priorities (NMC 2015)
- management of the service/logistical issues, for example location of storage of essential oils
- mentoring/supervision of those providing the therapy
- women who are eligible to receive the therapy
- indications for use of the therapy in pregnancy, birth or the puerperium
- contraindications and precautions/women who are ineligible
- specific issues related to individual therapies (especially when more than one therapy is offered)
- consent, confidentiality, record keeping
- evaluation of individual treatments
- audit of the service
- health and safety issues as appropriate, including protection of other mothers, babies, staff and visitors
- treatment protocols if appropriate to the therapy.

Adapted from Tiran (2014a, 2016a)

Midwives working in private practice offering complementary therapies

Increasingly, midwives in the UK are setting up in private practice offering maternity complementary therapies. These services are often provided in addition to continuing to work in mainstream midwifery, normally in the NHS, although many are moving to full-time freelance work in order to work with women more holistically, offering services which are not part of conventional maternity care, but for which women are prepared to pay.

Midwives moving into the commercial sector face two major problems: the transition from being employed to becoming self-employed and the need to differentiate between services which constitute midwifery and those which do not. It is not permitted for midwives in the UK to engage in private practice, offering antenatal and postnatal services which would normally be defined as midwifery-specific, unless they have adequate indemnity insurance cover. Practical and logistical issues need to be considered in terms of how the midwife wishes to work, for example as a mobile practice visiting women in their own homes, working from one's own home, renting rooms in an existing clinic or establishing a dedicated new clinic. Increasingly, changes in the NHS facilitate professionals in private practice wishing to contract their services to the NHS, especially if those services are not currently available, for example moxibustion for breech presentation.

Midwives working in private practice who also continue to work as employed midwives must ensure that there is no conflict of interest between their private and their NHS work. They are not permitted to promote private services whilst engaged in employed work. Further, they may not imply in advertising materials that being a midwife enhances the complementary therapy and other services that they provide in a private capacity. Where an individual works as an employed midwife in the same geographical area as her private practice, it can be particularly difficult to segregate the two aspects of the work, especially if a client attending for private treatment is also receiving midwifery care from the practitioner. When marketing one's private practice the NMC requires midwives to "make sure that any advertisements, publications or published material…produced for [their] professional services are accurate, responsible, ethical, do not mislead or exploit vulnerabilities and accurately reflect [their] relevant skills, experience and qualifications" (2015: 21.4).

There are also legal issues to be resolved in setting up a business, including whether the midwife chooses to act as a sole trader, in partnership with others or to establish a limited company, the latter normally being advised for larger enterprises. Dealing with Her Majesty's Revenue and Customs (HMRC, formerly the Inland Revenue) can be daunting, and those who choose to set up a limited company also have to register with Companies House which brings more legal requirements. There are even regulations pertaining to the name of the company set up by a midwife: in the UK it is not permitted to use the statutorily protected title of "midwife" or the word "midwifery" in a company name unless the midwife has obtained from the NMC a "Certificate of No Objection". As with normal midwifery practice, it is essential to maintain comprehensive records of treatments provided for women, adhering to the Data Protection Act if these records are held on computer.

In private practice, insurance cover for personal professional indemnity insurance for clinical negligence is required but it is important also to have public liability insurance for buildings accessed by clients. Those working at home need to adjust their home contents and building insurance, whilst those who are peripatetic must notify their motor insurance company that they are using their vehicle for business purposes. Anyone selling products which they have produced themselves will need Product Liability insurance, and midwives intending to dispense herbal, homeopathic, aromatherapy or other natural medicines must comply with national and international (currently the European Union) legislation relating to natural medicines.

Professional code of practice for maternity complementary therapies

To summarise the professional issues pertinent to the use of complementary therapies in pregnancy, during labour or after the birth of the baby, it is useful to consider a code of practice to which all practitioners should adhere. This code applies to midwives, doctors, doulas, antenatal teachers, maternity support workers, complementary therapists of all disciplines, physiotherapists and any others working in a professional capacity offering complementary therapies for pregnant and childbearing women. Whilst there are specific issues for each professional group, the code below is intended to cover the main principles relevant to all those using or advising on complementary therapies and natural remedies in maternity care. It should be used in conjunction with the legal and professional requirements set by the practitioner's primary regulatory or registering body.

The "use of complementary therapies" refers to direct administration of a therapy by the practitioner and the teaching of women about aspects of complementary therapies, as well as to the provision of information and advice relating to the self-administration of natural remedies. This code relates only to the care provided for women and excludes the use of complementary therapies for neonates (although the same principles generally apply). Table 3.3 provides a code of practice for maternity complementary therapies (Tiran 2014b).

Table 3.3 Professional code of practice for maternity complementary therapies

1 Education and training	• All professionals using or advising on complementary therapies and natural remedies for pregnancy and birth must have undertaken appropriate theoretical and practical education to enable them to practise competently and safely.
	• Courses should be facilitated by lecturers with substantial academic knowledge and clinical experience of conventional maternity care *and* maternity complementary therapies/natural remedies.
	• Courses should include, or build on, practitioners' current knowledge of relevant complementary therapies including mechanisms of action, indications, contraindications and precautions, healing reactions and side effects specifically related to maternity care.
	• Practitioners should have a comprehensive, working knowledge of pregnancy, birth and postnatal physiology, potential pathology, conventional antenatal, intrapartum and postnatal care and the roles and responsibilities of those working in the maternity services.
	• Practitioners must be able to relate the theory of complementary therapies and natural remedies to the bio-psycho-social condition of individual women.
2 Continuing professional development	• All professionals offering or advising on maternity complementary therapies and natural remedies must demonstrate competency through ongoing education and reflective practice, specifically relating to maternity complementary therapies.
	• Continuing professional development activities should be undertaken annually in order to remain up to date and competent to offer safe care based on contemporary research evidence.
3 Indemnity insurance	• All healthcare professionals must possess personal professional indemnity insurance cover pertinent to each area of their practice.
	• Practitioners of maternity complementary therapies are advised that their indemnity insurance should specifically cover working with women during the antenatal, intrapartum and postnatal periods, or parts thereof, depending on training and the parameters of personal practice.
	• Private practitioners intending to accompany women in labour should ensure that their indemnity insurance covers them for the use of complementary therapies in labour.
	• NB Conventional maternity services providers may require independent practitioners to sign a disclaimer form confirming that the practitioner has personal indemnity insurance and will not attempt to invoke the vicarious liability insurance of the institution in the event of a legal case of potential negligence.

4 Disclosure and barring check	• All professionals working with vulnerable clients including expectant mothers and their babies are required to be in possession of current clearance from the Disclosure and Barring Service (police check).
5 Parameters of practice	• Practitioners of maternity complementary therapies must adhere to the parameters of their specific area of practice. • Midwives offering private complementary therapies must not provide midwifery-specific care unless they are also insured to do so. • Therapists, doulas and antenatal teachers must defer to the midwife who remains legally accountable for the woman and her baby; any issues of conflict must be resolved discreetly and professionally.
6 Consent to treatment	• Practitioners must obtain fully informed consent of the woman by providing comprehensive, evidence-based, unbiased information on complementary therapies and/or natural remedies. • The woman's consent to treatment, whether given verbally or in writing, must be recorded in the clinical notes. • Practitioners should not attempt to persuade a woman to take a particular course of action relating to complementary therapies and/or natural remedies which is based on the individual practitioner's personal beliefs.
7 Confidentiality	• Practitioners of maternity complementary therapies should ensure complete confidentiality for women and their babies. • Independent practitioners must seek consent to liaise with the woman's midwife or doctor, if this is deemed necessary.
8 Record keeping and communication	• Midwives and doctors are legally required to retain maternity records for 25 years (Civil Liabilities Act 1976). Given the high number of obstetric litigation cases, it is recommended that doulas, therapists and others providing complementary therapies in a professional capacity, particularly in labour, also retain their records for 25 years. • Comprehensive records of maternity complementary therapies should be maintained contemporaneously. • Independent practitioners are not permitted to write in the standard maternity notes but should maintain their own records. • Inter-professional communication is essential to avoid untoward effects of inappropriate use of complementary therapies and natural remedies. • Women should be encouraged to inform their midwife about their use of complementary therapies and natural remedies in pregnancy, labour or the early postnatal period.
9 Evidence-based care	• All healthcare should be based on currently available research evidence or authoritative discourse. This is particularly relevant to the use of complementary therapies and natural remedies since practitioners may be challenged to justify their practice.

10 Deviations from normal in pregnancy, labour or after birth	• Practitioners of maternity complementary therapies must be able to differentiate between possible healing reactions to the complementary therapy treatment, normal physiological effects of pregnancy and emerging pathological conditions.
	• In the event of any deviation from the norm, treatment with complementary therapies or natural remedies should be avoided or discontinued until the woman has been fully assessed by the midwife/doctor and/or her condition has returned to normal.
	• Practitioners should assess clients at each appointment to ensure that complementary therapy treatment is appropriate.
	• Those using several complementary therapies in combination must be able to differentiate between effects deriving from each therapy and between these and normal physiological effects of pregnancy and birth.

Conclusion

The practice of complementary therapies by midwives, doulas and other care providers requires attention to the professional issues pertinent to integrating new – and somewhat alternative – strategies into mainstream maternity care. It is paramount that the introduction of one or more therapies is set in the context in which standard antenatal, intrapartum and postnatal care is delivered. Midwives and others must be able to apply the principles of the specific therapy to the practice of that therapy within the NHS (or other environment in which maternity care is provided). They are bound by local, national and even international laws, directives and policies pertaining to maternity care and also to the particular therapy they practise. Failure to address these issues risks the safety of mothers and babies and jeopardises the individual's professional registration.

CHAPTER 4

Complementary Therapies for Nausea and Vomiting in Pregnancy

Nausea and vomiting is one of the most troublesome symptoms experienced by women during pregnancy. In some women it commences only a few days after conception and it is commonly the first symptom that alerts women to a possible pregnancy. Unfortunately the problem, particularly the constant nausea, has a profound impact on the woman's physical and mental wellbeing, her day-to-day life and her ability to care for the family and to continue working.

This chapter will consider how midwives, doulas and other maternity caregivers can help women to cope with nausea and vomiting in pregnancy (NVP). The use of self-help strategies such as ginger and acupressure wristbands is discussed, with a focus on safety. The benefits and effectiveness of other therapies to which women could be referred, for example acupuncture and osteopathy, are also discussed.

This chapter includes:

- introduction

- NVP: a syndrome

- hyperemesis gravidarum

- conventional management of NVP

- nutritional management

- ginger

- peppermint and other herbal remedies

- aromatherapy

- homeopathy

- acupuncture/acupressure

- sound therapy

- osteopathy and chiropractic

- hypnotherapy

- conclusion.

Introduction

NVP is one of the earliest, commonest and most distressing conditions to affect expectant mothers. Significant symptoms occur in at least 50 per cent of women in early pregnancy but may occur to a lesser extent in up to 90 per cent (Lee and Saha 2011). Kramer *et al.* (2013) found the incidence to be 63.3 per cent in the first trimester and 45.5 per cent in later pregnancy, often exacerbated by social or occupational factors or psycho-emotional disturbances. Lacasse *et al.* (2009) showed that over 78 per cent of women in the first trimester and 40.1 per cent in the second trimester experienced NVP and associated problems such as hyper-salivation, with Caucasian women suffering – or at least reporting – greater symptoms than black and Asian women. Psychological issues prior to or during early pregnancy may increase the severity, and women who experience NVP may be at greater risk of postnatal depression or even post-traumatic stress disorder (Christodoulou-Smith *et al.* 2011). It is also known that severe NVP can adversely affect the fetus, including a higher than normal risk of neural tube defects, particularly when medication is required to manage the condition (Lu *et al.* 2015).

Commonly, and somewhat spuriously, termed "morning sickness" due to frequent hypoglycaemia-induced nausea on waking, many women experience symptoms all day, intermittently or continuously, with some even suffering during the night. Less than 2 per cent of women have morning-only symptoms. However, some women experience a return to the nausea and vomiting as they approach term, possibly in response to fluctuating hormone levels in preparation for labour. A few even continue vomiting into labour, with the condition miraculously and instantaneously resolving on the birth of the baby.

NVP is attributed to endocrine changes, primarily the high fluctuating levels of human chorionic gonadotrophin (hCG), oestrogens and progesterone. Thyroid hormones may be implicated (Buyukkayaci Duman, Ozcan and Bostanci 2015), as may impairment of the immune system (Fessler 2002) and alterations in serotonin, dopamine and histamine (Flake, Scalley and Bailey 2004). Effects on the vestibular apparatus in the ear are also thought to play a part, with many women reporting that any sensory stimulation, especially motion, provokes vomiting (Sinha *et al.* 2011). Some women are so debilitated that they are almost unable to lift their heads from the bed, and changes of position can either alleviate or increase symptoms.

The condition is often exacerbated by tiredness and anxiety, food cravings, aversions or preconceptional dietary deficiencies (Haugen *et al.* 2011) or by exposure to distinctive aromas. A personal or a family history of the condition, particularly in the woman's mother or siblings, appears to predispose her to more severe symptoms including an increased risk of hyperemesis gravidarum (Annagür *et al.* 2014). Smoking may add to the problem in some (Sinha *et al.* 2011), although Kramer *et al.* (2013) and Källén, Lundberg and Aberg (2003) suggested it may confer a degree of protection from more severe symptoms. Increased body mass index may also contribute to the problem (Sinha *et al.* 2011).

NVP: a syndrome

NVP is a bio-psycho-social syndrome affecting not only the woman but the whole family.

Physiologically, many women report associated symptoms, including heartburn, diarrhoea or constipation, headaches, backache, hyper-salivation and more. The paternalistic approach of many doctors is often to dismiss these as normal and temporary, but this is not helpful when the woman is feeling wretched. As with pain, nausea is a subjective symptom and is as severe as the woman perceives it to be.

Socially, NVP may interfere with the woman's ability to work and accounts for almost one third of sickness absence from work amongst pregnant women in the first trimester (Källén *et al.* 2003). Caring for other children may be difficult. Cooking meals may be almost impossible, particularly if nausea is worsened by exposure to meat, milk or other foods, a feature possibly related to the immunosuppression required to prevent fetal rejection (Fessler 2002). The partner may find it difficult to cope and the woman may worry about her lack of libido: it is known that men are most likely to have an extra-marital affair during the partner's first pregnancy (Haltzman and Foy DiGeronimo 2008).

Emotionally, anxiety and fear, frustration and guilt increase cortisol levels; severe stress is more likely to lead to hyperemesis gravidarum (Leeners, Sauer and Rath 2000). As with cancer chemotherapy, experience of excessive NVP in previous pregnancies can trigger anticipatory nausea in the current pregnancy (Kamen *et al.* 2014). Personality also plays a part: some women may be full of self-pity or demanding constant attention, whilst others attempt to override their symptoms in order to continue their daily life with fortitude.

Some women are so overwhelmed by their condition that they yearn for an end to the pregnancy and it is estimated that 1000 pregnancies may be terminated annually as a result (Pregnancy Sickness Support 2013).

Hyperemesis gravidarum

Hyperemesis gravidarum (HG) is defined as excessive vomiting (more than three daily episodes of expulsion of stomach contents) accompanied by weight loss of more than 3kg or 5 per cent of the pre-pregnancy weight, and/or dehydration (ACOG 2004), and affects around 0.3 to 2 per cent of the population (Goodwin 2008). It is, however, essential to differentiate a subjective claim of excessive NVP from the true pathological nature of HG. Celebrity pregnancies and media sensationalism of the condition have blurred women's – and some professionals' – understanding of HG and resulted in the popular notion that all NVP is HG. Indeed, over-medicalisation of the physiological syndrome can have adverse psycho-social effects and may impact on maternal-infant bonding (personal clinical experience).

In true clinical HG, the maximal number of daily vomiting episodes correlates closely with the maximal weight loss. Hospital admission is required only for those who have lost more than 3kg or 5 per cent of the booking weight and who require intravenous rehydration, although this may also be possible in the home setting. There may be an increased risk of intrauterine growth retardation if weight loss is excessive, since fetal growth patterns are disturbed by alterations in maternal metabolism. Other clinical signs and maternal symptoms of HG may include sunken eyes, dry mouth, ketotic, offensive-smelling breath, reduced skin elasticity and, in very severe circumstances, bradycardia, hypotension and oliguria with dark urine containing ketones, bile, sugars and protein, with a high specific gravity. The mother may exhibit signs of anaemia, alterations in vitamin B12, folic acid and vitamin C levels and disturbance in the electrolyte balance, with hyponatraemia, hypochloraemia, hypokalaemia, low urea levels and a raised haematocrit. Liver function tests may show abnormalities, and abnormal thyroid function (normally thyroxine deficiency) may be revealed.

It is vital to validate the woman's experience as being significant to the progress of her pregnancy and her ability to cope with the demands of becoming a mother. Although vomiting can be measured in terms of its effect on weight, hydration and ketosis, symptomatic nausea is more difficult to assess. There are various validated tools to assess NVP, including the Rhodes Index of Nausea, Vomiting and Retching (Rhodes and McDaniel 1999), the McGill Nausea Questionnaire (Lacroix, Eason and Melzack 2000), the Pregnancy-Unique Quantification of Emesis and nausea (PUQE) system (Ebrahimi *et al.* 2009) and the Health-related Quality Of Life for nausea and vomiting in pregnancy (NVP-QOL). These can be helpful in excluding physio-pathological aspects of HG (Dochez *et al.* 2016), but most fail adequately to address maternal perceptions of the syndrome. A simple Likert scale, using a measurement of one to ten, may assist in this process (Tiran 2004, p.11). It is the woman's perception of severity and, after treatment, of any improvement, which is important to her overall wellbeing, together with a professional validation of her symptoms.

Assessing the woman for the possibility of a differential diagnosis is important when considering appropriate treatment. HG and coincidental medical conditions must be excluded and, if necessary, treated; it is easy to assume that any nausea and/or vomiting, especially in early pregnancy, is solely due to gestational reasons. On the other hand, obstetricians generally feel that excessive vomiting after 16 weeks gestation is less likely to be pregnancy related and may indicate more serious pathology, which should be investigated, but care must be taken not to dismiss ongoing physiological NVP.

Thyroid hormones may be affected by NVP or, conversely, the NVP may disturb thyroid hormone balance, either scenario potentially triggering gestational thyrotoxicosis (Buyukkayaci *et al.* 2015) or previously undiagnosed preconceptional thyroid disease. If severe NVP symptoms remain unresolved with anti-emetics, thyroxine levels may need to be assessed and, if deficient, thyroxine medication can be offered. Other conditions which may cause vomiting, usually in conjunction with other signs and symptoms, include gastroenteritis and gastrointestinal disease, hepatitis, pyelonephritis, hiatus hernia and reflux oesophagitis occurring as a feature of other pathology. Hypercalcaemia, acute fatty liver and benign intracranial hypertension are less common but equally significant problems. Helicobacter pylori has been implicated, although this theory is controversial and research is inconclusive (Golberg, Szilagyi and Graves 2007). Genetic incompatibility between the mother and fetus, or epigenetic factors such as the effects of substance misuse on the woman's system, could increase symptoms or, indeed, raise new pathology. For example, pregnant women who are habitual cannabis users may develop apparently intractable NVP, but if accompanied by abdominal pain and the unusual classic feature of obsessive bathing or showering, it may indicate cannabinoid hyperemesis, which is treated by discontinuation of the drug (Alaniz *et al.* 2015).

Conventional management of NVP

Most women initially attempt to manage their symptoms themselves, only asking for professional help when the problem persists. Traditional advice has been to eat little and often to maintain blood sugar levels and to eat a dry biscuit or toast before rising to combat early-morning hypoglycaemia. Unfortunately, this is largely ineffective and depends on the precise nature of the woman's symptoms. Various dietary recommendations are made, such as avoiding fatty, spicy or strong-smelling or flavoured foods and eating small protein-dominant meals. This traditional advice in the UK may however no longer be appropriate in today's multicultural society, since experience suggests that women resort to their cultural "comfort foods" when nauseated. In reality, women need to experiment to find which foods suit them best and it is more important that they eat foods that are more likely to be retained, providing some calorific content, than that they try to eat foods considered to be most nutritious. Adding feelings of guilt about their poor diet to the physical and emotional distress already experienced as a result of this debilitating condition is unrealistic, inappropriate and unkind. Women should, however, be encouraged to maintain an adequate fluid intake, especially when vomiting frequently.

Rest and sleep are important to reduce the impact of fatigue and, if feasible, women may need to take time off work or be advised to adapt their work schedule, perhaps altering start times to avoid commuting in the rush hour, or working from home occasionally. A recognition that health professionals empathise and appreciate the impact of NVP will go a long way towards influencing the mother's perception of her condition, even though the amount of nausea and the frequency of vomiting may be very little different from before.

Women consulting their midwives or doctors for more specific assistance will probably, although not exclusively, be at a stage where they have tried many of the self-help suggestions (see below) but feel that they cannot cope any longer. Vitally, the specific cause of the problem should attempt to be sought prior to treatment. It is not sufficient to dictate a general course of action because this will not be effective for all women. Doctors commonly prescribe medication such as antihistamines (e.g. cyclizine, promethazine), vitamin B6 (pyridoxine), sometimes in combination with antihistamines (e.g. diclectin), phenothiazines (e.g. prochlorperazine), steroids (e.g. prednisolone) or the relatively new ondansetron. These may be available in suppository form for those women who vomit after ingesting them or who are unable to swallow them. However, whilst these are usually effective in reducing the severity of vomiting, they are frequently reported by women as being ineffective at adequately reducing the unremitting nausea, a symptom which is often worse than the actual vomiting (Fejzo *et al.* 2013). Further, some women do not wish to take medication, although the evidence of any possible teratogenicity appears to be unfounded. Conversely, Fejzo *et al.* (2013) found that, in a group of previously hyperemetic women with poor antenatal and labour outcomes including gestational hypertension, at least 50 per cent had taken medication, most commonly antihistamines, leading them to suggest an urgent need to address the safety of antihistamines in pregnancy.

Admission to hospital should only be considered for women with true hyperemesis, and there is a move towards day case treatment in specially designated clinics (Dean and Marsden 2017), as recommended in the green-top guidelines from the Royal College of Obstetricians and Gynaecologists (2016). This strategy has been shown to be more acceptable to women with hyperemesis and may represent a considerable cost saving to the NHS. The use of complementary therapies for hyperemesis is inappropriate and unlikely to be effective in treating the problem until the dehydration has been addressed and the woman has returned to eating sufficiently to enable her to continue gaining weight. Once she has recovered from the severe effects of the hyperemesis she may well appreciate relaxation therapies to ease stress, enhance her wellbeing and facilitate her coping mechanism.

Dean and Marsden's study (2017) indicated that women are generally dissatisfied with their treatment for NVP across the UK. This extends to the lack of information they receive, a despair that all health professionals seem to advocate the use of ginger (see below) irrespective of the severity of their condition, and the common dismissal and lack of validation of the problem by midwives and general practitioners. These factors persuade women to try various self-help and complementary and natural methods to deal with the sickness and its associated symptoms.

Nutritional management

Women frequently experiment with different foods in an attempt to alleviate their NVP, either by increasing their consumption of certain foods thought to be helpful, or eliminating others that exacerbate the problem. Some nutrients are implicated in the development and severity of NVP, including deficiency of vitamin B6, zinc and magnesium. Nutrition advice for NVP is considered an element of conventional management, with women being given information about what foods they may find useful to alleviate symptoms. Unfortunately, an in-depth knowledge of nutrition as therapy is often lacking amongst midwives. However, whilst complementary medicine incorporates a group of therapies loosely defined as "nutritional therapies", it is not the intention here to debate in any detail the more alternative or obscure modalities focusing on using foods as medicines. Maternity caregivers can be of help to women with NVP simply by developing a greater knowledge and understanding of how common foods can contribute to easing the symptoms.

Vitamin B6 (pyridoxine) is primarily needed to aid the metabolism of protein and amino acids; consumption of large amounts of protein requires increased levels of B6. The vitamin also helps in the metabolism of histamine, serotonin and hydroxytryptamine, and inadequate serum B6 contributes to mood disturbances. In pregnancy, B6 is needed for development of the embryonic neurological system, and contributes to brain development and cognitive function in the child. The metabolism of sugars and fatty acids and the formation of vitamin B3 from the amino acid tryptophan is also dependent on vitamin B6, as is the functioning of magnesium and zinc. The contraceptive Pill may interfere with the absorption of pyridoxine; women are usually advised to take a vitamin B supplement whilst taking the Pill. Those who become pregnant very shortly after discontinuing the Pill may embark on pregnancy with a clinical deficiency of the vitamin, potentially increasing the risks to the developing baby. Pregnancy, stress hormones (notably cortisol) and oestrogens also increase the risk of B6 deficiency due to an increase in tryptophan activity.

Zinc is also vital for a range of bodily processes, not least in reproduction. It is necessary for the transport of pyridoxine across the cell membranes, and inadequate levels may impair cellular immunity and other necessary functions during organogenesis. Zinc also aids in the metabolism of proteins, carbohydrates and phosphorus and facilitates the release of stored vitamin A. It is essential for the normal growth of the skin, hair and skeleton, a healthy immune system and repair of tissues throughout the body, including wound healing. Zinc requirements increase by up to 30 per cent in pregnancy to provide for development of the fetal central nervous system, and by up to 40 per cent in breastfeeding mothers. Calcium, vitamin B12, vitamin C, copper and other trace elements are needed to facilitate absorption of zinc from foods, which can be inhibited by excessive stress, consumption of tea, coffee and alcohol, processed grains and phytates found in bran and some cereals. Zinc absorption is also reduced by concomitant use of certain medications including the contraceptive Pill and iron tablets.

Magnesium metabolism is closely linked with that of calcium and phosphorus. Magnesium is essential for various metabolic processes including the distribution of sodium potassium and calcium across cell membranes, as well as vitamin B1 and B6 metabolism. There is a fair body of evidence on the use of magnesium, particularly in conjunction with vitamin D, to prevent pre-eclampsia, but there appear to have been few studies, particularly in recent years, on supplementation with magnesium to treat NVP.

Harker, Montgomery and Fahey (2004) argue that it is not appropriate to treat all pregnant women experiencing NVP with a single nutritional supplement (most commonly vitamin B6) and that individual assessment is required in order to determine precisely the nutrients in which they are deficient. Despite this, many general practitioners and obstetricians persist in routinely advocating vitamin B6 for women with NVP who are presumed to be deficient. Indeed, Wibowo et al. (2012) found that there was little statistically significant difference in NVP scores in women who took pyridoxine compared to a control group. Many studies compare vitamin B6 to ginger (see below) or to a prescribed anti-emetic or a placebo. These studies are generally taken from the perspective that vitamin B6 is a standard – and apparently successful – treatment; thus the conclusions usually promote the success of ginger as being at least as effective as pyridoxine, rather than as an investigation of the success of pyridoxine (Firouzbakht et al. 2014; Sharifzadeh et al. 2017).

Rather than taking commercially produced supplementation to replace vitamin B6, zinc, magnesium and other nutrients, it is far preferable if the woman is able to eat foods that contain these elements. However, it must be remembered that many women are unable to eat when nauseated, or unable to keep food from being regurgitated from the stomach, so empathy and diplomacy must be employed when advising women about dietary means of reducing their symptoms. Table 4.1 summarises some of the foods that contain the various elements discussed here.

A recent trial comparing vitamin B6 with the consumption of quince fruit (*Cydonia oblongata*) which is high in vitamin C suggested that quince may be more effective than pyridoxine in reducing NVP (Jafari-Dehkordi *et al.* 2017). In this study women were encouraged to eat the fruit. This is interesting since the purported therapeutic actions of quince, namely that it is pharmacologically antioxidant, antibacterial, antifungal, anti-inflammatory, hepatoprotective and antidepressant, relate to chemical constituents in the seeds which are usually discarded. One of the main active components in quince is mucilage, a soft fibre which can impair the absorption of oral medications, so women should be advised not to eat quince if they are taking prescribed anti-emetics.

Table 4.1 Foods containing nutritional elements that may ease nausea and vomiting

Vitamin B6	Zinc	Magnesium
• avocado	• beans: green, lima	• green leafy vegetables
• bananas	• carrots	• nuts
• egg yolk	• chicken	• prawns
• fish, especially tuna	• corn	• soya beans
• green leafy vegetables	• egg yolk	• tap water (hard water)
• meat, especially poultry breast, beef	• green peas	• whole grains
• nuts, especially pistachio	• herbs and spices: ginger, garlic, parsley	
• pinto beans	• meat, pork chops, beef	
• potatoes, sweet potatoes	• milk, raw	
• seeds	• nuts: brazils, hazelnuts, walnuts, almonds	
• tomatoes	• oats, rye	
• wholegrain cereals	• oysters	
	• potatoes	
	• wheatgerm	
	• wholemeal bread	
	• yeast	

Ginger

Ginger is one of the most popular self-help strategies used by women with NVP. However, the common practice in the UK of eating ginger biscuits is largely ineffective as there is insufficient ginger in commercially produced biscuits to have a therapeutic effect, although some temporary relief may be obtained, most probably due to the carbohydrate content alleviating hypoglycaemia. Unfortunately, this is usually followed by a reactionary slump in blood sugar, causing a resurgence of symptoms. Crystallised ginger may also work in the short term, as may ginger beer or ale. Traditionally brewed ginger beer may contain as much as 11 per cent alcohol and there is a high sugar content in most commercially produced brands, provoking a reactionary effect similar to that with ginger biscuits. More significantly, artificial sweeteners, such as Aspartame™, are used in some types of ginger beer, which can be potentially detrimental to the fetus (Portela, Azoubel and Batigália 2007). One Iranian study claimed successful treatment of pregnancy sickness with ginger biscuits (Basirat *et al.* 2009). However, the biscuits used in this study were specially formulated to contain a therapeutic dose of ginger and the study should not be interpreted as evidence that commercially produced ginger biscuits are effective at resolving symptoms.

Ginger, when taken in therapeutic doses, acts pharmacologically and should therefore be used with the same caution as applied to drugs. Ginger root is a common – and powerful – medicinal agent used in traditional systems of healthcare in many eastern cultures such as Chinese, Korean and Indian Ayurvedic medicine. It is important to use the correct species of ginger root for therapeutic use, namely *Zingiber officinale*, the common type offered for culinary use in most western markets and shops. Thai ginger (*Alpinia galangal*, technically a form of galangal), wild ginger (*Asarum*), wall ginger (*Alpinia*) and particularly green ginger (*Artemisia absinthium*) contain different chemical constituents which may be unsafe in pregnancy.

The balance of therapeutic chemicals varies according to whether the ginger is fresh, semi-dried or fully dried. It is best ingested as a tea made from grated fresh root ginger steeped in boiling water, to be sipped throughout the day. Chewing and then swallowing raw ginger root is not appropriate as poor mastication may lead to intestinal obstruction. The anti-emetic action of ginger is not yet fully understood but may be due to gingerols or shogaol, the dehydrated products of gingerols, and zingiberene, which antagonise serotonin (5-HT) and suppress vasopressin, reducing gastric activity (Lete and Allué 2016). The balance of gingerols to shogaols differs according to whether the remedy is made from fresh or dried ginger, and gingerols are known to be chemically unstable in certain circumstances (Giacosa *et al.* 2015). There is currently no consensus between countries on the maximum safe dose of ginger, but it is generally felt that doses should be no more than 1gm per day in divided doses of 250mg (Lete and Allué 2016).

There are many studies demonstrating that ginger, in therapeutic doses, is effective as an anti-emetic, for nausea and/or vomiting, in pregnancy, during chemotherapy, post-operatively and due to motion sickness (Lindblad and Koppula 2016; Panahi *et al.* 2012; Ryan *et al.* 2012; Thomson, Corbin and Leung 2014), although many advocate caution, as the safety of ginger has not yet been clarified. Viljoen *et al.* (2014) found that ginger appeared to reduce nausea but was not significantly effective in reducing episodes of vomiting. However, this increasing evidence for effectiveness has led NICE irresponsibly to recommend that advice about ginger can be offered as standard to women with NVP, despite the fact that it is not classified as a medicine and has therefore not been evaluated in terms of safety (NICE 2017a).

Unfortunately, the numerous studies that appear to demonstrate anti-emetic effectiveness vary considerably in terms of research methodology, making it difficult to interpret the results and draw firm conclusions, a fact which does not appear to have been acknowledged by the NICE working party. For example, some studies compare fresh or dried ginger or commercially prepared ginger capsules with vitamin B6 (Chittumma, Kaewkiattikun and Wiriyasiriwach 2007; Ensiyeh and Sakineh 2009; Firouzbakht *et al.* 2014; Haji Seid Javadi, Salehi and Mashrabi 2013; Sripramote and Lekhyananda 2003). Others compare it with a placebo (Nanthakomon and Pongrojpaw 2006; Ozgoli, Goli and Simbar 2009) or to various anti-emetic prescription drugs such as metoclopramide or dimenhydrinate (Pongrojpaw, Somprasit and Chanthasenanont 2007). Saberi *et al.* (2013) further complicated the picture by using a combination of ginger and acupressure at the Pericardium 6 acupoint (see below). Some studies did not identify which species of ginger was used, although most used *Zingiber officinale*. There is also inconsistency in the dosages, the form of ginger used (fresh or dried root, syrup, etc.) and the frequency and duration of administration (Lete and Allué 2016).

Significantly, in virtually all studies, the precise cause of symptoms in different subjects has not been identified, a fact which can seriously skew success rates. For example, ginger with vitamin B6 may successfully treat women with NVP due to pyridoxine deficiency but may be ineffective for NVP related to other aetiology. Furthermore, the outcome measures of most studies focus on the effect of ginger in stopping or reducing vomiting, whereas nausea is significantly more distressing for most women, occasional vomiting often bringing temporary relief (personal communications with women).

However, ginger, like all herbal medicines, is a pharmacological agent containing a wide range of chemical constituents with specific therapeutic actions, as well as possible side effects when used inappropriately. Shawahna and Taha (2017) purport that the pharmacokinetics of conventional NVP medication can be adversely affected by gestational alterations in gastric motility, glomerular filtration and plasma volume and the absorption, distribution, metabolism and excretion of drugs. These physiological issues would also, of course, affect the metabolism of other pharmacologically active substances such as herbal remedies, including ginger, suggesting perhaps that ginger and prescribed medication for NVP should not be taken concurrently.

There is, for example, evidence of the considerable anticoagulant effects of many herbal remedies, including ginger (Abebe 2002; Shalansky *et al.* 2007; Spolarich and Andrews 2007; Ulbricht *et al.* 2007), although Jiang, Blair and McLachlan (2006) dispute this. As there is a moderate risk of bleeding, women on anticoagulants, anti-platelet drugs, non-steroidal anti-inflammatories such as aspirin, or other drugs or herbs with an impact on blood clotting should avoid ginger, and all other herbal remedies with a similar action. Prolonged use may interfere with clotting factors; thus ginger is contraindicated in women with a history of miscarriage, vaginal bleeding or coagulation disorders. Women who regularly ingest therapeutically applicable doses of ginger for more than about three weeks should have blood taken to test for clotting factors, since prolonged duration may thin the blood. Marx *et al.* (2015) suggest there is some evidence for the action of ginger on platelet aggregation, although they accept that more research is needed to substantiate this.

Ginger can irritate the stomach and trigger oesophagitis; it is contraindicated if the woman is already suffering heartburn and should be discontinued if heartburn develops whilst taking it. Ginger may increase bile secretion and must not be taken by women with a history of gallstones (Yamahara *et al.* 1985), although Hu *et al.* (2011) dispute this. The gastric irritant effects also suggest that ginger should be avoided if there is a history of irritable bowel syndrome or duodenal ulcer. Swallowing masticated ginger root, as advocated in some cultures, is particularly inadvisable as the fibrous nature of the root may cause gastrointestinal blockage. Ginger lowers blood pressure and may interact with anti-hypertensive medication (Ghayur and Gilani 2005). Ginger may also, theoretically, cause cardiac arrhythmias and should therefore be avoided by anyone on calcium channel blockers such as nifederpine (Young et al. 2006). (NB Pregnant women with major cardiac disease should avoid all herbal remedies.)

The potential for ginger to interact with prescribed drugs is well documented, including anticoagulants as previously mentioned, barbiturates, benzodiazepines, beta blockers and herbs with similar actions, such as garlic, gingko biloba, ginseng, red clover and turmeric (Ulbricht et al. 2007). Further, since ginger is known to lower blood sugar, it should be avoided in women with diabetes mellitus which is controlled by medication or insulin (Mozaffari-Khosravi et al. 2014). Vaginal spotting has been observed in one study, and as ginger may inhibit thromboxane synthesis and platelet aggregation in vitro, concern was expressed by the researchers that continued administration at term could increase the risk of postpartum haemorrhage (Heitmann, Nordeng and Holst 2013), although, due to the changes in viscosity of the blood at this time, this is probably more a theoretical possibility than a real risk.

No substantive evidence could be found to indicate that ginger is teratogenic or mutagenic, although Finland and Denmark have taken steps warning pregnant women against antenatal use of commercial ginger-containing products. Furthermore, Finland specifically advises against ingestion of ginger and many other herbal remedies during pregnancy since it is not known which constituents could adversely affect the mother or fetus (Evira Finnish Food Safety Authority 2016). Conversely, more recent Norwegian research demonstrated no increased risk of fetal abnormalities when women ingested ginger when compared with a control group (Heitmann et al. 2013). A Korean study by Choi et al. (2015) found no greater incidence of fetal malformations in women who used dried ginger but there was a slight increase in stillbirths. However, the researchers noted that many women concomitantly used other herbal remedies, a factor that may have had a bearing on these results.

Ginger has been shown to be weakly cholinergic (stimulates acetylcholine) (Ghayur and Gilani 2005). This corresponds to the traditional Chinese medicine approach, in which ginger is considered a "hot" or "Yang" remedy. Its warming effects are therefore unhelpful in women whose internal energies are already too "hot" or "Yang". This would include those who feel hot, are constantly thirsty, wanting cold drinks to cool them down, red-faced, perhaps "hot tempered" or irritable (see Chapter 2, Acupuncture).

In conclusion, it is beholden on healthcare professionals to dispel the myth that ginger is a universal anti-emetic remedy for NVP, because there are many women in whom it may be, at best, inappropriate, possibly exacerbating their NVP symptoms, or worse, unsafe according to their personal medical or obstetric history and current condition. A simple checklist can be used to aid prescription and eliminate contraindications (see Table 4.2). Whilst inadvertent use of ginger-containing foods and drinks are unlikely to cause harm in most women, it is necessary to remember that ginger is a pharmacological agent which should be prescribed individually. It is not merely a food supplement or a "natural" remedy, but a powerful tool which may reduce the severity of NVP symptoms in some women when used appropriately. Its risk-benefit profile has only recently started to come to light and there is a need for considerably more research into safety to balance the evidence we already have on its efficacy.

Table 4.2 Contraindications to use of ginger for nausea and vomiting in pregnancy

Effects	Obstetric contraindications	Medical contraindications	Medications which may interact with ginger
Anticoagulant	History of miscarriage/ antepartum haemorrhage Current vaginal bleeding	Clotting disorders Elective surgery within next 2 weeks	Anticoagulants Anti-platelets Non-steroidal anti-inflammatories, e.g. aspirin Gingko biloba All herbs with anti-coagulant action
Cholagoguic (stimulates bile secretion)	Cholestasis of pregnancy	Gallstones, obstructive jaundice, acute liver disease	Ursodeoxycholic acid or other gallstone medication
Cardiovascular, hypotensive	Tendency to mid-trimester fainting and dizziness	Hypotension Cardiac disease	Anti-hypertensives
Potentiates sedatives, hypnotics	Fulminating pre-eclampsia	Epilepsy	Anti-epileptic drugs, benzodiazepines, barbiturates
Hypoglycaemic	Gestational diabetes, insulin-dependent or unstable	Diabetes mellitus, insulin-dependent or unstable	Insulin, oral anti-diabetic medication

Cholinergic: "yin-yang" balance	Hot, sweating, thirsty for cold drinks, irritable	Pyrexia, infection	NB Try peppermint instead of ginger (unless cardiac disease)
Gastrointestinal	Heartburn, flatulence, diarrhoea	Inflammatory bowel disease Duodenal ulcer Irritable bowel disease	Antacids
Interference with iron absorption	Gestational anaemia	Pre-existing iron deficiency anaemia	Iron therapy
Allergy	Pruritus	Inflammatory skin conditions Allergic susceptibility	

Peppermint and other herbal remedies

Mint has long been heralded as an effective remedy for sickness. However, there are many different types of mint, some of which are not safe in pregnancy, and there are variable methods of administration. Peppermint (*Mentha piperata*), usually taken as a tea, is a popular alternative to ginger and is sometimes more appropriate for women, particularly for those who are more "yin" (see above and Chapter 2, Acupuncture). It has long been used in traditional medicine to treat a variety of gastrointestinal conditions. When administered orally as a tea or in capsule form, it can be effective for irritable bowel syndrome (Cappello *et al.* 2007) through an effect on gastric emptying (Inamori *et al.* 2007). Peppermint is also sometimes used for respiratory infections, headaches, neuralgia and toothache, for menorrhagia and dysmenorrhoea (Masoumi *et al.* 2016) and as a stimulant.

Peppermint essential oil is the only natural product included in the *British National Formulary* and is used in post-operative care for paralytic ileus and as an antispasmodic during procedures such as barium enema. There is also some suggestion that it may help with preventing cracked nipples in breastfeeding mothers (Sayyah Melli *et al.* 2007), although any oil should be washed from the skin of the breasts before the baby suckles. When used in combination with ginger essential oil, peppermint has been found to be effective for post-operative nausea (Hunt *et al.* 2013; Sites *et al.* 2014), including post-Caesarean section (Lane *et al.* 2012). However, ginger essential oil should be avoided in pregnancy as it is thought to have an effect on uterine activity (Calvert 2005).

Peppermint essential oil is a complex mixture of compounds, including 35 per cent to 70 per cent menthol, 15 per cent to 30 per cent menthone and 4 per cent to 14 per cent menthyl acetate, although pharmaceutical grade oil is typically standardised to contain at least 44 per cent menthol. Peppermint oil contains between 1 per cent and 4 per cent pugelone, which is neurologically and hepatically toxic, although various processes are used to reduce the pugelone content in commercial peppermint to below 1 per cent. When taken orally in large doses, peppermint oil can cause gastrointestinal symptoms including additional nausea and vomiting, as well as headache, allergic reactions and perianal irritation. Drinking the oil can cause mouth ulceration and gastric irritation. Animal research suggests that peppermint oil may adversely affect cytochrome P450s (Unger and Frank 2004), impacting on the metabolism of some drugs. Drinking large quantities of peppermint tea may affect iron absorption and interfere with drugs that are metabolised via the liver, including the anti-emetic ondansetron (Akdogan, Gultekin and Yontem 2004). It is also known to be a cardiac stimulant and to cause relaxation of smooth muscles in the bronchial tract (Balakrishnan 2015; Meamarbashi and Rajabi 2013), and hence also probably in the uterus, although this may be dose-dependent. Topically, strong percentages of the oil cause dermatitis.

A Middle Eastern randomised, double-blinded controlled trial of 60 women with NVP treated with peppermint oil obtained results that were not statistically significant (Pasha *et al.* 2012). Unusually, the treatment, conducted prior to night-time sleeping, consisted of placing a bowl of water containing four drops of peppermint oil on the floor by the beds of the women in the trial group, whilst the control group had bowls of water with four drops of normal saline added. This would not be the normal course of action for midwives providing aromatherapy to women, not least because sickness primarily commences in the mornings and the effects of the peppermint oil would not be sustained throughout the night as it would evaporate. In addition, women admitted to hospital are likely to be suffering more severe NVP requiring medication, and the placing of bowls of water on the floor in a ward area contravenes health and safety regulations. Furthermore, the type of mint used was not specified in this study, the oil being described only as "pure" peppermint which was specially prepared for the trial. This is of concern since certain types of mint are contraindicated in pregnancy, particularly in essential oil form as they contain high levels of constituents that should be avoided during organogenesis.

Roman chamomile

Roman chamomile (*Anthemis nobilis*) is one member of the Asteracea/ Compositae family that is considered relatively safe to use during pregnancy, unlike German chamomile (*Matricaria chamomilla*) which may have oestrogenic effects (Zangeneh *et al.* 2010). Chamomile is a traditional remedy taken orally as a tea for nausea and other gastrointestinal problems and is used topically in essential oil form for wound healing and inflammation, including sore nipples. Chamomile tea is also known to aid sleep, although excessive doses may have the opposite effect. Chamomile has been used orally to stimulate uterine contractions in women with post-dates pregnancy and there is some suggestion that it may be sufficiently uterotonic to be abortifacient in the first trimester (Gholami *et al.* 2016). Chamomile tea may also be useful for lactation (Silva *et al.* 2017). Chamomile studies are variable and do not always identify the type of chamomile used; some involve the ingestion of teas, which are more dilute than prescribed tablets, or occasionally essential oils administered dermally. One paper reported the apparent effect of chamomile consumption in pregnancy on premature closure of the ductus arteriosus in the fetus. Alarmingly, this paper, published in the journal *Ultrasound in Obstetrics and Gynecology*, erroneously identified the tea consumed by the women as chamomile (from the Asteracea family), yet the authors' discussion centred on *Camellia sinensis*, an evergreen shrub from the Theaceae family (Sridharan, Archer and Manning 2009). There are various reports on the possible adverse reaction of contact dermatitis from chamomile oil or even the tea, although this tends to be from *Matricaria chamomilla* rather than Roman chamomile (Anzai *et al.* 2015; Paulsen and Andersen 2012). At least one case of anaphylaxis from chamomile tea has been reported (Andres *et al.* 2009), and women (and caregivers) with sensitivity to members of the Compositae plant family, including chamomile and arnica, should avoid chamomile teas, essential oils, creams and other products (Paulsen, Chistensen and Andersen 2008).

Slippery elm bark

Slippery elm bark (*Ulmus rubra*), usually in lozenge form and more commonly used for constipation, is quoted on some websites as a suitable remedy for pregnancy sickness; indeed it may be prescribed by qualified medical herbalists. However, self-administration is not recommended because slippery elm has a reputation as an abortifacient, possibly due to certain chemicals in the outer bark. However, it is usually the inner bark that is used for medicinal purposes, and virtually no studies appear to have been undertaken on its safety in pregnancy.

Nettle

Nettle (*Urtica urens*) tea is also advocated for sickness and constipation. Stinging nettle leaves contain high levels of iron, vitamins, potassium, calcium and carotene and may be advised by herbalists as a tonic during pregnancy. Herbal remedies are produced from the above-ground parts of the plant and from the root. Traditionally, the most common use for nettle is as a diuretic and for urinary problems such as nocturia, dysuria, frequency of micturition and retention of urine, as well as benign prostatic hyperplasia. It may also have a role to play in reducing blood pressure and heart rate (Qayyum *et al.* 2016). Taken to excess in tea form, nettle can cause diarrhoea, sweating and skin irritation, and a case of a woman who attempted to suck the leaves resulting in severe tongue oedema has been reported (Caliskaner, Karaayvaz and Ozturk 2004). There is risk of interaction with anti-diabetic and anti-hypertensive medication and with warfarin (Edgcumbe and McAuley 2008).

Aromatherapy

There is increasing interest in the use of aromatherapy as a treatment for pregnancy sickness. A recent Iranian randomised controlled trial of 100 women suggested that inhalation of lemon essential oil may ease NVP (Yavari Kia *et al.* 2014), although smelling fresh lemons may be a cheaper, easier and safer method of easing the nausea. The use of peppermint (*Mentha piperata*) oil has been discussed above. However, since there is some suggestion that NVP may be related to olfactory hyper-sensitivity (Cameron 2007; Erick 1995), aromatherapy may not be the most suitable treatment, although Cameron (2014) now disputes this olfactory link. However, the effect of odours on the severity of women's experiences of NVP appears to be similar to that found in migraine patients, and is possibly linked to genetic factors (Heinrichs 2002). The close association between the senses of smell and taste also need to be taken into account, as women commonly crave or become averse to specific foods (Schachtman *et al.* 2016). In cases where a woman suffering NVP wishes to receive aromatherapy, percentages should be kept possibly to as low as 0.5 per cent, using a single essential oil.

Light refreshing citrus oils can be pleasant for some women, including lemon (*Citrus limon*), lime (*Citrus aurantium*) or bergamot (*Citrus bergamia*).

Homeopathy

No formal evidence for the use of homeopathic remedies for NVP could be found when searching the literature. A randomised double-blinded controlled study in France by Pérol *et al.* (2012) – in which breast cancer patients were given either standard anti-emetics, a homeopathic remedy combined with anti-emetics or a placebo – proved inconclusive as a means of treating chemotherapy-induced sickness, but no other trials on nausea and vomiting of any aetiology could be found. The main issue is that, in homeopathic terms, the symptom of sickness cannot exist on its own; rather the person experiences sickness as part of a whole symptom picture and therefore the woman must be treated holistically (see Chapter 2).

On the other hand, many women, especially those who are already familiar with the concept of homeopathy and homeopathic prescribing, like to use these remedies to alleviate nausea, vomiting and associated symptoms and there is considerable anecdotal clinical evidence that homeopathy can help. As with any other condition, homeopathic remedies must be prescribed according to the precise nature of the woman's symptoms. No other therapy highlights so completely the complex nature of NVP; a focus on all symptoms experienced by the woman, however trivial or apparently inconsequential, will enable the practitioner to determine the most appropriate remedy.

There are several commonly used remedies that may be effective, but many more may be preferable if the characteristics of the woman's condition dictate them. Only one remedy should be taken at a time and they should not be used concomitantly with aromatherapy essential oils or with certain strong drugs (see Chapter 2). Women who are familiar with self-prescribing of homeopathic remedies may be able to identify the most appropriate remedy for themselves. However, the complex nature of NVP suggests that women with no knowledge of this therapy should be encouraged to consult a qualified homeopath, because over-use of a remedy, or choosing one that is not appropriate, can trigger a reverse proving. Box 4.1 summarises a small selection of homeopathic remedies that may be of use for women with NVP.

BOX 4.1

Suggested homeopathic remedies for nausea
and vomiting in pregnancy

- *Ipecacuanha* – constant nausea unrelieved by vomiting; profuse saliva, vomits food, bile frequently exacerbates nausea; dislikes smell of food or tobacco

- *Nux vomica* – constant nausea, often worse immediately after eating but relieved by vomiting; worst in morning; craves stimulants, e.g. coffee, tea, alcohol; "workaholic"

- *Pulsatilla* – nausea, worst in morning, unrelieved by vomiting; bitter taste in mouth; desires sour, fresh food; averse to fatty food, milk, meat, bread; changeable mood, easily moved to tears; fresh air, cold drinks improve symptoms, but exacerbated by hot drinks, stuffy room

- *Sepia* – intermittent nausea, with empty, dragging sensation in abdomen; craves vinegar, sour foods, sweets; averse to bread, fatty food, milk; exacerbated by exertion, smell and thought of food; worst before breakfast and between 1500 and 1700 hours

- *Arsenicum* – woman feels "deathly"; profuse frequent vomiting of food, bile, water, causing sweating; burning sensation in stomach; may crave coffee; symptoms are better with warmth; worse after cold food or drinks, particularly afternoons; dislikes smell of food

- *Colchicum* – most appropriate remedy when predominating feature is motion; particularly symptomatic in car, but in severe cases may be unable even to lift head from pillow

- *Cocculus* – most appropriate remedy when predominating feature is smell or sight of food, particularly eggs, fish

- *Kreosotum* – particularly valuable when there is excessive salivation

Acupuncture/acupressure

During the first trimester of pregnancy when nausea is usually at its worst, women would benefit from being informed about the inexpensive commercially produced wristbands that are available. Although popularly used for travel sickness, these wristbands can be self-administered and may enable a woman to continue with her daily life without becoming debilitated. The wristbands have a small press stud on the inner aspect which is positioned over a specific acupoint, the Pericardium 6 or Neiguan point.

The Neiguan point is on the bilateral Pericardium meridian lines that start deep inside the chest; one branch on each side then descends into the abdomen through the diaphragm, whilst another branch emerges on the skin just below the axilla, proceeds down the inner aspect of the arm to the elbow and wrist, ending at the tip of the middle (third) finger. In Chinese medicine the connection with the diaphragm is vital as the diaphragmatic muscle is associated with the pericardium. The sixth point on the Pericardium meridian (Pericardium 6) is termed the "inner gate", allowing access to the heart and controlling the diaphragm and other organs such as the stomach and uterus. The function of Pericardium 6 is to release, relax or unbind the chest area to harmonise the qi, calming the heart rate and respiration. Its mechanism in controlling the diaphragm also acts to steady stomach activity, reducing the tendency to vomit. Other acupuncture points also influence these organs; therefore Pericardium 6 is not always the most effective point for nausea, but it is useful for motion and gestational sickness, various abdominal organ conditions and possibly also immediately postpartum if the mother bleeds abnormally and feels dizzy. Figure 4.1 shows the location of the Pericardium meridian and Figure 4.2 shows the location of the Pericardium 6 acupoint.

It is important that the woman is advised on the correct positioning of the wristbands to ensure that the stud on the inside is located directly over the Pericardium 6 acupuncture points on both wrists. The Pericardium 6 point is located three finger breadths up from the wrist crease on the inside of the forearm. The measurement should be assessed according to the breadth of the woman's own fingers. Adjustments should therefore be made by professionals demonstrating the position to take account of any differences in width of their own fingers. A dip is usually felt between the tendons which, when pressed deeply, is likely to feel tender, as if slightly bruised. The woman should be advised to position the bands on both wrist points prior to sitting up in bed on waking so that there is no immediate alteration in blood pressure or blood sugar levels. If the woman is admitted to hospital with worsened NVP requiring intravenous rehydration, care should be taken to relocate the wristbands to the correct position if they are moved to accommodate insertion of a cannula.

There are numerous studies on the stimulation of the Pericardium 6 acupoint, either by needling or applied pressure (Moore and Hickey 2017). As far back as the mid-1980s, good quality studies were undertaken on Pericardium 6 stimulation for nausea and vomiting of various aetiologies (Dundee *et al.* 1986; Dundee, Ghaly, Bill *et al.* 1989; Dundee, Ghaly, Fitzpatrick *et al.* 1989; Ghaly, Fitzpatrick and Dundee 1987). The effectiveness and cost-effectiveness of acupressure in particular, with few apparent side effects or risks, has meant a continued and prolific interest in using acupoint stimulation for gestational, post-operative, motion and radiotherapy-induced sickness, yet it is interesting to note that there is only limited use of this technique in conventional healthcare. As an alternative, it would be relatively easy to teach midwives how to use TENS, applied to the Pericardium 6 acupoints: an Australian study by Chu *et al.* (2013) on healthy volunteers with simulated flight sickness demonstrated increased sympathetic and decreased parasympathetic activity with reduced nausea. Study of the use of acupressure wristbands has also proved positive (Can Gürkan and Arslan 2008), although a systematic review by van den Heuvel *et al.* (2016) showed inconclusive results. A Cochrane review found that Pericardium 6 acupuncture was comparable to anti-emetics in relieving post-operative nausea and vomiting (Lee, Chan and Fan 2015), whereas a meta-analysis by Helmreich, Shiao and Dune (2006) suggested that electro-acupuncture is the most successful strategy.

The duration and frequency of treatment also needs consideration. Zhou *et al.*'s randomised controlled study of gastric cancer patients undergoing chemotherapy (2017) found that 30 minutes of acupuncture given daily for two weeks had a significant effect on nausea and vomiting as well as other gastrointestinal symptoms, greatly improving patients' quality of life. However, in keeping with traditional Chinese medicine, in addition to the Pericardium 6 acupoint four other points were used for these treatments, providing a more holistic approach than simply using a single point. In a study carried out in the intensive care unit, three 20-minute Pericardium 6 stimulation treatments were given to patients experiencing nausea and pain, with good effect (Feeney *et al.* 2017). However, this type of regime would be impractical for expectant mothers not admitted to hospital and would be costly in terms of staff time. In addition, the relatively chronic nature of sickness in pregnancy requires therapy from which the effect is sustained as much as possible between treatment sessions.

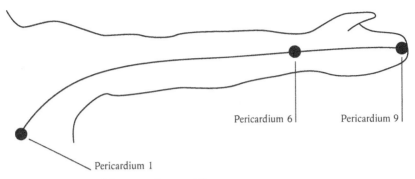

Pericardium 6   Pericardium 9

Pericardium 1

Figure 4.1 Location of the Pericardium meridian

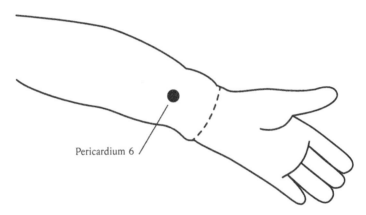

Pericardium 6

Figure 4.2 Position of Pericardium 6 wristbands for nausea and vomiting

Sound therapy

The conventional view of the aetiology of NVP focuses on hormonal changes, immunological or metabolic factors and, increasingly, an appreciation of possible genetic and epigenetic factors. There have also been some suggestions that anatomical factors may play a part. Women whose NVP is worsened by movement of any kind may have issues relating to the vestibular apparatus in the inner ear, and Black (2002) debated the possibility of the vestibular apparatus impacting on neurochemical parameters.

Harnessing sound as a therapeutic intervention has been part of traditional systems of medicine for thousands of years, including Chinese and Ayurvedic medicine. In modern complementary medicine, however, the use of sound has recently become more recognised as a therapy in its own right. Sound is a vibrational energy consisting of three inter-related elements: pulse, wave and form. Evidence of the vibrational effect of sound can be seen in the shattering of a glass with the resonance of an opera singer's voice. Sound therapy is based on creating a sound frequency and vibration appropriate to the necessary healing process and has spawned a new scientific specialism, psycho-acoustics, which is the study of the effects of sound on the neurological system. It is based on the principle that all matter vibrates at specific frequencies, and nausea, depression, stress and other symptoms cause human vibrations to reduce in frequency. Using tones (sound waves) to promote recovery and healing is said to encourage DNA repair, thus returning the body to homeostatic balance. Contemporary practitioners commonly use tuning forks to elicit the required vibrations and resonance which activates the brainwaves to overcome the clinical problem being treated. Acupuncturists also sometimes use tuning forks to encourage vibration at specific acupoints, as an alternative to electro-stimulation.

Much of the current sound therapy research is based on the early work of the biophysicist Gerald Oster. Oster demonstrated that when a tone is played in one ear and a different tone is played in the other ear, the brain reacts by creating a third, internal tone, called a binaural beat. This is thought to synchronise the brain waves in both cerebral hemispheres, a process which has been termed "brain wave entrainment", although a study by Solcà, Mottaz and Guggisberg (2016) suggests that the effect is more one of binaural integration rather than training. This synchronicity facilitates a deeper focus, changing electrical activity within the brain to impact on the symptom being experienced by the client (Romei *et al.* 2016), and a systematic review by Huang and Charyton (2008) found a reasonable level of evidence to support the use of sound waves as therapy. The neurophysiology behind brainwave entrainment is complex. Evidence shows that it slows down electrical conductivity (measured quantitatively in hertz) to facilitate rest, relaxation and sleep through a reduction in cortical activity (Schweimer *et al.* 2011).

A simple means of using sound waves for NVP is the commercially produced downloadable *Morningwell*™ application ("app") for mobile telephones (or there is a compact disc version). This system involves a programme of music, underlying which a series of frequent pulsations tap into the vestibular apparatus of the ear, which are then transmitted to the brain. The music is simply to make the application or compact disc pleasant to listen to, but it is important that the woman uses personal headphones so that the pulsations (vibrations) effectively bounce on the vestibular apparatus of both ears. These pulsations rebalance the vestibular apparatus by interrupting the passage of emetic signals between the brain and gastrointestinal tract. The music is not intended for relaxation and, as there are no spoken words, the system is not based on hypnotherapeutic suggestions. A trial undertaken in a maternity unit in Hampshire, UK (Mayo 2001), claimed to be up to 90 per cent effective in relieving or reducing the symptoms of nausea; personal clinical experience of this author would support this. Golaszewski *et al.* (1995) used a similar system for women with hyperemesis gravidarum, with good effects. However, the effectiveness of the *Morningwell*™ system may be relatively short lived: women have reported that several weeks of continual use can trigger a Pavlovian association of the music with sickness, causing a return to more severe symptoms (communications with pregnant women). On the other hand, this system may offer an inexpensive, self-administered method of relieving nausea and vomiting that is sufficient for many women.

Osteopathy and chiropractic

Musculoskeletal misalignment is thought to trigger and exacerbate the symptoms of the NVP syndrome. It is known that relaxin has a significant impact on the musculoskeletal system (Aldabe *et al.* 2012), contributing to pelvic girdle pain, backache and sciatica in later pregnancy, but kinetic and motor control factors also play a part. Women with a history of musculoskeletal injury or congenital deviations may be particularly at risk. If one considers the skeleton as the body's main supporting framework, with the soft tissue organs within and without, it can be surmised that any impact to the skeleton will disturb the homeostatic anatomy of the whole body, with a consequent effect on the whole. Spinal and neck problems place excessive strain on the entire system, causing compensatory alterations in other parts of the body.

Women with a history of whiplash injury seem to be particularly vulnerable to severe NVP: it is noticeable that those who experience trauma between pregnancies will often suffer greater NVP in subsequent pregnancies (Tiran 2010b). Cervical vertebral trauma places tension on the vomiting centre in the brain and on the vagus nerve, whilst associated strain or unusual force exerted lower down the spine and across the shoulder and pelvic girdle areas are likely to cause heartburn and other gastrointestinal symptoms, as well as problems such as carpal tunnel syndrome. Other potential causative factors include coccygeal injury from a fall or previous dislocation during childbirth, or pelvic or leg fractures, perhaps following a skiing or road traffic accident. Traumatic dental surgery such as removal of grossly impacted wisdom teeth, or a previous jaw fracture, may place strain on the neck and throat, leading to a risk of accompanying hyper-salivation during pregnancy.

When musculoskeletal factors are present, osteopathy or chiropractic can effectively treat nausea and vomiting, heartburn and hyper-salivation. However, despite clinical successes, the formal evidence is sparse. Cuthbert (2006) explored the use of chiropractic for people with motion sickness and found spinal and cranial manipulative techniques to be effective in alleviating sensory, motor and proprioceptive issues associated with the condition. While the aetiology of motion sickness is different from that of NVP, it is possible to draw some conclusions about how manipulative therapy may be of use for these women. Some chiropractors also believe that liver congestion from the need to detoxify toxins and debris produced as the trophoblastic cells of the fertilised ovum digest the endometrium to allow implantation. Treatment focuses on manipulative techniques to facilitate homeostatic balance in the liver and associated organs.

Women who experience severe NVP that can be traced back to musculoskeletal issues may also be prone to malposition or malpresentation later in the pregnancy due to abnormal pelvic diameters caused by overall spinal deviations. In the experience of this author, breech presentation is common in these women because of an accentuated angle of inclination of the pelvic brim preventing the fetal head from entering the cavity. (See also Chapter 6.)

Hypnotherapy

Hypnosis for NVP is less well used and somewhat controversial, although it is known that NVP can be exacerbated by stress, anxiety and other psychological factors (Chou *et al.* 2008). Simon and Schwarz (1999) expressed concern that hypnotherapy is usually sought only after conventional treatment and common self-help strategies have proven ineffective. They argue that, since some women may be unconsciously ambivalent towards their pregnancies, early hypnotherapy can effectively improve wellbeing. It is believed that the deep sense of relaxation achieved through hypnosis decreases the stimulation of the sympathetic nervous system, whilst the use of cues, with suggestions for changing the ways in which the woman perceives the sickness, may help. For example, she can be helped to change her view of NVP as a negative issue to one in which she recognises that NVP ensures that high hormone levels maintain the pregnancy. Other cues may focus on anatomical relaxation of the throat and stomach muscles with a view to reducing nausea, gagging, retching and vomiting. Operative conditioning may also play a part (Quinn and Colagiuri 2016).

Several studies on hypnosis for NVP were undertaken in the 1980s and 1990s but little contemporary evidence could be found. This may be due to the fact that current obstetric hypnotherapy research trends tend to focus around birth preparation and tocophobia. There are, however, several case reports. Beevi *et al.* (2015) reported on a woman with first and second trimester hyperemesis gravidarum and concomitant hyper-salivation who responded well to a course of hypnotherapy up to 36 weeks gestation. However, whilst this may have achieved an eventual resolution, it could be argued that ongoing contact with a sympathetic professional may have contributed to the overall effect. Where midwives and other maternity professionals offer hypnotherapy for NVP, this can have a significant effect on the relationship, the woman's self-confidence and her overall ability to cope with her symptoms. Four successful cases were also presented by Madrid, Giovannoli and Wolfe (2011). McCormack (2010) undertook a systematic review of 45 studies, of which six trials met the inclusion criteria. They found promising evidence for using hypnosis for NVP but, as usual, suggested that further research is needed in order to demonstrate how effective hypnosis may be.

Psychotherapy may also be helpful, although, again, it is unclear whether any positive effects arise from the specific mindfulness techniques used or the impact of time spent talking with a professional (Faramarzi, Yazdani and Barat 2015). Interestingly, the Royal College of Obstetricians and Gynaecologists (RCOG) guidelines on NVP (RCOG 2016) advocate counselling and medication as suitable strategies for NVP.

Conclusion

Despite being a largely physiological effect of pregnancy, nausea and vomiting can be debilitating and affect the woman's day-to-day life and that of her family, friends and colleagues. Women try to deal with the condition by experimenting with various self-help approaches, and tend only to seek medical help when symptoms become intractable. There are many natural ways of reducing the severity of nausea and the frequency of vomiting, but these must be used cautiously and correctly.

Maternity care providers are in an invaluable situation to advise women about diet and simple strategies such as wristbands and to give correct and comprehensive information about ginger, other herbal remedies and homeopathic medicines. Midwives and doulas who practise complementary therapies such as acupuncture or clinical hypnosis may be able to provide treatment specifically to curtail the symptoms experienced by the woman. If the woman is prepared to pay for private treatment, referral to another qualified practitioner, such as an osteopath, chiropractor, acupuncturist or hypnotherapist, may offer a dynamic and successful solution. Indeed, helping women to cope with, and possibly to resolve, nausea and vomiting in the early part of the pregnancy may have a positive impact on the remainder of the pregnancy.

CHAPTER 5

Back Pain in Pregnancy

Backache, sciatica and pelvic pain are common physiological discomforts in the antenatal period because of the impact of pregnancy hormones on the musculoskeletal system. As the expectant mother's weight increases and postural compensations occur, back pain can become extremely debilitating, often necessitating absence from work. Whilst physiotherapy can be helpful, the current state of the maternity services may mean that women experience a long waiting time for appointments, and increasingly they turn to complementary therapies for a solution. There are several notable therapeutic strategies that can be used to help these women, most notably osteopathy, chiropractic and acupuncture. Natural remedies are less effective and less popular as they can only be, at best, palliative.

This chapter includes discussion on the following aspects:

- introduction

- conventional management of back pain

- exercise strategies

- complementary therapies

- massage, aromatherapy and reflexology

- osteopathy and chiropractic

- acupuncture

- natural remedies

- conclusion.

Introduction

Low back pain and related pelvic pain, particularly in the region of the symphysis pubis, are significant issues during and after pregnancy, occurring in at least 50 per cent of women (Malmqvist *et al.* 2012). A Cochrane review by Liddle and Pennick (2015) suggested that as many as 60 per cent of expectant mothers experience generalised lumbosacral back pain, with 20 per cent suffering pelvic pain, either concomitantly or separately, while Mogren and Pohjanen (2005) found an incidence of 72 per cent. Sibbritt, Ladanyi and Adams (2016) revealed that, in a population of over 1800 pregnant Australian women, almost 40 per cent experienced backache, 16 per cent suffered pelvic pain and 12 per cent reported neck pain. Conversely, a Nigerian study found a higher incidence of pelvic, rather than lower back, pain (34.3% and 57.4% respectively), with an incidental finding of urinary incontinence in many of the women (Usman *et al.* 2017). Lumbar pain is frequently accompanied by sacroiliac joint pain and/or sciatica, as well as groin and buttock discomfort. Back and pelvic pain can be debilitating, often impacting on daily life, work and sleep, with not only physical but also psycho-social effects.

Physiologically, relaxation of the muscles, ligaments and tendons occurs during pregnancy, mainly due to the action of the hormone relaxin, as well as progesterone. Biomechanical factors also play a part, with pre-existing or gestational musculoskeletal misalignment increasingly being acknowledged (Fishburn 2015; Tiran 2010b). Micronutrient deficiencies may contribute to overall compromise to the musculoskeletal system, including loss of bone mass density and an epigenetic effect on the fetal skeleton, suggesting that there is justification for the use of vitamin D supplementation before and during pregnancy (Moon, Harvey and Cooper 2015). Weight increases and postural adaptations to accommodate the changing centre of gravity cause an increased lumbar lordosis (concave curvature) and a correspondingly accentuated thoracic kyphosis (convex curvature).

Pre-existing back or neck pain, sciatica or other musculoskeletal issues appear to exacerbate the physiological discomfort (Padua *et al.* 2002), which often causes an increased angle of inclination of the pelvic brim to compensate, leading to an accentuated lumbar lordosis beyond that normally expected in pregnancy. Excessive increase in the size and weight of the breasts in pregnancy can also lead to upper back, shoulder and neck pain and may predispose the woman to other shoulder girdle problems such as carpal tunnel syndrome. Pressure from the general weight gain causes abduction of the knees in later pregnancy, potentially adding to the problem, although Padua *et al.* (2002) found no correlation between back pain and higher body mass index. Low back pain and pelvic girdle pain are usually viewed by medical practitioners as two separate conditions but they are inter-related and one may lead to the other. Katonis *et al.* (2011) suggest that pelvic girdle pain is four times more prevalent than lumbosacral pain, whilst a combination of the two conditions is amongst the most common reasons for sickness absence from work during pregnancy. Women who have suffered back pain in previous pregnancies are highly likely to experience problems in subsequent pregnancies due to ligament stretching, which may be worsened in women whose earlier deliveries were difficult. Also, the musculoskeletal system takes considerably longer than soft tissue systems to recover from the hormonal and physical upheavals of pregnancy, birth and lactation, and some women may continue to experience back pain and pelvic girdle pain for more than a year after the birth (Bergström, Persson and Mogren 2016). Persistent difficulties may occur in some women or musculoskeletal compromise may predispose some to the development of new longer-term problems.

Back pain tends to be exacerbated by tiredness, poor posture during day-to-day activities, positions adopted whilst sleeping and by inappropriate or inadequate exercise, whereas women who undertake regular pre-pregnancy exercise routines tend to experience fewer problems (Mogren 2005). It has been shown that abdominal muscles become thinner during pregnancy under hormonal influences (Weis *et al.* 2015), predisposing women who are obese or who have a large fetus, multiple pregnancy or poor pre-conceptional abdominal muscle tone to increased discomfort. However, this theory remains somewhat controversial as a later study found no real variation in abdominal muscle thickness in women who had back pain compared to those who did not (Weis *et al.* 2017).

The almost universal practice amongst mothers of balancing an infant on one hip, at a time when the musculoskeletal system may not yet have fully recovered from the pregnancy, can cause a permanent misalignment in the pelvis which, together with over-stretched ligaments, often exacerbates back pain in subsequent pregnancies. Women may attempt to deal with the pain by over-exaggerating the natural postural compensation, possibly predisposing them to continuing problems in the postpartum period (Stapleton, MacLennan and Kristiansson 2002), and morbidity can continue for up to three years after delivery (Norén *et al.* 2002). Unremitting pain can also be psychologically distressing (Field *et al.* 2012), an increase in stress hormones heightening the mother's perception of pain and adversely affecting her ability to cope. Clinical experience suggests that some women's experience of back pain in pregnancy is so debilitating, especially if they require crutches or a walking frame to remain mobile, that they request elective Caesarean section in order to put an end to their symptoms.

Conventional management of back pain

As with many other physiological discomforts, expectant mothers frequently attempt to self-manage their back pain, perhaps because they have no real faith in conventional methods to resolve the problem (Close *et al.* 2016a). One study found that only 12 per cent of women experiencing symptoms actually sought professional help (Chang, Jensen and Lai 2015). Similarly, Sibbritt *et al.* (2016) found that around 30 per cent of women do not inform their midwife or consult their doctor or another professional such as a physiotherapist. Of the remaining 70 per cent, only 22 per cent request medical help, whereas 32 per cent opt to consult massage therapists or other complementary practitioners (27%). When there is accompanying sciatica, women may, however, be more likely to seek medical help at an earlier stage (Hall, Lauche *et al.* 2016). Unfortunately, Hall, Cramer *et al.*'s meta-analysis (2016) found limited robust evidence for the effectiveness of complementary therapies for back pain, although they acknowledge that the client-therapist relationship and the accessibility of a practitioner over a sustained period of time may play a part in some subjective relief of symptoms.

In the UK, conventional treatment for antenatal back pain has not been well researched. Mens *et al.* (2006) demonstrated that the wearing of a pelvic girdle or belt decreases sacroiliac joint hypermobility, but exercise appears to have variable results. However, women frequently report additional discomfort from wearing belts. In Belgium, Bertuit *et al.* (2017) found that women who used belts had greater relief of backache and increased mobility than a control group, but suggested that wearing them for short periods helped to avoid the chafing and discomfort of the belt itself. Gutke *et al.* (2015) suggest that there is little evidence to support the use of supportive belts, although van Kampen *et al.* (2015) consider they may be effective as a preventative measure. However, this is counter-intuitive to dealing with the problem as relaxin and progesterone levels rise, as it is virtually impossible to prevent some degree of pregnancy back pain. Treatment can only be palliative since symptoms tend to worsen as pregnancy progresses and weight and postural adjustments increase. Conventional options for the management of back pain, sciatica and pelvic girdle pain is limited, and midwives feel impotent to help. Some suggestions for advice that may help women are given in Table 5.1.

Table 5.1 Suggestions which professionals can offer on self-care for back pain in pregnancy

Daily living	• Stand up straight and tall, point chin down to prevent head tilting back. Pace walking to avoid straining ligaments further
	• In bed, use pillows for support; keep thighs parallel to prevent top leg twisting across body (modified recovery position). The mattress should be turned regularly and changed if more than seven years old
	• Get out of bed by rolling onto one side, push up to a sitting position, stand slowly; do not come to a sitting position directly from lying down – including when arising from an examination couch in the antenatal clinic
	• Ask toddlers to climb up rather than bending down to lift them. *Never* carry a toddler on one hip – causes permanent musculoskeletal misalignment
	• Ask for help with housework and chores: iron sitting down or press just a few items at a time. Ask a family member to empty the dishwasher to avoid constant bending, to clean the bath and vacuum the floor to avoid overstretching. Use a trolley when shopping; carry small bags in both hands rather than one large one. Ask for help to lift, carry or reach for things on high shelves
	• Wear comfortable shoes with broad supporting heels. Ensure maternity bra is properly fitted – breasts supported by wide straps and adequately sized cups, to avoid extra strain on shoulders and rib cage
At work	• Ask someone to vacate a seat on the bus, train or tube to avoid the need to stand for the entire journey. Negotiate to change working hours to travel off-peak
	• When driving, sit tall and comfortable – *then* adjust rear view mirror. Mirror may need adjusting each morning and evening as posture changes during the day
	• Use extra cushions for support or ask for an orthopaedic chair if sitting for long periods of time. Keep both feet on the floor and avoid crossing legs. Leave desk regularly to move about
	• Readjust computer screen to avoid poor posture over keyboard. Place mouse mat close enough to avoid stretching
	• If work involves standing, try shifting from one foot to the other to ease aches, and sit down when possible
Exercise	• Walking and stretching may relieve stiffness and pain
	• Swimming – if using breast stroke, face must be in the water to keep neck and spine straight
	• Water-based exercise, yoga, tai chi, Alexander technique or relaxation classes may ease discomfort – ensure teacher is aware of pregnancy
	• Regular exercise can be continued but adapt techniques as necessary, sip plenty of water and avoid becoming over-heated

The NICE guideline on antenatal care (CG62: NICE 2017a) advocates water-based exercise, massage therapy and back care education, either individually or in groups, but does not recommend the use of any complementary therapies. This is consistent with the NICE guideline on the management of back pain in the general adult population (NG59: NICE 2016) which suggests exercise but discourages the wearing of corsets and belts. Unlike the antenatal guideline, however, the NG59 guideline recommends the use of massage and other manual therapies, as well as psychological therapies. Unfortunately, in a change from the previous version of this guideline, NICE now discourages the use of acupuncture and transcutaneous electrical nerve stimulation due to an apparent lack of robust evidence.

Exercise strategies

Women are commonly referred to an obstetric physiotherapist for advice and education on home-based exercises. However, in the UK, there is often a long waiting list for women to access an NHS obstetric physiotherapist, and practitioners may not be able to provide the necessary ongoing treatment for the duration of the pregnancy, perhaps only offering a course of three to six weeks (Bishop *et al.* 2016). Twice-weekly aerobic and resistance exercises performed at home, plus brisk daily walking for 30 minutes, may reduce the pain and associated disability (Sklempe Kokic *et al.* 2017), and longer courses of 12-week group-based exercise classes have proved successful in Norway (Mørkved *et al.* 2007). Third trimester exercise has been found to reduce pain intensity, but it does not reduce lumbar lordosis and may contribute significantly to reduced spinal flexibility which may have a direct impact on birth outcomes (Garshasbi and Faghih Zadeh 2005).

Water-based exercise may be more effective than land-based techniques (Granath, Hellgren and Gunnarsson 2006; Pennick and Liddle 2013; Waller, Lambeck and Daly 2009) and may contribute to improved sleep, indirectly affecting subjective pain perception (Rodriguez-Blanque *et al.* 2017). Progressive muscle relaxation exercises may help, especially when accompanied by music (Akmeşe and Oran 2014), although it is difficult to extrapolate which modality may be the more effective, with both aiming to aid relaxation, either physical or emotional. Kanji (2000) suggested that other forms of relaxation, such as autogenic training, may also be of value. Research suggests that autogenic training encourages changes in stress markers such as salivary amylase (Kiba *et al.* 2017), thus promoting enhanced coping strategies.

Yoga

Yoga has been shown to be an effective intervention for back pain in the general population, including that caused by specific spinal deviations such as spondylitis (Field 2016b; Manik *et al.* 2017; Sutar, Yadav and Desai 2016), and may reduce sickness absence from work (Brämberg *et al.* 2017). Yoga can be adapted for pregnancy and appears to be more effective than postural exercises (Babbar and Shyken 2016; Kinser *et al.* 2017; Martins and Pinto e Silva 2014). Pilates exercise may also ease discomfort and help to prevent falls (Mazzarino *et al.* 2015; Uppal, Manley and Schofield 2016; Wells *et al.* 2014).

Alexander technique

The Alexander technique may benefit people with chronic low back pain (Yardley *et al.* 2010) and could be adapted to help women with antenatal and postnatal symptoms. The Alexander technique is a way of learning to move and use one's body mindfully, correcting habitual postures, movements, coordination and balance, as well as the patterns of accumulated tension which interfere with the innate ability to move easily and efficiently. It is an empowering self-help strategy that, once taught, should ideally become a way of life, but it can be used in the short term for specific problems such as back pain, especially in pregnancy. Daily activities – sitting, lying, standing, walking, lifting and other physical activities – become easier by using the body in a more efficient manner, with less risk of pain and discomfort. The Alexander technique is energising because the client learns how to move with less energy expenditure, thus promoting an enhanced sense of wellbeing. Unfortunately, although the Alexander technique is popular amongst actors to assist optimal positioning for voice projection (it was devised by an actor), its use as a general complementary therapy has declined in recent years and it may be difficult for expectant mothers to access a local teacher of the discipline.

Complementary therapies

There is a reasonable amount of literature to support the use of various complementary therapies to treat back pain in the general public. It is accepted that most complementary therapies will have some effect, particularly when the condition is chronic, but patients may need prolonged courses of treatment to achieve long-term relief. In pregnancy, since the symptoms are relatively transitory, even though they often persist and worsen as pregnancy progresses, some women will be prepared to pay for private complementary therapy treatments to alleviate their distressing symptoms. Manual therapies come into their own for musculoskeletal problems, whilst natural remedies tend to be used less and are possibly less effective anyway.

However, one of the issues for women seeking manual treatments is that they may need to commit to a prolonged course of treatment, which can prove costly in terms of time and money (Bernard and Tuchin 2016). Added to this may be the logistical difficulty in attending a clinic, since mobility may be considerably reduced. A study of acupuncture treatment for chronic low back pain in otherwise healthy non-pregnant adults (Bishop *et al.* 2017) found that adherence to treatment and compliance with suggestions for home-based strategies such as exercise were dependent on patients' beliefs in the chosen therapy, the relationship with the individual practitioner and the practicalities of attending for multiple appointments. Non-attendance at subsequent appointments was, as can be expected, also affected by patients' wellbeing, although early improvements in symptoms did not appear to affect attendance adversely. Similar effects on compliance and attendance could be expected amongst pregnant women. On the other hand, women's experiences of back pain can be so profound that they are often committed to doing anything they can to relieve the severity of their symptoms.

Massage, aromatherapy and reflexology

Massage may be helpful for antenatal, intrapartum and postnatal backache, particularly where there is associated muscular strain or tension or if the woman is distressed and tired, making it difficult for her to cope with the symptoms (Oswald, Higgins and Assimakopoulos 2013). Women are more likely to consult a massage practitioner for their back or neck pain, but less so for pelvic pain (Sibbritt *et al.* 2016), perhaps because they view the former as relatively normal but pelvic girdle pain as significantly more problematic. Although massage cannot, of course, reduce skeletal pain, its benefits lie in reducing corresponding tension in the erector spinae muscles either side of the vertebrae. In addition, as has been discussed elsewhere in this book, massage has a profound relaxation impact on most women.

Massage tends to have an accumulative effect without significant adverse effects (Farber and Wieland 2016), and could be taught to partners so that they can continue the treatment at home. Simple effleurage (stroking) techniques can ease discomfort in the lower back, upper back and neck regions and over the sacroiliac joint areas of the pelvis. Care should, however, be taken, before 37 weeks gestation, not to over-stimulate the sacral foramen in the lower back, as these correspond to acupuncture points that may stimulate contractions. This means avoiding the excessive use of petrissage movements (kneading with finger and thumb tips) deep into the "dimples" either side of the lower lumbar vertebrae.

There is some evidence to support the use of massage for back pain in the non-pregnant population, although Rothberg and Friedman (2016) suggest that manual treatment is no more effective than conventional medical strategies. Many different styles of massage have been used with a moderate-to-good, albeit sometimes temporary, effect, including Ayurvedic massage (Kumar *et al.* 2016), Iranian traditional massage (Hashemi *et al.* 2016) and Thai massage (Buttagat *et al.* 2016). Women's perceptions of the benefits of complementary therapies, particularly massage, may enhance the effectiveness of treatment, particularly amongst better-educated women over the age of 40, living in urban areas (Kavadar *et al.* 2016). As with non-pregnant patients, the fact that expectant mothers autonomously choose to self-refer for massage may contribute to its value in alleviating pain. Receiving real-time video feedback of the back during massage may exert a psychological analgesic effect (Löffler *et al.* 2017). Massage can also be effective in relieving lumbar pain in the early postpartum period, for example after intrapartum epidural anaesthesia (Lee and Ko 2015).

Aromatherapy essential oils may be used to complement the massage treatment. One study (Shirazi *et al.* 2016) used rose oil (*Rosa damascena*), applied topically, to treat a group of women experiencing third trimester backache. However, the safety of rose oil in pregnancy has not been established; Tiran (2016a) suggests that it should not be used until at least 35 weeks gestation as some types of rose oil contain higher levels of chemicals that may initiate uterine contractions. Black pepper oil (*Piper nigrum*) blended with other, less aromatically potent oils may have a greater analgesic effect and would be safer in earlier pregnancy. Lavender (*Lavandula angustifolia*) is also an effective analgesic oil, although it is difficult to extrapolate definitively from the limited studies whether this is due to the chemistry of the lavender or the use of massage and other manual techniques such as acupressure (Yip and Tse 2006).

Although this author has had good success in employing specific reflex zone therapy (reflexology) techniques in the treatment of lumbosacral and pelvic girdle pain, as well as neck pain and carpal tunnel syndrome, there is little research evidence, if any, for the effectiveness of reflexology in treating women with these conditions (see Tiran 2010b). Poole, Glenn and Murphy (2007) found little value in using reflexology for a group of non-pregnant patients with back pain. A more recent study by Close *et al.* (2016b) suggests there is some benefit to using reflexology for pregnant women, but acknowledged methodological problems with their pilot study, in which a footbath was offered as the sham treatment which, in itself, may have had some effect. Additionally, as with reflexology studies for other conditions, the diversity of styles may mean that different treatment techniques are used by different researchers, further confounding the variables. It is probable that in some studies the treatment intervention is little more than an adapted foot massage, giving rise to the debate on whether any effectiveness is similar to that gained from other touch modalities including basic massage (see Chapter 2).

A study by Dalal *et al.* (2013) explored the potential effectiveness of treatment for back pain by investigating two groups of non-pregnant subjects, one without symptoms and one with backache. The team attempted to confirm a relationship between the spine reflex zones on the feet and the intensity of pain and discomfort felt over these zones by the subjects with back pain. The team demonstrated an interesting scientific correlation that may confirm the location of the reflex zones for the spine, from a clinical perspective. However, this does not address the holistic treatment that may be required for someone with back pain, because the spinal reflex zones would not be the only areas of the feet to be treated. In a pregnant woman, for example, it would be normal to include reflex zones on the feet corresponding to the entire musculoskeletal system, including those for the spinal vertebrae, spinal musculature, bony pelvis, symphysis pubis, sacroiliac joint and sciatic nerves, as well as the reflex zones for the upper musculoskeletal system – the shoulder girdle, arms, wrists and hand areas, and specific relaxation points.

Osteopathy and chiropractic

Osteopathy, chiropractic and craniosacral therapy offer probably the most dynamic treatment options for women with lower or upper back pain, pelvic girdle pain or any other musculoskeletal problems in pregnancy such as carpal tunnel syndrome and shoulder girdle pain. Expectant mothers commonly choose to consult practitioners such as osteopaths for backache (Frawley, Sundberg *et al.* 2016). Lavelle (2012) suggests that musculoskeletal realignment not only eases discomforts in pregnancy but also rebalances homeostasis, potentially facilitating greater normality in childbirth.

A longitudinal follow-up of 115 women who received chiropractic for back pain in pregnancy indicated a 52 per cent improvement after one treatment, with steadily increasing rates of improvement with longer courses of treatment, particularly when continued postnatally for up to a year (Peterson *et al.* 2014). It is, however, difficult to determine the validity of this study which was not matched to a control group, thus offering no comparable information about the rates for symptom improvement over a similar time-frame for women who did not receive chiropractic. In countries such as Canada, where chiropractic is accepted as being complementary to conventional healthcare, women with musculoskeletal symptoms can receive care which is genuinely shared between the obstetrician and the chiropractor (George *et al.* 2013), but in the UK, chiropractic is a definite "alternative" option for women able to pay for private treatment. Chiropractic can be effective for symphysis pubis discomfort, easing pain and improving mobility and stability but, as above, the course of treatment should ideally be continued into the postnatal period (Howell 2012; Murphy *et al.* 2009). A study by Schwerla *et al.* (2015) offered twice-weekly osteopathic manipulative therapy to 80 postnatal mothers with continuing back pain, achieving significant improvement in reported pain and mobility, but concluded that longer term studies are needed.

Unfortunately, the evidence from robust trials of chiropractic and osteopathy is lacking, with most papers being case reports or non-controlled evaluations. A controlled, single-blinded multicentre study was undertaken in Sweden, in which women with pelvic girdle pain were randomly assigned to receive either standard care or craniosacral therapy plus standard care (Elden *et al.* 2013). However, whilst improvements were greater in the intervention group, the treatment effects were relatively minor and the authors of the report suggest caution in interpreting the results. A recent meta-analysis (Hall, Cramer *et al.* 2016) found insufficient evidence for the efficacy of manipulative manual techniques for low back pain. Conversely, Peterson, Haas and Gregory (2012) suggest that spinal manipulation and exercise are preferable to the neuro-emotional technique, a mind-body tool aimed at rebalancing neurological imbalances caused by stress.

Many women report success in alleviation of symptoms following manipulative therapies, although it is unclear whether this is due to the effectiveness of the therapy or perhaps the inadequacy of conventional treatment modalities. It may also be related to increased time, both in single sessions and in the accumulative effects of repeated sessions of treatment. Perception of reduced pain could also be due to the nature of the relationship that builds between the woman and her individual practitioner, which may be very different from the relationship she has with an NHS physiotherapist, particularly when antenatal back care is often dealt with in groups.

Hensel *et al.* (2015) established the Pregnancy Research on Osteopathic Manipulation Optimizing Treatment Effects (PROMOTE) study to evaluate the efficacy of osteopathic techniques for musculoskeletal pain in late pregnancy. Four hundred pregnant women were randomly allocated to receive standard care, osteopathy with standard care or placebo ultrasound treatment with standard care. Both osteopathy and the placebo treatment achieved some improvement in symptoms reported by participants, although osteopathy was significantly more effective. This was one of the largest trials ever conducted on the effectiveness of osteopathic manipulations in pregnancy, although it was interesting to note a high attrition rate, stated as being due to missed appointments and the onset of labour before 40 weeks gestation in some women. As with much other complementary medicine research, the need to use a standardised treatment regime rather than individually tailored clinically relevant programmes of treatment may have affected the ultimate efficacy of treatment.

Acupuncture

Acupuncture is an increasingly popular modality for treating back pain, although, somewhat surprisingly, physiotherapists who are trained in acupuncture seem to be reluctant to use it on pregnant women, perhaps due to a lack of confidence and a fear of initiating miscarriage or preterm labour (Bishop *et al.* 2015; Waterfield *et al.* 2015). Although many research trials have been undertaken in China, there is increasing interest in using acupuncture for back pain and related problems in the UK, both in the general population and for pregnant women.

In 2006 Lund *et al.* undertook a study in which they provided ten acupuncture treatments for women with second and third trimester pelvic pain with good effect, reducing pain intensity at rest and during daily activities as well as improving emotional wellbeing and energy levels. The results were consistent, irrespective of whether superficial or deep needling was used. However, the effectiveness of this study indicated that treatment must be individually designed, a fact that gave clinically significant results but not statistically significant outcomes. This poses the question of the validity of the evidence in terms of clinical versus statistical results or, indeed, the precise acupoints used during treatment. Further, whilst most studies investigate the impact of needling the acupoints, other Chinese medicine techniques may also bring positive results. For example, cupping to a specific acupoint, Bladder 23, has been shown to reduce back pain, the effect of which may be extended into the puerperium (Akbarzadeh *et al.* 2014).

Pennick and Young (2007) reviewed eight randomised controlled trials of acupuncture treatments for backache and pelvic girdle pain. They concluded that acupuncture was effective for pelvic girdle pain alone or when combined with low back pain, but it was less effective for low back pain in isolation. However, they did conclude that the results should be viewed with caution as there was a high risk of bias in some studies. Richards *et al.* (2012) also undertook a systematic review of four studies involving 566 women and found that back pain and pelvic girdle problems respond well to acupuncture. Similarly, Elden *et al.* (2005) demonstrated that acupuncture was superior to both standard care and stabilising exercises, whilst a later study on 115 women with pelvic girdle pain (Elden *et al.* 2008) found true acupuncture to be no more effective than sham acupuncture.

The EASE Back pilot study (Bishop *et al.* 2016; Foster *et al.* 2016) aimed to determine the feasibility of conducting a randomised controlled trial in which acupuncture is added to standard care for women with back pain in pregnancy. Survey questionnaires were distributed and focus groups held of both expectant mothers and professionals (midwives and physiotherapists) to determine women's experiences and current practice. The feasibility was explored of assigning women to receive standard care plus a booklet on the self-management of back pain, or standard care plus either true acupuncture, physiotherapy or sham (non-penetrating) acupuncture. A full randomised controlled trial is in progress at the time of writing to compare standard care with both true and sham acupuncture for women with low back pain, with or without pelvic girdle pain. The "usual care" group is given an information leaflet about back pain, tips for self-help and referral to a physiotherapist if appropriate; the other two groups are given the information booklet, the usual care delivered by physiotherapists and either acupuncture to appropriate acupoints (between six and ten bilateral needle insertions) or usual care and the information booklet plus non-penetrating acupuncture to up to four bilateral acupoints.

Shiatsu has also been used to reasonable effect in a group of non-pregnant clients (Brady *et al.* 2001), although the integration of massage techniques within this study may have skewed the results. Silva *et al.* (2016) suggest that acupressure is a simple, non-invasive and inexpensive technique that can be effective for back pain and other discomforts in pregnancy and labour and advocate its inclusion in the training of nurses and midwives. The application of ear studs at the auricular acupressure points (Purepong *et al.* 2015) could also easily be incorporated into the management of antenatal backache.

TENS has been proposed as an effective treatment. Keskin *et al.* (2012) conducted a prospective, randomised, controlled trial of 79 women who were at least 32 weeks gestation. They were allocated to one of four groups: a control group, an exercise group, a group which received oral analgesia (paracetamol) and a group which used TENS. Although all three interventions resulted in reduced pain compared to the control group, the TENS group had greatest effect on the level of back pain. However, whilst the research team claimed that TENS is both effective and safe, care must be taken with this strategy. Women who are less than 37 weeks gestation should generally not use TENS to relieve back pain. This is because the TENS transducers are normally positioned over the lumbosacral foramen of the pelvis, an area served both by the uterine nerves and related to specific acupuncture points known to trigger contractions (see Chapters 2 and 8). This suggests that injudicious use of TENS to treat back pain prior to term may pose a slight risk of preterm labour in susceptible women.

Natural remedies

Herbal and homeopathic medicines tend to be less well used for back pain, perhaps because the problem is generally acknowledged to respond better to manual therapies. Many of the herbal remedies traditionally used for pain relief, such as capsicum, comfrey, Devil's claw and willow bark, may be safe enough in small amounts, perhaps applied topically in cream form to the back, but oral use should be avoided (see Chapter 2, Herbal medicine). Several abstracts of homeopathic usage for low back pain were found, mostly in German language journals, but little research has been conducted. Homeopathic arnica may be useful for backache exacerbated by excessive exercise (Barkey and Kaszkin-Bettag 2012), but routine or sustained use of arnica (or any other homeopathic remedy) is inadvisable as it would likely lead to a reverse proving (see Chapter 2, Homeopathy).

Conclusion

Women with back pain in pregnancy may turn to complementary therapies to resolve or relieve the discomfort, but ongoing treatment tends to be needed for the duration of the pregnancy and into the postnatal period. There is a reasonable amount of evidence to support the use of acupuncture and massage, but rather less so in the case of osteopathy and chiropractic, and very little research or clinical use of natural remedies. Midwives and doulas can advise that women seek help from experienced practitioners, but in current UK practice, these are generally working in the private sector, meaning that those less able or willing to pay may be deprived of effective palliative treatment for their musculoskeletal aches and pains.

CHAPTER 6

Complementary Therapies for Breech Presentation

Breech presentation can be a worrying diagnosis for the expectant mother, given the limited options for conventional obstetric care. Many women want to avoid Caesarean section or external cephalic version, and few are given the option of a vaginal breech birth. Moxibustion, a traditional Chinese medicine technique, has become a popular, inexpensive and empowering alternative for these women and is now fairly well known in the west, although its availability on the NHS is negligible.

This chapter addresses moxibustion treatment in detail, with an exploration of the mechanism of action and research into the effectiveness and safety of the technique. A brief discussion on other complementary therapies for women with breech presentation is also included.

This chapter includes:

- introduction
- moxibustion
- other alternative options for women with breech presentation
- conclusion.

Introduction

The incidence of breech presentation at term is around 3 to 4 per cent (Mitchell and Allen 2008) and may be associated with stillbirth and adverse perinatal outcomes including oligohydramnios, fetal growth restriction, gestational diabetes and congenital anomalies (Macharey *et al.* 2017). Standard obstetric practice is to offer women external cephalic version (ECV) or Caesarean section to minimise the risks to mother and baby (RCOG 2017). Vaginal breech birth is not currently offered as a standard option in the majority of UK maternity units, except in the case of a late admission or an undiagnosed breech presentation, because of the perceived risks such as fetal asphyxia and neonatal trauma. ECV and Caesarean section are, however, also associated with significant risks (Hunter 2014). Questions have been raised about the ability of obstetricians to perform Caesareans safely (Glezerman 2011), although the phenomenal operative delivery rates in many countries suggest that they are exceptionally experienced in the surgical procedures involved. This may, of course, be one of the reasons why vaginal breech birth is not viewed favourably by obstetricians, as their skills have developed in operative delivery, but this also means that midwives have also largely become de-skilled.

Guittier *et al.* (2011) found that women undergo a complex decision-making process on being informed that they have a breech presentation. They need time to discuss their concerns in a supportive environment in order to maintain control over the experience (Warriner, Bryan and Brown 2014). The limited conventional options available have led women to seek alternative ways to attempt to turn a breech-presenting fetus to cephalic in an effort to facilitate normal birth.

Moxibustion is by far the most well-known complementary therapy for breech presentation, with almost two thirds of women now prepared to try it, rather than submitting to ECV and/or Caesarean section (Guittier *et al.* 2012). Practitioners of other therapies such as hypnotherapy, reflexology and homeopathy may also be consulted by women with an abnormal presentation. Some therapies can also be used to assist in achieving the optimal position for the fetus when the presentation is cephalic.

Moxibustion

Moxibustion is a technique used in traditional Chinese medicine, the mechanism of action of which can be difficult to understand for those trained in conventional anatomy and physiology. Traditional Chinese medicine is based on the concept of holism, with the notion of a branching tree-like structure of internal subcuticular energy lines, called meridians, which convey the body's life force and link one part of the body to another (see Chapter 2, Acupuncture). Moxibustion is a technique used to stimulate heat and energy along these meridians where the internal energy is deficient. In China, moxibustion is used in the treatment of over 300 medical conditions (Deng and Shen 2013) and in maternity care has long been used as an alternative to, or alongside, ECV. In western medical research, there is increasing interest in the potential of moxa therapy to treat various conditions including irritable bowel syndrome (Bao *et al.* 2016), osteoarthritis (Choi *et al.* 2017) and dysmenorrhoea (Yang *et al.* 2017). Moxibustion is also often used in combination with acupuncture, to increase the heat stimulation to the acupoints.

In Chinese medicine theory, fetal malpresentations such as breech and malpositions such as occipito-posterior are thought to arise from a deficiency in the energy (qi) passing through the Kidney meridian, which is in close proximity to the uterus. The Kidney meridian is said to have a role in nourishing the fetus; disharmony in Kidney qi can lead to deficiency or stagnation of the qi in the uterus. Kidney meridian deficiency also affects uterine and fetal muscle tone, so the fetus is unable to maintain a cephalic presentation or possibly even a longitudinal lie. The Bladder meridian, which is closely linked with the Kidney meridian, is instrumental in reproduction, and Bladder qi also influences uterine function. This means that Kidney meridian qi deficiency can be corrected by working on the Bladder meridian, and this is relevant to the practice of moxibustion to convert a breech presentation to cephalic.

The bilateral Bladder meridians (sometimes called the Urinary Bladder meridians) start in the inner corner of the two eye sockets (these points being called the left- and right-sided Bladder 1 acupoints). They then pass up and over the head, down the back either side of the spine, around the kidneys, through the bladder and continue down the legs, around the lower edges of the outer ankle bones, along the outer edges of the feet and end in the outer corners of the little toes (see Figure 6.1). This final acupoint, Bladder 67 (also called "Zhiyin"), is the point at which the Bladder and Kidney meridians connect; thus treatment at this point helps to correct both Bladder and Kidney meridian energy.

The Zhiyin point is said to have a specific function in promoting downwards movement of the fetal head; it is considered one of the points contraindicated for use in earlier pregnancy, as it may trigger miscarriage or preterm labour. The Bladder 67 point also has an impact at the other end of the meridian and can be used to treat headache, migraine, eye pain, epistaxis and sinus congestion (in non-pregnant clients). Indeed, it is interesting to note that many women with a breech presentation suffer from sinus congestion in pregnancy. In maternity care, the acupoint is used to correct a malpresentation or malposition; needling of the point can aid a difficult or protracted labour and deal with a retained placenta (following appropriate training).

Moxibustion is performed using moxa, specially prepared sticks containing a compressed, dried herb, mugwort (*Artemesia vulgaris*). The sticks are used as a heat source applied to the Bladder 67 acupoints on the dorsal surface at the outer edges of the cuticles on the little (fifth) toes (see Figure 6.1). Locating the point can, however, be complicated by the shape of the individual's toenails, and can also be quite deep within the tissues. Inserting a sharp fingernail should elicit a sensation of tenderness on the correct point. It is for this reason that acupressure (applying finger or thumb pressure to the point) is generally ineffective in stimulating sufficient energy to cause conversion of the breech to cephalic presentation.

The aim of the treatment is to stimulate the deficient energy in the Bladder and Kidney meridians, increasing muscle tone and thus converting the breech to a cephalic presentation by harmonising the qi. In conventional physiological terms, the heat generated via moxibustion stimulates the adrenocortical system (adrenaline and noradrenaline), leading to changes in placental oestrogen and prostaglandin output, thereby increasing myometrial sensitivity and contractility. Moxa heat may also stimulate adenosine triphosphate (energy) (Hu *et al.* 2015), particularly in the fetus, so there is usually a slight, but normal, rise in the fetal heart rate during the treatment. A combination of extra "give" in the uterus from the hormonal changes and increased fetal activity may lead the fetus to turn itself to a cephalic presentation.

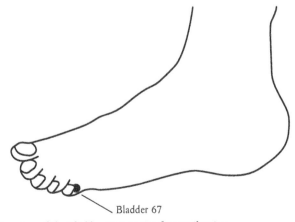

Bladder 67

Figure 6.1 Location of the Bladder 67 acupoint for moxibustion

Moxa sticks burn in a way which allows the acupoints to absorb the heat with less risk of burning the external skin than would be the case with another heat source (Pach, Brinkhaus and Willich 2009). It is thought that, in general Chinese medicine use, moxibustion has an effect on the superficial and deep tissues in the skin, which sends thermo-physical impulses from the focus acupoints along the meridians (Deng and Shen 2013). Using smoking moxibustion sticks, in which the flame has been extinguished but heat continues to be emitted, causes significant warming, leading to vasoconstriction at the precise acupoint, with vasodilatation around the point and an increased peripheral arterial blood flow and vascular permeability (Takayama *et al.* 2011).

Suitability for moxibustion

As with any clinical treatment, there are some women in whom moxibustion is contraindicated. Acupuncturists assess women in terms of their qi deficiency and stagnation and do not consider the normal physio-pathological issues which are part of mainstream clinical practice. However, where midwives, doctors, doulas or antenatal educators are advising women about self-administration of moxibustion, caution should be employed to ensure that there are no clinical contraindications. This is particularly important when clinicians incorporate a complementary strategy which is new to the management of breech presentation, particularly a technique which has a relatively poor evidence base (or one for which most research papers are in Chinese). Also, when the woman is carrying out the treatment at home, there are no facilities for emergency treatment in the event of complications, so extra safety considerations are paramount.

In simple terms, contraindications to moxibustion are essentially the same as those for ECV. In addition, any woman with current or previous essential or gestational hypertension should not receive the treatment, because the moxa heat may raise the blood pressure, although systematic reviews by Kim *et al.* (2010) and Yang *et al.* (2014) suggest that moxibustion is sometimes used to reduce blood pressure (in non-pregnant patients and applied to different acupoints). In addition, anyone with respiratory compromise such as asthma should avoid moxibustion as the smoke generated during burning of the moxa sticks contains numerous constituents that are inhaled by the client and anyone else present and may, in susceptible people, cause respiratory problems or allergic reactions (Li and Liu 2008). For these women, acupuncture would be a safer option.

If a woman has had a previous Caesarean section, this is a significant contraindication, although many women will be keen to try to achieve a vaginal birth. Further, they may perceive moxibustion as a natural – therefore, inherently "harmless" – technique which they assume to be safer than ECV. Whilst the woman should be advised against self-administering the technique at home, she could consult a qualified acupuncturist who can take the necessary Chinese medicine precautions and offer acupuncture treatment that helps to turn the fetus. Midwives offering moxibustion services within an NHS setting may conclude that women who have had a Caesarean section in the previous two years should avoid moxibustion (similar to ECV protocols), but consider as a precaution any woman whose Caesarean was performed more than two years previously. On the other hand, professionals working in private practice would be wise to decline to treat women with any previous uterine scar to avoid the slight possibility of scar dehiscence, although this risk is disputed by some acupuncturists.

Women due to have an elective Caesarean section for another medical or obstetric indication should refrain from using moxibustion as it may complicate the condition. Indeed, any major medical or obstetric complication is a contraindication to using moxibustion. Confirmed or suspected cephalopelvic disproportion may mean vaginal birth may not be feasible, and it would therefore be inappropriate to subject the fetus to the stress of moxibustion for no reason. It should not be performed by or for women with poorly controlled diabetes or if there is a risk of a large baby, although non-insulin-controlled diabetes mellitus is not, in itself, a reason to avoid moxibustion. Current vaginal bleeding, major placental abruption, known placenta praevia or low-lying placenta are logical contraindications in a compromised pregnancy. Pyrexia, with or without infection, is also a reason to decline, as moxa heat may increase the body temperature, although this is disputed by Dharmananda (2004).

If there has been threatened preterm labour in this or a previous pregnancy it may be wise to delay the use of moxibustion until at least 36 weeks gestation to avoid any risk of preterm contractions or membrane rupture (Djakovic et al. 2015), although this may reduce the chances of successful version. In the event of an unstable lie, it is highly likely that any conversion will revert to a breech presentation if moxibustion is performed too early, so delaying the procedure until almost term may prevent this. Moxa heat may exacerbate existing fetal distress and, in the case of intrauterine growth retardation or reduced fetal movements, may stress the fetus unnecessarily. Moxibustion is contraindicated in multiple pregnancy to avoid the risk of fetal or cord entanglement. In the case of abnormal liquor volume, moxibustion would be a precaution if polyhydramnios is present, although the fetal lie may be changeable in any case. The procedure is contraindicated with oligohydramnios as it may cause additional problems, particularly if the reduction in amniotic fluid is due to fetal abnormalities. In the event of intrauterine death, moxibustion is inappropriate as the loss of muscle tone will probably cause the fetus to revert and it is not known how moxibustion may affect clotting factors, which can be compromised after fetal death. See Table 6.1 for a summary of the contraindications to moxibustion.

Table 6.1 Contraindications to moxibustion for breech presentation

Obstetric contraindications	Fetal contraindications	Medical contraindications
Previous Caesarean section or uterine scar	Suspected or known cephalo-pelvic disproportion	Elective Caesarean booked for obstetric or medical indication
Antepartum haemorrhage	Fetal distress	Hypertension/pre-eclampsia
		History of fulminating pre-eclampsia/eclampsia in previous pregnancy
Multiple pregnancy	Intrauterine growth retardation	Asthma, hay fever or pre-existing respiratory disease
Preterm labour – current or previous pregnancy	Unstable lie	Diabetic mother
Preterm rupture of membranes	Intrauterine fetal death	Pyrexia or known infection
Abnormal liquor volume		

The moxibustion treatment

It is vital to ensure that the moxibustion sticks used to treat women with breech presentation are labelled as *mild* moxa sticks, as there are several types, some of which would be inappropriate for expectant mothers because they contain other substances in addition to the mugwort. Two types of mild moxa are available. The original sticks are made from dried *Artemisia* which is compressed, rolled and wrapped in paper. When using these sticks it is necessary to remove about a centimetre of the paper around the top of the sticks before each treatment, to enable them to burn down (but removing too much paper can result in the sticks continuing to burn, therefore wasting the moxa). The other type of moxa stick is made from charcoal impregnated with moxa and it is claimed that these are smokeless and will not trigger institutional fire alarms. Certainly the paper-wrapped original sticks produce a considerable amount of smoke (with a grassy aroma similar to cannabis), although they are easier to light and to extinguish and appear to be more successful in turning the breech to cephalic (personal clinical experience). Some acupuncturists agree with this and suggest that there is little evidence to indicate that smokeless moxa is more effective. Although there are no obstetric studies, a clinical trial to compare conventional and smokeless moxa for the treatment of patients with knee osteoarthritis is currently in progress (Zhu *et al.* 2017).

Certain precautions should be taken when moxa sticks are used. Women should be made aware of the risk of fire, keeping clothing and other flammable items clear of the sticks when lit. It is preferable that the woman is assisted by her partner or a friend or family member so that the risk of burning if the moxa sticks come into contact with the skin is minimised. Smoke alarms may be very sensitive to the smoke emitted from the moxa sticks (which can be considerable) and it may be best for the treatment to be carried out near an open window or door, or even outside, weather permitting. Moxibustion treatment is not directly pharmacological, but the moxa itself, from the *Artemisia* leaf, contains over 600 chemical constituents including 1,8-Cineole, camphor, borneol and other chemicals, as well as tannins, flavonoids, sterols, polysaccharides, trace elements and other ingredients (Kobayashi 1988). A Korean study of moxa safety concluded that concentrations of carbon oxides, nitrogen oxides and various other volatile organic compounds emitted during the burning of moxa remain within safe limits and concluded that almost 2.5 grams of moxa would need to be burned in order to become potentially risky (Kwon *et al.* 2017).

According to Chinese medicine, the optimum gestation to perform moxibustion is between 33 and 35 weeks but the treatment can be done at any time up to term. This author has even seen it to be successful in a woman at 40 weeks gestation awaiting Caesarean section for breech presentation, who then progressed to a normal vaginal cephalic birth. However, acupuncture (needling of the Bladder 67 points) tends to be more successful from about 38 weeks gestation (Betts 2006). For midwives introducing moxibustion into NHS care of women with breech presentation, protocols may dictate that treatment is delayed until 36 or 37 weeks; in practice, it would be ideal to commence a course of treatment at about 36 weeks gestation, which is completed immediately prior to a scheduled ECV. If the treatment is unsuccessful, the woman can then be encouraged to have the ECV and it is possible that the moxibustion may improve the chances of success of the medical procedure.

Once a breech presentation has been confirmed, preferably by ultrasound scan, the woman and her partner can be taught how to perform the procedure by a midwife, empowering them to carry out the treatment at home. This avoids the risk of setting off institutional fire alarms caused by the smoke if treatment is performed in the maternity unit or a clinic and minimises the risk of air pollution from successive women being treated in the same place (Lu *et al.* 2016). Facilitating the couple to use the technique at home also avoids the need for them to travel to the clinic frequently, as the treatment is performed for about 30 minutes, twice daily, for five to seven days (10 to 14 treatments).

NB Midwives and doulas working in private practice in the UK will be unable to obtain professional indemnity insurance to perform moxibustion unless they are fully qualified acupuncturists. Insurance cover for antenatal education will suffice if the couple is taught how to perform the procedure for themselves. The practitioner should not physically light the sticks and perform the treatment but can observe the partner carrying it out to ensure that it is done correctly.

In preparation for the treatment, the mother should empty her bladder, loosen her clothing and be seated comfortably in a semi-reclining position, allowing space within the abdominal cavity for the fetus to move. It is for this reason that it is not practical for the woman to treat herself, since bending down to access her feet would compress the abdominal cavity. The sticks of moxa are lit with a match or lighter, ensuring that the round end of the stick is completely alight. The flame is then extinguished and the stick continues to glow and emit smoke (although there is less smoke with the moxa-impregnated charcoal sticks). It is best for the partner, or whoever is carrying out the treatment, to position the moxa stick about one centimetre away from the skin at the relevant point: the mother should feel the warmth of the moxa without it being uncomfortably hot. The glowing stick is alternated between the two points, changing to the opposite foot after about 30 seconds and then back again until the full 30-minute treatment has been completed. The fetus can become quite active during the treatment and for some hours afterwards, and the woman should be informed of this so that she does not worry about the change in the pattern of fetal movements. The fetus tends to become more active as the course of treatment continues, and conversion to cephalic presentation most commonly occurs after five or six treatments (personal clinical experience). Conversely, there is some suggestion that the fetal heart rate may reduce during moxibustion (Neri *et al.* 2004).

On completion of each treatment, the moxa sticks should be extinguished fully by tapping the end inside a glass jar or on the surface of a kitchen sink, although it is important to avoid getting the stick damp as the wet portion cannot be used for subsequent treatments, particularly with the paper-wrapped type. Some moxa sticks can re-ignite if incompletely extinguished, so they should be left in a safe place in case this occurs (such as in the glass jar). If the fetus is thought to have turned within a few sessions, the full course of ten treatments must still be completed, because continuing application of heat to the Bladder 67 acupoint will encourage further descent and may aid engagement of the fetal head (Dharmananda 2004). However, if no conversion has occurred, moxibustion can be continued for another two days (14 treatments in total).

Success of moxibustion

Early studies in China showed rates of successful conversion of a breech to cephalic presentation of between 80.9 per cent and 90.3 per cent (Cooperative Research Group of Moxibustion Version of Jangxi Province 1984), although these were essentially audits of practice rather than randomised controlled trials. Later, Cardini *et al.* (1991) showed a 66.6 per cent rate between 30 and 38 weeks gestation, with 34 weeks being considered the optimum time to perform moxibustion (Cardini and Marcolongo 1993; Cardini and Weixin 1998). Kanakura *et al.* (2001) achieved cephalic version in 92 per cent of women treated with moxibustion, but the inclusion of women between 28 and 33 weeks gestation caused a significant number of reversions, as could be expected.

The 1998 study by Cardini and Weixin was possibly the first randomised controlled trial to come to the notice of western authorities and demonstrated increased fetal activity and reduced incidence of breech presentation at term, with better outcomes at delivery, when compared to a control group. This initial study was carried out in China, whereas a later study (Cardini *et al.* 2005) was undertaken in Italy. The results of the 2005 trial were less statistically significant, but the researchers attribute this to problems with cultural compliance, given that moxibustion was unfamiliar to women in Italy, compared to those in China for whom traditional medicine sits alongside conventional strategies. They also concluded that there were issues in educating the Italian women to use the moxa sticks, particularly as some women were deemed to be less well educated than others. The study was interrupted and its underpowered calculations did not enable the researchers to draw any conclusions as to the effectiveness of moxibustion for breech presentation. Two occurrences of early membrane rupture leading to preterm birth were not thought to be directly due to the moxibustion, but it was suggested that further studies should investigate the impact on pregnancy progress and fetal wellbeing.

It is difficult to conduct blinded trials on moxibustion, although some researchers now use "sham" moxa devices (Zhao *et al.* 2014), but these are not without some methodological difficulties. Other studies combine moxibustion with acupuncture. Neri *et al.* (2004) undertook a randomised controlled trial in Italy on women between 33 and 35 weeks gestation using moxibusion at the Zhiyin point with acupuncture at other selected points. This study achieved a 53.5 per cent conversion to cephalic presentation by term in the trial group, compared to 37.7 per cent in the control group, without any significant complications of the treatment. In a later study (Neri *et al.* 2007) a comparison of moxibustion versus acupuncture versus moxibustion with acupuncture was undertaken. There was an 80 per cent overall success rate, 28 per cent with acupuncture and 57 per cent with moxibustion combined with acupuncture. However, this was a small study and the authors concluded that further research with larger sample sizes is warranted. Do *et al.* (2011) suggest that the optimum sample size for future studies is 381 women.

A prospective study by two UK midwives (Manyande and Grabowska 2009) found that moxibustion performed prior to ECV increased the likelihood of successful version leading to vaginal birth. There was a 40.8 per cent success rate after moxibustion and, of the remaining women who then underwent ECV, 43.3 per cent also achieved a cephalic presentation. The intervention was more successful in multiparous women, a feature common to several other studies.

Vas *et al.* (2009) conducted a systematic review and meta-analysis of trials to date and found that moxibustion appeared to be at least as safe as standard care and offered a positive experience for women, either alone or in combination with other approaches. Vas *et al.* (2013) later undertook a study in which moxibustion at the Bladder 67 acupoint was compared with moxibustion at a "non-specific" acupoint (Spleen 1) and a control group which received standard care only. Moxibustion was shown to be 58.1 per cent successful in turning the breech to cephalic, whereas "non-specific" moxa was 43.4 per cent, and standard care, 44.8 per cent.

Van den Berg *et al.* (2008) also carried out a systematic review of studies investigating the effectiveness of "acupuncture-type" interventions versus expectant management which found them to be largely effective, although some women were seen to have withdrawn from some studies due to adverse respiratory effects from the moxa smoke. However, further work by van den Berg *et al.* (2010) found that moxibustion was a cost-effective option, with a mean saving of 450 euros per woman compared to expectant management.

Li *et al.* (2009) reviewed ten randomised controlled trials and seven clinical trials and concluded that moxibustion, acupuncture and laser acupoint stimulation of the Bladder 67 acupoint were effective in converting a breech presentation to cephalic but, like others, commented on the number of studies, the low participant numbers and the variability of treatments offered. Do *et al.* (2011) reported similar findings, although they describe their sample size as underpowered. More recently, a Danish trial (Bue and Lauszus 2016) found no significant effects of moxibustion treatment to correct breech presentation. Other European studies have also shown no demonstrable effects (Coulon *et al.* 2014). Personal experience of this author, and communication with other practitioners of moxibustion, indicates that the technique is less successful when the fetus presents with extended legs, although most of the studies do not reflect on this aspect.

Adverse effects

The incidence of complications from moxibustion appears to be less than that for ECV, although this may represent a difference in reporting practices, together with a greater use of cephalic version within conventional western obstetrics. In addition, many women seeking moxibustion now purchase their own moxa sticks to undertake treatment at home, sometimes without informing their midwife or doctor. Others consult independent acupuncturists, who may not report any adverse effects to a centralised information-gathering service. Ewies and Olah's review (2002) suggests that moxa is a safe, painless, inexpensive and easily administered option, but again highlight the small sample sizes of most studies, with lack of randomisation.

There have been some reports of minor adverse reactions, such as burns (Bensoussan, Myers and Carlton 2000), although these generally refer to moxibustion used to treat non-obstetric medical conditions. Also, although there is no direct contact with the moxa in the sticks, allergic reactions and dermal irritation have been recorded with some moxibustion treatments for other clinical indications (Park *et al.* 2010), so it is wise to avoid dropping loose moxa from the paper-wrapped sticks on to the skin. Park *et al.* (2010) also cite other papers in which adverse reactions such as itching, blistering, headache, fatigue and gastric upset have been reported. Coughing and adverse respiratory effects, as well as nausea and vomiting, may also occur (Xu, Deng and Shen 2014), although the emission of toxic metabolites from moxibustion smoke has been demonstrated to be within safe limits (Kwon *et al.* 2017).

In obstetric terms, no adverse fetal effects or abnormal uterine action during or after treatment were found by Neri *et al.* (2002), although Xu *et al.* (2014) suggest that fetal distress and preterm birth are possible consequences of moxibustion. In Do *et al.*'s small study (2011) two babies were admitted to the neonatal intensive care unit, although it is not clear if this was related to the effects of moxibustion. Engel *et al.* (1992) reported on a single case of a primigravida at term in whom feto-maternal blood transfusion was revealed during an emergency Caesarean section for fetal distress following moxibustion. However, unlike the potential for ECV to force an unwilling fetus to turn to cephalic presentation, moxibustion will only stimulate fetal activity, which may have increased spontaneously, and it is difficult to attribute the above case solely to the use of moxibustion.

Guittier *et al.* (2008) carried out a randomised controlled trial in which cardiotocography was used to monitor wellbeing, with no side effects or significant adverse effects demonstrated in either maternal or fetal health. Moxibustion was generally found to be acceptable to the women, making compliance good. However, a later study (Guittier *et al.* 2009) showed no statistically significant effect of moxibustion to turn breech presentation to cephalic (18% success rate, compared to 16% spontaneous version in the control group). Lee *et al.* (2011) investigated moxibustion for various medical conditions, including breech presentation, and found inconclusive evidence for the safety (or otherwise) of moxibustion. Xu *et al.* (2014) argue that other factors, such as the position and wellbeing of the woman, the distance between the moxa stick and the skin, the duration of treatment, proficiency of the practitioner performing the treatment and the effects of the smoke, may all affect the perceived safety (and effectiveness) of moxibustion. It is, however, considered to be cost effective and may reduce the costs of cephalic version, Caesarean section and other aspects of care such as longer inpatient stays and admissions to the neonatal unit (García-Mochón *et al.* 2015).

Whilst some studies on the use of acupuncture for breech presentation have combined needling with moxibustion, it is also possible to use acupuncture as a modality in its own right. The principles of rebalancing deficient qi in the Kidney and Bladder meridians via the Bladder 67 acupoint are the same as when moxibustion is used, but acupuncturists assess women more holistically and may include additional acupoints. Some studies focus on the Bladder 67 point but use moxa at the end of a needle ("fire needling") for greater effectiveness. In France, Sananes *et al.* (2016) conducted a randomised, single-blinded, sham-controlled study of 259 women who were allocated to receive either acupuncture with moxa needling or a sham control treatment. Cephalic version occurred in 37.7 per cent of the trial group and 28.7 per cent of the control, which was deemed not to be a statistically significant difference.

Midwives who do not themselves engage in assessing and teaching expectant parents how to perform moxibustion may wish to refer women to an acupuncturist. Treatment may be successful, although it can be expensive as acupuncturists in the UK generally perform the full course of treatment themselves rather than teaching the couple how to do this at home. In Australia and New Zealand, where moxibustion is a common strategy for women with breech presentation, 90 per cent of acupuncturists approve of women self-administering the moxa and agree that smokeless, odourless moxa sticks should be used (Smith and Betts 2014). Some acupuncturists apply auricular acupuncture needles, using tiny needles on plasters taped into the ears at the relevant points so that the woman can apply finger pressure at regular intervals. This is relatively common in practice, although only one research study could be found on the use of auricular acupuncture, with an 83 per cent success rate, but this study was old and does not appear to have been replicated (Qin and Tang 1989).

It is, however, fair to conclude that moxibustion and/or acupuncture may have a part to play in the management of breech presentation and in offering an alternative option for women but, as always, there is a need for larger, more robust studies on both effectiveness and safety.

Other alternative options for women with breech presentation

Postural techniques and musculoskeletal realignment

Optimal fetal positioning, including commercially available antenatal classes teaching specific movement and posture, may assist in encouraging a cephalic presentation with an occipito-anterior position. Yoga has become very popular with many pregnant women in recent years and certain postures are thought to encourage a cephalic presentation and descent of the fetal head into the pelvis (Oakley and Evans 2014). The relaxation effects of yoga and the proven reduction in cortisol and other stress hormones (Chen *et al.* 2017; Kusaka *et al.* 2016) may assist in reducing tense muscles, having an indirect effect on the fetal presentation and also helping the woman to cope with the situation. The rebozo technique and specialist antenatal classes focusing on movement to encourage optimal fetal positioning may also be of help (Cohen and Thomas 2015).

Unfortunately, systematic reviews suggest that there is insufficient evidence to support the inclusion of these strategies in conventional maternity care (Hofmeyr and Kulier 2012). On the other hand, it has been argued that a more sedentary lifestyle, with frequent sitting, together with a more mechanised approach to many aspects of daily life, has contributed to a greater incidence of malpresentation and malposition than occurred perhaps 50 years ago. Women no longer need to exert as much energy or adopt positions that traditionally helped fetal positioning (for example, cleaning the kitchen floor on hands and knees) and many spend much of their daily lives sitting in ergonomically inappropriate positions, such as at computers or driving. Given that these strategies are non-medical, the paucity of evidence to support optimal fetal positioning may be due more to lack of interest by researchers looking for paternalistic medical options to offer women than to any real evidence that the techniques do not work.

Realignment of the musculoskeletal system with osteopathy or chiropractic has been advocated and may be useful for women with a history of musculoskeletal trauma, disease or genetic conditions. Problems such as previous pelvic or leg fractures, sacrococcygeal injury or spinal disc protrusions may impact on the pelvic girdle. In pregnancy the effects of progesterone and relaxin on the pelvic joints and ligaments accentuate the problems, further detracting from optimal descent of the fetal head. These issues potentially cause an exaggerated angle of inclination of the pelvic brim into which the fetal head cannot pass, or a tilting of the pelvis to one side, with one leg shorter than the other, adversely affecting the diameters throughout the brim, cavity and outlet of the pelvis.

Roecker (2013) reported the unsuccessful case of a primigravida with breech presentation for whom the chiropractic Webster technique was used (sacral manipulation and abdominal effleurage). Treatment was performed over a period of three weeks, with little effect. Conversely, a survey of

US chiropractors (Pistolese 2002) revealed that of 112 questionnaires returned 82 per cent of practitioners had success with the Webster technique, particularly when undertaken at around 36 weeks gestation when external cephalic version has been unsuccessful.

Edwards and Alcantara (2014) describe the case of a multiparous woman with breech presentation and placenta praevia who received a course of chiropractic treatment which successfully corrected the fetal presentation to cephalic. Of interest in this case is the fact that the treatment appeared to minimise the issues pertaining to the placenta praevia by realigning the musculoskeletal structure with trigger point release movements, chiropractic adjustments and a series of exercises which the woman was encouraged to practise. The authors argue that these techniques facilitated an improvement in the structural and neurological environment so that the placenta appeared to "migrate" to a more favourable location following correction of a pelvic tilt causing round ligament tension. Obviously the placental insertion in the decidua did not physically move, but post-treatment ultrasound examination indicated that the placenta was no longer in a compromised position in relation to the cervical os.

Hypnotherapy

Deep relaxation with hypnotherapy may reduce maternal stress levels, helping the woman's coping abilities and potentially easing muscular tension that may have a bearing on fetal presentation and position. It may also improve the success rates of ECV. A study by Mehl (1994) compared 100 women with breech presentation at term with a matched control group. The hypnosis suggestions focused on general relaxation, reduction in fear and anxiety and visualisation on the reasons why the fetus was presenting by the breech. Women in the intervention group demonstrated an 81 per cent cephalic version rate following hypnosis, compared with just 48 per cent in the control group. The researcher postulated that psychological and physiological factors can impact on fetal presentation, offering a possible explanation for the success of hypnotherapy.

More recently, Reinhard, Peiffer et al. (2012) conducted a prospective randomised controlled study to compare clinical hypnosis with neurolinguistic programming prior to external cephalic version at term. Similar success rates for external cephalic version were found in the two trial groups (40.5% and 44.7% respectively) compared to a control group (27.3%). It is important here to differentiate clinical hypnosis and other complementary psychological interventions from the popular "hypnobirthing" for birth preparation, although it stands to reason that simple relaxation strategies may also assist in cephalic version.

Reflexology

Many women, midwives and even reflexologists erroneously believe that reflexology will convert a breech to cephalic presentation. This is probably due to confusion over the fact that both reflexology and stimulation of the Bladder 67 acupuncture point are performed on the feet (personal communications with midwives and reflexologists). However, whilst it is possible to apply manual thumb pressure to the Bladder 67 acupoint, this is not reflexology, which is based on the theory that each part of the two feet corresponds to a specific organ or area of the body. There is no reflexology zone on the feet that relates specifically to the fetus, even though an experienced midwife-reflexologist may be able to identify from the feet the position or presentation of the fetus within the uterus. However, it would be highly dangerous to perform a technique on the part of the feet corresponding to the reflex zone for the uterus in the misguided belief that this could turn the fetus, similarly to ECV. This is more likely to cause placental separation than to turn the fetus and should be avoided completely.

Some practitioners may legitimately undertake foot-applied acupressure to the Bladder 67 acupoint but must, in professional and academic terms, differentiate this from "reflexology" even though they may explain it as part of a foot-based reflexology treatment to the woman. The relaxation component of a reflexology treatment may, in any case, be sufficient to help. On the other hand, it is of grave concern that some therapists presume to over-step their boundaries without adequate knowledge of what they are doing. Midwives referring women with breech presentation for complementary treatments should advise that women try to find therapists who are experienced in maternity therapy, who do not guarantee to turn the breech to cephalic and who appreciate the difference between reflexology and acupressure.

Conclusion

Moxibustion is the most commonly used complementary strategy for the treatment of breech presentation. It could easily be taught to midwives in order that they can advise women and teach them how to use the procedure safely. Incorporating moxibustion into a standard NHS clinic for women with breech presentation may contribute to reducing the need for ECV and Caesarean section, thus increasing the normal birth rate and avoiding the risks of the long-term sequelae of operative delivery and offering a safe, relatively effective and cost-effective option for women.

There remains, however, limited evidence for effectiveness and safety on other complementary options, particularly for osteopathy and chiropractic, hypnotherapy and reflexology. This does not mean that they are without some merit, and anecdotal evidence suggests that they can be very effective strategies, not least by relaxing the woman and empowering her to make her own decisions about the "waiting time" which may indirectly lead to spontaneous version to cephalic presentation.

CHAPTER 7

Complementary Therapies for Post-Dates Pregnancy

Many women are anxious to avoid medical induction of labour simply because they are "overdue" but feel pressurised by defensive obstetric practices influenced by a professional desire to prevent late intrauterine deaths and to avoid litigation. There is considerable social pressure on women to give birth as close to their estimated due date as possible, and many women become so desperate to expedite labour that they try every strategy they know to trigger uterine contractions. Unfortunately, these attempts to initiate labour, sometimes even before term, coupled with women's lack of understanding that any intervention may cause a "cascade of intervention", can lead to adverse effects on the mother, fetus or the physiological progress of labour. Conversely, there is an increasing interest amongst midwives to assist women in avoiding medical induction of labour and many are now investigating the use of complementary therapies for "natural induction".

This chapter explores the vast range of self-help and natural means of triggering contractions, focusing on the evidence for effectiveness and safety. It also debates the growing trend for midwives to establish post-dates pregnancy clinics using various complementary therapies.

This chapter includes:

- introduction

- women's desire to self-initiate labour

- self-help methods to aid cervical ripening and dilatation

- self-administration of pharmacologically active plant remedies

- consumption of fruit to aid labour onset

- homeopathic remedies

- acupuncture and acupressure

- professional use of complementary therapies and natural remedies for women with post-dates pregnancy

- conclusion.

Introduction

There is considerable debate on precisely what constitutes "post-dates" pregnancy and on the justification for the various medical options for initiating labour in women whose pregnancies progress beyond the estimated date of delivery (EDD). The accuracy of the EDD calculation is highly debatable, with only 5 per cent of births occurring on the given estimated date (Khambalia *et al.* 2013), but it is not the purpose of this chapter to analyse current debate on how "term pregnancy" is determined. Suffice it to say that professionals advise women that they will normally give birth by 42 weeks gestation but suggest that induction of labour is offered between 41 and 42 weeks gestation to "avoid the risk of prolonged pregnancy" (NICE 2008: CG70). In practice, however, this is often discouraged by professionals whose advice may be biased, although this may be unintentional. Women who are pressurised are often subjected to a degree of "emotional blackmail" about the dangers of continuing pregnancy beyond 41 weeks gestation, and have been shown to be significantly more likely to have labour induced, sometimes even without clear clinical indications (Jou *et al.* 2015).

Induction of labour is one of the most widely used obstetric interventions, the most common indication being for post-dates pregnancy (Humphrey and Tucker 2009), although the reasons given can be somewhat spurious. In 2014–2015, the labour induction rate in England was 26.8 per cent, with an increasing upwards trend since then (NHS Digital 2015). It is suggested that the risk of adverse fetal outcomes increases significantly after 42 weeks gestation, leading to the recommendation that all women between 41 and 42 weeks gestation should be offered induction to reduce perinatal mortality and morbidity (NICE 2008). Induction of labour may be by membrane sweep alone or in combination with other methods, such as intravaginal misoprostol or dinoprostone (Propess™), artificial membrane rupture and/or intravenous oxytocin. Propess™ has become increasingly popular, with some maternity units even offering this as an out-patient service for 24 hours.

However, induction by any method poses risks to the woman, her baby and the progress of the labour (Smith, Crowther and Grant 2013). Artificially forcing the woman's body to start labour may adversely affect her perception of pain, leading to an increased need for epidural anaesthesia, with a consequent risk of requiring instrumental or operative delivery, although Wood, Cooper and Ross (2014) concluded that induction may actually *reduce* the need for Caesarean section. Irrespective of the mode of birth consequent to induction, the procedure is costly to the maternity services in terms of time, hospital bed use and possible iatrogenic complications requiring further medical care (the so-called "cascade of intervention"). It also has a negative effect on women's satisfaction with their birth experiences and may cause psychological issues in subsequent pregnancies (Gammie and Key 2014; Gatward *et al.* 2010; Jay 2015; Murtagh and Folan 2014).

Empowerment of women in the decision-making process is important and may even contribute to the success of any method used to start labour artificially, either medically or naturally. Women should not be directed towards a particular method, but should be given adequate comprehensive information to enable them to make informed choices about their care (NHS England 2016). This should include the option *not* to have labour induced, the pros and cons of continuing pregnancy beyond a certain gestation and a full, evidence-based discussion on the benefits and risks of medical methods of induction.

Women's desire to self-initiate labour

Hall, McKenna and Griffiths (2012) undertook a systematic review on the commonly used natural methods for induction of labour and found, unsurprisingly, that these are mostly recommended on the basis of traditional knowledge but that they lack scientific evidence to support their incorporation into maternity care. Whilst there appeared to be some evidence to support the use of breast stimulation or acupuncture, very few other methods were shown to be valid or safe, including raspberry leaf, castor oil, evening primrose oil and blue cohosh.

In the UK, NICE does not advocate the use of natural means of inducing labour, such as herbal supplements, acupuncture, homeopathy, castor oil, hot baths, enemas and sexual intercourse, as there is insufficient evidence of effectiveness and safety (NICE 2008: 1.4.2). On the other hand, women's satisfaction and audits of the results of "natural induction" services set up by midwives are very positive (Pauley and Percival 2014; Weston and Grabowska 2013).

There is, however, a difference between professionals advocating these methods once trained to use them safely and the fact that many women will try natural ways to initiate labour if they wish to avoid medical induction. It is vital to remember that *any* means of inducing labour is an intervention in the normal physiological process of the onset of birth. Indeed, the concept of "natural induction" is somewhat of an oxymoron, since the process of induction is, by definition, unnatural. The woman's body is designed to start the process of expulsion of the fetus at a time when maternal and fetal factors dictate. Whilst much is written about the potential risks of artificial oxytocin, membrane rupture or prostaglandins, many women – and professionals – fail to appreciate the dangers of inappropriate, uncontrolled use of natural methods to stimulate contractions. Women are often so keen to initiate labour in order to end the discomforts of pregnancy, particularly when there is social and medical pressure to give birth close to the time of the EDD, that they will try anything. Of even more concern is the fact that they also frequently combine several methods, which can be extremely dangerous, most especially when commenced before term.

This desperate desire to start labour seems to be an almost universal practice across the world. In South Africa, for example, Zulu women drink a herbal concoction called *Isihlambezo*, thought to contain as many as 55 different plant extracts, many of which have strong uterotonic effects (Brookes 2004). Concomitant undeclared self-administration of *Isihlambezo* with misoprostol has been shown to cause uterine hypertonia, meconium-stained liquor and fetal distress (Essilfie-Appiah and Hofmeyr 2005), a feature which can be seen with other multiple-method self-administered attempts to start labour. Plants combined with crushed ostrich eggshell have also been used (van der Kooi and Theobald 2006). Elsewhere in Africa, up to 75 Ugandan plants used by pregnant women have been identified as being uterotonic, but many are also potentially toxic (Kamatenesi-Mugisha and Oryem-Origa 2007). The use of a porridge combined with herbal oxytocic-like plants, together with other methods to expedite labour, is considered to be a major cause of maternal mortality in Malawi (Maliwichi-Nyirenda and Maliwichi 2010). Natural, reputedly uterotonic, medicines are also used in many parts of Asia and South America (Michel, Caceres and Mahady 2016). (See also de Boer and Lamxay 2009; Martinez 2008; Ososki *et al.* 2002; Ticktin and Dalle 2005; Wang, Nankorn and Fukui 2003.)

Whilst indigenous plants may be the only accessible alternative to biomedicine in many remote areas of some countries, urbanisation, emigration and the Internet have increased the western public's access to traditional medicines. In addition, in western maternity units with a high proportion of mothers from ethnic minority groups, midwives frequently care for women using traditional medicines to aid labour onset and progress, although often the women do not inform their midwives, and occasionally refuse to impart information about remedies being used (personal communications with midwives and mothers).

A case is known to this author in which an expectant mother, recently arrived from the Asian sub-continent, continually sipped at a glass of water, on the surface of which was floating a flower, which was eventually discovered to be hibiscus, a plant known to cause smooth muscle contraction (Da Costa Rocha *et al.* 2014; Kuriyan, Kumar and Kurpad 2010). The woman and her own mother declined to reveal the identity or purpose of the drink, but every time the woman took a sip, significant fetal heart decelerations occurred and the contractions increased in intensity. She continued to drink the water despite the midwife's advice against it, and eventually she required an emergency Caesarean section for severe fetal distress and meconium-stained liquor. Whilst the pathology cannot definitely be attributed solely to the herbal mixture, it is highly likely that it contributed to the situation. Other similar situations have also been disclosed.

Adverse effects of natural remedies are often precipitated by combining them with prescribed pharmaceuticals, uterotonic infusions or pessaries, or with other herbs with similar pharmacological properties, by taking excessively high or prolonged doses, or by administration at an inappropriate gestation. Professionals should advise women to refrain from combining methods, particularly if they are at home with intravaginal Propess™ *in situ* or, in hospital, once the induction process has commenced. Combining natural remedies with other manual strategies to induce contractions can also be problematic, but it is the pharmacologically active herbal remedies which cause most concern because women fail to appreciate that they act like drugs and can interact with or potentiate medical means of induction.

A search of various Internet sites revealed over 70 suggestions for self-inducing labour, including many that were not based on any real physiological foundation and some that were extremely dangerous. One suggestion, found on several American websites, was that women should fast to the point of dehydration. This was explained as the increased production of anti-diuretic hormone from the posterior pituitary gland stimulating oxytocin production and may be based on an old German paper (Suranyi and Nagy 1957) in which dehydration was considered "harmless" as a means of induction. Several more recent papers, particularly from Muslim countries, have examined the impact of dehydration and fasting during Ramadan on the incidence of preterm labour, possibly suggesting a link between low food and water consumption on uterine activity. It would, however, seem unethical and contrary to good practice to advocate an unproven method of self-induction which could have serious consequences for mother or baby, particularly as it is known that dehydration during labour impairs uterine activity.

Unfortunately, access to this online information – and mis-information – means that westerners often make leaps of assumption about the effectiveness of particular remedies and their application to pregnancy and childbirth. There is a misconception that natural remedies known to be abortifacient (capable of causing miscarriage) will help to induce labour, or that those considered emmenagoguic (capable of causing bleeding per vaginam) are also uterotonic. However, the physio-pathology of uterine action during miscarriage or late-pregnancy placental bleeding is very different from that of physiologically normal uterine action during term labour in which myometrial contraction and retraction influences the polarity between the upper and lower uterine segments. Similarly, the endocrine factors that trigger miscarriage or third trimester antepartum haemorrhage are noticeably different from the hormonal changes occurring at the onset of term labour (Gruber and O'Brien 2011). It must also be recognised that natural remedies or complementary strategies which act systemically may not only cause contraction of uterine muscle but of all areas of the body that contain smooth muscle, including the circulatory and gastrointestinal systems, indicating that caution is needed in women with specific medical conditions such as hypertension, vascular impairment or irritable bowel syndrome.

It is the injudicious use of self-help methods of starting labour which are so disquieting, especially when women commonly do not inform their midwives or doctors. Professionals should make a point of discussing with women the various techniques or remedies they intend to use to prepare for, initiate or aid progress in labour. Midwives and doulas must be able to advise on complementary therapies and natural remedies which women choose to self-administer, treatments for which they may consult a complementary practitioner, or strategies which may be offered by midwives in some maternity units. Only *one* method should be used at any one time, unless a combination is used under appropriate professional supervision. Patient information leaflets on induction of labour should stress that it may be inappropriate to consume herbal teas, use aromatherapy oils or apply other natural remedies in conjunction with medical methods of inducing labour.

Midwives and doulas who are not adequately trained to advise on self-help methods should refrain from doing so. Indeed, the safety issues arising from women injudiciously using self-help and natural methods indicate an urgent need for this subject to be included in midwifery and doula education in order that they can respond with correct, comprehensive and, where possible, evidence-based information (Tiran 2011). This author is aware of many situations in which incorrect or incomplete information is offered in an attempt to act as the mother's advocate, but which risks complications occurring from injudicious use. (See also Chapter 3 on professional issues.)

Conversely, since many women will seek treatment from independent complementary practitioners, often urging them to start labour, therapists should also have up-to-date knowledge and understanding of contemporary methods of medical induction, as well as the indications, contraindications and precautions related to the use of their own therapies as strategies for natural induction. Furthermore, we need to emphasise to women that babies are born when they are "ready" and that any attempt to expedite the normal physiological process can lead to problems.

Self-help methods to aid cervical ripening and dilatation

Sexual activity

The reasoning behind engaging in sexual activity towards term is that nipple stimulation and orgasm decrease cortisol and increase posterior pituitary gland oxytocin production. Penetrative sex causes a local release of prostaglandins from around the cervical opening and initiates natural contractions of the uterus, particularly during orgasm, whilst semen is a rich source of prostaglandins in its own right (Jones, Chan and Farine 2011). Nipple stimulation has also long been advocated to increase oxytocin levels and may encourage cervical ripening (Singh *et al.* 2014) and reduce the incidence of medical induction and other interventions (Demirel and Guler 2015; Mozurkewich *et al.* 2011), although it should be done with care and probably avoided before term if there is a history of preterm labour.

Although most authorities believe that no harm will occur in women with low-risk pregnancies who engage in sexual activity towards term, it is generally considered that there is no real evidence to support its use as a formal means of inducing labour (Kavanagh, Kelly and Thomas 2001). Sex does not appear to have any direct effect on the Bishop score, the onset of labour, incidence of Caesarean section or neonatal outcomes (Jones *et al.* 2011). Conversely, Tan *et al.* (2006) found a correlation between sexual activity at term and a reduction in pregnancy continuing beyond 41 weeks gestation, with a reduced need for induction of labour. However, Omar *et al.* (2013) found no evidence that advising women to engage in coitus at term facilitated labour onset or reduced the need for induction.

Balloon catheter

The insertion of an extra-amniotic balloon catheter into the cervix is standard obstetric practice in some countries, and the procedure is growing in popularity in some maternity units in the UK to the extent that NICE (2008) considers there is enough evidence to support its use in obstetrics (Amorosa and Stone 2015; Lim, Ng and Xu 2013). Mozurkewich *et al.*'s systematic review (2011) found that balloon catheters were less likely to cause uterine hyper-stimulation but may be associated with maternal or neonatal infection. There is evidence to demonstrate that it can be an effective means of cervical ripening and may encourage more rapid cervical dilatation in early labour than misoprostol, although establishment of active labour is somewhat slower (Tuuli *et al.* 2013). Some authorities use single balloon catheters; others use double balloons (Pennell *et al.* 2009; Salim *et al.* 2011). However, it is the injudicious, unsupervised self-use of balloon catheters by women at home that gives rise to concern. Balloon catheters can be purchased via the Internet and are advocated on several maternity consumer websites. Possible risks include infection, vaginal bleeding and pain, and the use of balloon catheters may be inappropriate for some women.

Laminaria

Similarly, *Laminaria* (kelp), a type of seaweed native to Japan, has traditionally been used topically to aid cervical ripening, particularly in primigravidae, and to facilitate labour, either alone or in conjunction with prostaglandins. It remains popular in the Americas but is less so in the UK. It was also used professionally in the 1970s and 1980s prior to procedures such as dilatation and curettage, termination of pregnancy, removal of intrauterine devices and to facilitate uterine placement of therapeutic radium, although it is no longer recommended as a medical strategy (Lin *et al.* 2006).

The seaweed is hygroscopic, in that it has the ability to form a viscous colloidal solution of gel in water, which is effective as a bulk laxative. This suggests it can aid dilatation of the cervix using laminaria "tents" inserted intra-cervically. These "tents" absorb ambient moisture, gradually swelling to a diameter of 1cm over four to six hours. Its mechanism of action may be due to the presence of a foreign body in the cervix initiating prostaglandin release, or possibly due to a high content of arachidonic acid, a prostaglandin precursor.

Women using laminaria "tents" may experience pelvic cramping and cervical bleeding, and there may be an increased risk of maternal and neonatal infection (Kazzi, Bottoms and Rosen 1982), although this is rare when commercially produced laminaria is used (Lichtenberg 2004). It has also been associated with fetal hypoxia and intrauterine death, and the "tents" can fragment and be retained in the cervical or vaginal canals, causing cervical wall rupture and infection (Borgatta and Barad 1991).

Laminaria should not be taken orally as there have been reports of adverse effects on the thyroid gland due to the high iodine content (Eliason 1998), allergic reactions (Kim *et al.* 2003; Knowles *et al.* 2002) and even arsenic poisoning, because the plant accumulates arsenic from the sea, although the concentration of arsenic may vary (Amster, Tiwary and Schenker 2007; Norman *et al.* 1988; Pye *et al.* 1992). Oral use may cause interactions with certain drugs including potassium supplements and some diuretics, and the high potassium level may cause hyperkalaemia. There is, however, very little evidence of effectiveness or safety; many references are from the latter part of the 20th century, perhaps because the technique was then more acceptable to medical practitioners (Jonasson et al. 1989; Kazzi et al. 1982).

Laminaria does not seem to be significantly effective in ripening the cervix. It may reduce the need for medical induction of labour, but it does not reduce the incidence of Caesarean section (Boulvain et al. 2001), although lack of blinding in the studies may have influenced the results. Conversely, there does not appear to be an increased risk of Caesarean in studies comparing laminaria with placebo, oxytocin, extra-amniotic infusion or prostaglandins (Boulvain et al. 2001). Studies on the use of laminaria prior to mid-trimester termination of pregnancy are also inconclusive (Almog et al. 2005), although there appears to be no increased risk to subsequent pregnancies (Jackson et al. 2007). More recent trials have evaluated laminaria versus misoprostol and mifepristone, demonstrating similar rates of efficacy, but finding increased costs, induction times and reported pain (Borgatta et al. 2005; Darwish, Ahmad and Mohammad 2004; Edelman et al. 2006; Prairie et al. 2007).

Self-administration of pharmacologically active plant remedies

Oral administration of natural remedies derived from various parts of different plants is by far the most commonly used means of attempting to self-induce labour. Even herbal teas contain active constituents which may be therapeutic or harmful, depending on the dose, frequency, gestation and method of administration. There are some herbal remedies which can be used to good effect by medical herbalists when prescribed appropriately, but it is the unwise self-prescription and ingestion of some of these same substances which can lead to maternal or fetal complications. NB *All self-help remedies carry the risk of disproportionate or incoordinate uterine action and fetal distress if taken to excess.*

NICE (2008) identifies that there is a lack of robust evidence on natural remedies to start labour. One of the problems of researching plant medicines is the ethics of testing them on pregnant humans when insufficient information is known about their risks. Studies on animals may contribute to the overall body of knowledge, but the physiology of human parturition is distinctly different from any other mammal. In vitro studies involving strips of myometrial tissue are controversial, not least because of the ethical issues involved in obtaining samples, but also because the impact of herbal medicines in human labour is not isolated to the uterine myometrium.

It is especially worrying to note that NICE erroneously categorises herbal supplements as "non-pharmacological" methods of induction of labour (NICE 2008: 1.4.2.1). NICE also separates castor oil from "herbal" remedies, despite it originating from a plant and having pharmacological properties.

The following sections explore some of the plant remedies commonly used by women in the UK, Australia and the United States. It is appreciated that professionals in other countries may also be aware of remedies used by their clients that are derived from local indigenous plants. It is hoped that the debate will enable midwives and birth workers in areas where different plant remedies are used to apply the principles discussed here to their own practice and to take steps to discover in more detail information on their local plants so that they can advise women on safety.

Raspberry leaf (Rubus idaeus)

This is probably the most popular of all the natural remedies used by women in the UK to avoid post-dates pregnancy and the threat of medical induction of labour. Although the ingestion of raspberry leaf, as a tea or in capsules, during the third trimester of pregnancy is relatively safe when taken under appropriate professional supervision, it is the injudicious over-use by women with little knowledge of its effects which makes it so problematic in contemporary maternity care. Expectant mothers and many midwives incorrectly believe that raspberry leaf can be used to trigger the onset of labour. This author is aware of several maternity units where guidelines suggest that midwives actively advise women to start taking their raspberry leaf tea at term to avoid induction (personal communications with midwives). However, medical herbalists consider that raspberry leaf is a *preparation for birth* to be taken during the third trimester and should not be commenced at term. Inappropriate use at this late stage is more likely to trigger hypertonic uterine action and fetal distress rather than aiding the onset of labour. There are also many women for whom raspberry leaf is contraindicated. (See Chapter 8 for more information on using raspberry leaf as a preparation for birth.)

Clary sage essential oil (Salvia sclarea)

This is, in the opinion of this author, excessively over-used and inadvertently abused by pregnant women and, to a lesser extent, by midwives. As with raspberry leaf, this misuse is largely due to lack of knowledge and understanding that clary sage, like all essential oils, acts pharmacologically, and may have therapeutic or harmful effects, depending on the appropriateness of its use. Its popularity has increased in the last 15 years, possibly as a result of studies on labour aromatherapy, such as Burns *et al.* (2000), in which clary sage was used by midwives to good effect to augment contractions. One only has to read the various Internet consumer discussion groups to see the huge number of questions about clary sage and the alarmingly inappropriate "advice" from mothers who have used it in their own labours to appreciate the size of the problem – and occasionally some incorrect and potentially dangerous comments from midwives.

Clary sage is a member of the Labiatae family which also includes common garden sage (*Salvia officinalis*). Both common sage and clary sage are contraindicated in pregnancy in essential oil or capsule form, although a small amount of common sage occasionally used as a culinary herb is acceptable. However, it is vital that, if *Salvia sclarea* is considered appropriate for stimulation of contractions, it must not be confused with *Salvia officinalis* oil which contains far more potentially harmful, emmenagoguic chemicals and is completely inappropriate in the preconception, antenatal, intrapartum or early postnatal periods (see Tiran 2016a).

There is very little evidence of the safety of clary sage as a medicinal substance. The debate in this chapter is based on the author's research and clinical experience of over 30 years, combined with numerous anecdotal reports, particularly in recent years, from midwifery colleagues who have cared for women using clary sage. From anecdotal evidence, clary sage certainly appears to have a contractile effect on the uterus. This may be due to the high sclareol content of the oil which is thought to mimic oestrogen, although Tisserand (2010) disagrees with this. However, it is generally held that the oil should not be used or inhaled by women with a history of oestrogen-dependent tumours (and care should be taken by non-pregnant menopausal women, including care providers, who are taking hormone replacement therapy). Conversely, Noori, Hassan and Salehian (2013) suggest that the sclareol content may act as an immunosuppressant and therefore offer some potential for enhancing cancer treatments.

Experience of the impact of clary sage on uterine contractions indicates that it should *never* be used before term (see Tiran 2016a). Midwives coming into contact with women in ostensibly idiopathic preterm labour should question them about their use of any herbs or oils which may have an effect on the uterus: many women have been found to have used clary sage prematurely (i.e. before 37 weeks gestation), administered via inappropriate methods and in excessive doses (for example, massaged neat into the abdomen from 30 weeks of pregnancy).

Clary sage appears to reduce cortisol (Lee, Cho and Kang 2014) and may also possess anti-depressive capabilities, possibly through the modulation of dopamine (Seol *et al.* 2010). However, it should be avoided by pregnant women with depression and is not a replacement for, or an adjunct to, antidepressant medication. It also appears to have some anticonvulsant activity in animals and may potentiate the effects of anticonvulsant medication; therefore it should not be used by women taking these drugs (pregnant women with epilepsy should avoid *all* natural remedies unless prescribed by a qualified practitioner – see Chapter 2). It helps to lower blood pressure, so women on anti-hypertensive medication or those with an epidural *in situ* should avoid it (Seol *et al.* 2013). It may also potentiate the effects of alcohol and can lead to vivid dreams and difficulty in sleeping, so caregivers who have worked with women using clary sage in labour should be circumspect about their consumption of alcohol.

Conversely, for midwives, clary sage may be a useful essential oil to incorporate into a "post-dates pregnancy" treatment (see below), but it is contraindicated in any women with uterine compromise, including previous Caesarean section, precipitate labour, multiple pregnancy or placental issues such as placenta praevia or abruption. An aromatherapy treatment which includes clary sage oil may be effective, although it is difficult to determine whether contractions arise as a result of the chemical constituents of clary sage or other oils used, the relaxation effects of the massage by which they are administered which reduces cortisol levels and facilitates an increase in oxytocin, or the specific massage techniques that may be used, such as acupressure stimulation (see below). Table 7.1 summarises the contraindications to clary sage (*Salvia sclarea*).

Table 7.1 Contraindications and precautions to the use of clary sage in late pregnancy

Do not use before 37 weeks gestation – risk of preterm labour

Do not use in established labour – risk of hypertonic uterine action, fetal distress

Obstetric contraindications/precautions	Medical contraindications/precautions
Previous Caesarean section	Anti-hypertensive medication
History of precipitate labour	Women with an epidural anaesthesia *in situ*
Placenta praevia or placental abruption	Women with epilepsy, particularly if on anticonvulsants
Multiple pregnancy	
Reduced fetal movements	Women on antidepressants
Abnormal or unstable lie or presentation	History of oestrogen-dependent tumours, fibroids or endometriosis
Suspected cephalopelvic disproportion	

Contraindications/precautions for midwives, doulas, other staff, woman's partner and visitors

NB Contraindications and precautions apply to everyone inhaling the aromas

Menstruating, particularly if menorrhagia	Epileptic
Fibroids, particularly if causing uterine bleeding	Taking antidepressants, anti-hypertensives, barbiturates
History of oestrogen-dependent tumours, endometriosis	Alcohol
Attempting to conceive, undergoing fertility treatment, pregnant or newly birthed (lochia)	Avoid prolonged exposure in clinical practice – may induce drowsiness

Evening primrose oil (Oenothera biennis)

Evening primrose oil contains up to 16 per cent gamma-linolenic acid (GLA), over 65 per cent linolenic acid and vitamin E. It is commonly used for premenstrual syndrome, menopausal symptoms and endometriosis, as well as a range of skin and inflammatory conditions (Gartoulla *et al.* 2015). Evening primrose oil has long been recommended by American nurse-midwives to be taken orally in pregnancy to shorten the duration of labour, for post-dates pregnancy induction and to prevent pre-eclampsia (McFarlin *et al.* 1999). Many women use evening primrose oil capsules, often inserting them into the vagina for a period of time approaching term. It is generally considered safe (Bayles and Usatine 2009) and is well tolerated (Bendich 2000; Hardy 2000).

The evidence for the effectiveness of evening primrose oil as a means of stimulating contractions at term is varied. Early work suggested that it does not appear to aid labour onset nor shorten the duration of labour (Dove and Johnson 1999; Laivuori *et al.* 1993). More recently, several studies have found it effective for cervical ripening prior to hysteroscopy and postulated that it offered a more acceptable and cost-effective option (Bastu *et al.* 2013; Tanchoco and Aguilar 2015), and Ty-Torredes (2006) suggests that careful use may increase the Bishop score and reduce the need for medical induction.

However, in addition to the possibility of requiring instrumental delivery, evening primrose oil may increase the risk of other complications, including delayed rupture of membranes, the need for oxytocin augmentation and obstructed labour (Dove and Johnson 1999). There is one old case report of a woman experiencing convulsions associated with the use of a combination of evening primrose oil, black cohosh and chasteberry (*Vitex agnus castus*) to stimulate labour (Shuster 1996), although it is not clear which of the three herbs may have contributed to the condition. Evening primrose oil has also been linked to a case of extensive but transient petechiae and ecchymoses in a newborn infant whose mother took 6.5 grams a week before giving birth (Wedig and Whitsett 2008).

Women with epilepsy have previously been advised to avoid evening primrose oil completely as it was thought to trigger convulsions, lower the seizure threshold or interact with anti-epileptic medication, notably phenothiazines (Spinella 2001), although more recent work appears to dispute this (Puri 2007). There is, however, considerable risk of interaction with anticoagulant and anti-platelet medication including warfarin and heparin, as well as non-steroidal anti-inflammatories such as diclofenac and ibuprofen (Riaz, Khan and Ahmed 2009). Women due for elective Caesarean section should, as with all herbal medicines, discontinue the use of evening primrose oil at least two weeks prior to surgery to avoid the risks of intraoperative bleeding – although it would be preferable to advise them to avoid it altogether.

Borage seed oil (Borago officinalis)

This is similar in action to, and is thought to be more powerful than, evening primrose oil as it contains more of the active gamma linolenic acids. It is used by some women to induce labour but is less popular than evening primrose oil. Although borage seed oil is considered generally safe when used appropriately, and has been used in several clinical trials of non-obstetric conditions, it may be dangerous if the product contains hepatotoxic pyrrollidines. These occur mainly in the root, but also in the leaf, flower and seed of the plant. Repeated exposure to low concentrations of hepatotoxic pyrrollidines can cause severe veno-occlusive disease; it is claimed that there are sufficient amounts of hepatotoxic pyrrollidines in some borage seed commercial products to cause significant toxicity (Chojkier 2003; Vacillotto *et al.* 2013). Women choosing to use borage preparations to induce labour should ensure that the product is labelled as hepatotoxic-pyrrollidine-free.

Although borage oil does not, in itself, seem to affect platelet aggregation, its gamma linolenic acid content suggests that it should not be used concomitantly with evening primrose oil, especially if taken by mouth. Alarmingly, several chat sites for pregnant women advocate concomitant oral and vaginal administration of either borage or evening primrose oil, in doses ranging from one to four 500–1000mg capsules from 37 weeks gestation, often with no identified precautions. As with evening primrose oil, borage should be avoided in women with coagulation disorders or taking anticoagulant and other medications with similar actions, and those awaiting elective surgery (Bamford *et al.* 2013). It is also contraindicated in women with liver conditions, as borage seed is metabolised via the liver and some of its metabolites can be harmful.

Castor oil (Ricinus communis)

This has long been used as a traditional remedy to induce labour (Mathie and Dawson 1959), to promote lactation and for constipation and bowel obstruction. It has also been used intravaginally as a means of natural contraception and intracervically as an abortifacient. Castor oil is a glyceride that can be absorbed from the intestine and metabolised as a fatty acid. It is hydrolysed in the duodenum by pancreatic lipase to release ricinoleic acid, which may have stimulant laxative effects. These factors have given rise to its popularity as a labour stimulant through a perceived reflex stimulation of the uterine emyometrium. Castor oil might also increase prostaglandin production, which stimulates uterine activity (Garry *et al.* 2000), due to prostaglandin-activating chemical constituents (Tunaru *et al.* 2012).

Self-administered doses of between 5 and 120ml have been recorded (McFarlin *et al.* 1999). A single dose of 60ml of castor oil appears to ripen the cervix, "spontaneously" establish labour within 24 hours and may reduce the incidence of Caesarean section (Azhari *et al.* 2006; Garry *et al.* 2000; Neri *et al.* 2017). However, Boel *et al.*'s large retrospective Asian study (2009) found no significant difference in the onset of labour between women who ingested castor oil and those who did not.

Castor oil should not be used before term, for example for constipation, as it could theoretically cause miscarriage or vaginal bleeding, but it is considered relatively safe in small amounts in women at term. Minor side effects of ingesting castor oil include nausea, partly due to its unpleasant taste, and abdominal cramps; dermatitis may occur with topical use (Mozurkewich et al. 2011). More seriously, it may cause fluid and electrolyte loss in large doses, particularly potassium, which can result in hypokalaemia and should certainly be avoided by women taking diuretics. There is some concern, admittedly from a single case report, that castor oil could cause amniotic fluid embolism (Steingrub et al. 1988), although no more recent reports of this possibility were found. Only the oil should be ingested; chewing whole seeds can cause severe toxic effects due to a poisonous substance, ricin, which is not present in the oil, and which has even been reported to cause death (Audi et al. 2005; Challoner and McCarron 1990). However, inappropriate or excessive use of castor oil by women desperate to start labour may trigger adverse effects, including meconium-stained liquor and fetal distress (Mitri, Hofmeyr and van Gelderen 1987), although Garry et al. (2000) considered that the incidence of meconium was no greater than in the control group.

Black cohosh (Cimicifuga racemosa)

Black cohosh is traditionally taken orally for symptoms of menopause, premenstrual syndrome and dysmenorrhoea and to induce labour. It is thought to have hormonal, menstrual and uterine-stimulating effects, which, theoretically, may increase the risk of miscarriage, and it should therefore be avoided in early pregnancy (Dugoua, Seely et al. 2006). There is little reliable information available on the safety of black cohosh and, although as many as 45 per cent of nurse-midwives in the USA use it to induce labour at term (McFarlin et al. 1999), there is no contemporary reliable clinical evidence of its effectiveness.

Orally, black cohosh can cause gastrointestinal disturbance (Whiting, Clouston and Kerlin 2003), headache, dizziness, breast tenderness and skin irritation. When used for menopausal symptoms, it may trigger vaginal spotting or bleeding (Wuttke et al. 2003). Several case reports of liver toxicity have been described in women taking black cohosh products alone, or in combination with other herbs, over a prolonged period of time, some requiring immediate liver transplantation (Chow et al. 2008; Cohen et al. 2004; Joy, Joy and Duane 2008; Lontos et al. 2003; Mahady et al. 2008;

Vitetta, Sali and Thomsen 2003). On the other hand, a more recent systematic review by Naser *et al.* (2011) disputed this risk.

Blitz *et al.* (2016) report the case of a woman who took several black cohosh capsules to expedite labour who then became lethargic, disorientated and non-verbal. She was transferred from home to hospital, where she was found to be extremely hyponatraemic. Following Caesarean section and correction of her sodium levels in the intensive care unit, she recovered with no apparent prolonged effects and was discharged home. There have also been case reports of severe complications, including convulsions, renal failure and respiratory distress in the baby of a mother who took an unknown dose of black cohosh and blue cohosh at 42 weeks gestation to induce labour (Baillie and Rasmussen 1997; Gunn and Wright 1996), although these effects are more likely to have been due to the blue cohosh (see below). Women with a history of hepatic or renal disease, epilepsy or vaginal bleeding in pregnancy should be advised to avoid black cohosh.

Blue cohosh (Caulophyllum thalictroides)

A traditional remedy, blue cohosh is primarily used to stimulate uterine contractions and to encourage menstruation. It has also been used as an antispasmodic, a laxative and for a variety of other conditions. However, there is little robust evidence on the effectiveness of blue cohosh to support its use at all in pregnancy or birth, despite the fact that many nurse-midwives in the USA have long used it to promote uterine action, typically in doses of 0.3 to 1gm/day (McFarlin *et al.* 1999).

There have been reports of severe poisoning and adverse effects such as hyponatraemia (Blitz *et al.* 2016) when taken orally. It is thought that blue cohosh has oestrogenic properties and may be potentially teratogenic in early pregnancy (Wu *et al.* 2010). When used at or near term, usually to induce labour, it can cause life-threatening toxicity in the baby, including stroke, acute myocardial infarction, congestive heart failure, multiple organ injury and neonatal shock, and it may negatively impact on mitochondrial activity (Datta *et al.* 2014; Finkel and Zarlengo 2004). Several older case reports have indicated respiratory distress, convulsions and renal failure in the babies of women who took blue cohosh (Edmunds 1999; Gunn and Wright 1996; Irikura and Kennelly 1999; Jones and Lawson 1998).

Adult adverse effects include diarrhoea, abdominal cramps, hypertension (Jalili *et al.* 2013) and hyperglycaemia (Rao and Hoffman 2002). Women on anti-hypertensive or diabetic medication should avoid blue cohosh, as well as those who are heavy smokers, as it contains nicotinic substances which may exacerbate the adverse effects of smoking. The oestrogenic constituents suggest that it should not be taken by women with a personal or family history of hormone-sensitive cancers. Other constituents (saponins and various alkaloids) may inhibit P450 cytochromes, potentially risking interactions with drug metabolism (Madgula *et al.* 2009). Dugoua *et al.* (2008) expressed concern about the adverse effects of blue cohosh in pregnancy and labour and suggested that it should be used with extreme caution, if at all. They recommended that blue cohosh should not be available to the general public and that it should be used only under strict medical or medical-herbalist supervision. The general feeling amongst most authorities is that blue cohosh should not be used at all for childbirth.

NB It is essential to differentiate between black cohosh (*Cimicifuga racemosa*) and blue cohosh (*Caulophyllum thalictroides*) to avoid confusion and inappropriate administration. It is also important to differentiate between the herbal (pharmacological) and homeopathic (energetic) use of these plants (see below and Chapter 2).

Licorice (Glycyrrhiza glabra)

Licorice is used by some women because it is thought to have laxative and oestrogenic effects. Glycyrrhizin is an inhibitor of cortisol metabolism, which may play a part in altering the cortisol-oxytocin balance at the end of pregnancy (Strandberg *et al.* 2001). However, excess antenatal consumption (250 grams per week, equivalent to 500mg of glycyrrhizin) may increase the risk of preterm birth (Strandberg *et al.* 2002). One study has also suggested that high maternal intake may have an epigenetic effect on the infant, increasing salivary cortisol levels, possibly due to increased hypothalamic-pituitary-adrenocortical axis activity, potentially predisposing the child to various illnesses in later life (Räikkönen *et al.* 2010). Swallowing the chewed fibrous licorice root can lead to intestinal blockage, and women with any chronic gastrointestinal condition should avoid it. However, the most significant adverse effect of excessive licorice consumption is the impact on the blood pressure due to very high sodium levels which can lead to hypokalaemia (Yasue *et al.* 2007). Women with hypertension or renal disease may be more sensitive to these effects and should avoid taking licorice in medicinal quantities (Sigurjónsdóttir *et al.* 2001). Its laxative effects may also cause diarrhoea, with over-use leading to potassium depletion (Yoshida and Takayama 2003); women requiring diuretics should avoid licorice to prevent potassium loss. There is also a major risk of interaction with warfarin (Mu *et al.* 2006) and possibly with metformin medication for diabetes mellitus (Awad *et al.* 2016).

Motherwort (Leonurus artemisia)

Another plant sometimes used to induce labour is motherwort, which appears to have uterine-stimulating effects. It is contraindicated in pregnancy but may be used by medical herbalists for women whose pregnancies are post-dates (de Boer and Cotingting 2014). It does not seem to be as popular as a self-help remedy as some of the other herbs discussed here, although it may be prescribed by a qualified medical herbalist attending a labouring woman. Several side effects can occur with prolonged or excessive doses, including gastrointestinal disturbance, uterine bleeding and allergic reactions (Oyedemi, Yakubu and Afolayan 2010). Motherwort used concomitantly with sedatives or antihistamines may potentiate the sedative and tranquillising effects of the drugs.

Consumption of fruit to aid labour onset

Pineapple

Pineapple (*Ananas comosus*) is not usually regarded as a herbal remedy, but any potential therapeutic action is certainly due to the pharmacological effects of its chemical constituents. Although little research has been found on its impact on the uterus in human parturition, women in some parts of the world are discouraged from consuming pineapple during pregnancy as it is traditionally thought to cause miscarriage. Any effect on uterine contractions at term is thought to be due to the bromelain content. Bromelain is a composite enzyme that is active in the relatively low pH of the stomach and intestines. As with castor oil, there may thus be a reflex effect on uterine muscle as a result of gastrointestinal stimulation; certainly excessive consumption can trigger diarrhoea or other gastrointestinal disturbance. However, more recent in vitro research suggests it may be due to serotonergic processes from 5HT and 5HT-like substances (Monji *et al.* 2016).

Bromelain is used for a variety of medicinal uses, including osteoarthritis, as an anti-cancer agent, and for its anti-inflammatory activity (Pavan *et al.* 2012), although the small number of studies available have sometimes used bromelain extract. This means that the active ingredient has been isolated from the whole plant. As with pharmaceutical preparations, isolation of a single component from the plant detracts from the overall interaction of bromelain with other chemicals in pineapple, many of which have a synergistically limiting effect on the overall risk of side effects. It is therefore difficult to extrapolate data which can be reasonably applied to labour physiology. When consumed as the fruit, the bromelain is destroyed by cooking, canning or juicing and the largest concentration is found in the fresh, raw central fibrous core which many people discard. Since bromelain acts in the gastrointestinal tract, oral consumption is the correct means of obtaining it, *not* per vaginam as this author has occasionally heard midwives advising.

There is insufficient bromelain in a single pineapple to have any impact on initiating labour, and women would probably need to eat several in order to ingest enough of the therapeutic chemicals. This poses a problem as immunoglobulin E-mediated allergic reactions to bromelain may occur when eaten in large quantities by susceptible women. These reactions include the possibility of cross-allergenicity between bromelain and foods such as wheat, celery, carrot and fennel, and to grass pollen, flowers from the *Compositae* plant family including chrysanthemums, marigolds, daisies and echinacea, and many other herbs (Nettis *et al.* 2001).

Bromelain may also have anticoagulant effects (Kaur *et al.* 2016; Taussig and Batkin 1988) and should therefore be avoided by women with any coagulation disorder, vaginal bleeding or taking anticoagulant medication, non-steroidal anti-inflammatories or other drugs or herbs with similar effects. There is also one case report of severe bruising apparently resulting from concomitant use of bromelain and naproxen (Bush *et al.* 2007).

Enzymes that are similar to bromelain are also found in *papaya* (pawpaw) and *mangoes* which contain papain, an aid to protein digestion, noticeably when the fruit is ripe (Cherian 2000). As with pineapple, women in many countries are also advised against eating these fruits during pregnancy as it is thought they may trigger miscarriage, particularly in high doses (Oderinde *et al.* 2002).

Dates

Dates (*Phoenix dactylifera*) have also become popular in recent years as a means of stimulating contractions. In some cultures, notably in Middle Eastern countries, tradition dictates that pregnant women should avoid eating palm dates as they may trigger preterm labour. In a prospective comparative study of 114 women, Al-Kuran *et al.* (2011) suggested that eating six large fresh dates daily for four weeks prior to the estimated delivery date facilitates spontaneous onset of labour (96% compared to 79% in the control group), requires less use of oxytocics, shortens the first stage of labour and is more likely to result in a normal vaginal birth. An Iranian randomised controlled study (Kordi *et al.* 2014) also found that women who ate up to 75 grams of fresh dates daily from 37 weeks gestation had increased Bishop scores and cervical dilatation on admission to hospital; where medical induction was required it was more successful than for women in the control group. The most recent study (Razali *et al.* 2017) also found good effects on cervical ripening and a reduction on the need for oxytocic augmentation, but did not appear to show an impact directly on the spontaneous onset of labour. It is useful to note here that these studies were all undertaken in the Middle East where dates grow naturally and are generally eaten fresh rather than dried and where, culturally, women appreciate the need to refrain from consuming dates in earlier pregnancy. These factors may all, in isolation or in combination, have had a bearing on the results.

Table 7.2 summarises some of the possible risks of various self-help remedies used to start labour contractions.

Table 7.2 Contraindications, precautions and possible side effects of the most commonly used natural remedies for post-dates pregnancy

Name	Contraindications, precautions, side effects	Side effects
Black cohosh	Hepatic disease	Nausea, vomiting, diarrhoea
Cimicifuga racemosa	Renal disease	Headache, dizziness, lethargy
	Epilepsy	Vaginal bleeding, breast tenderness
		Liver toxicity with prolonged use
		Serious neonatal effects
Blue cohosh	DO NOT USE FOR INDUCTION OF LABOUR	Poisoning
Caulophyllum thalictroides		Diarrhoea, abdominal cramps, fluid loss
		Hyponatraemia
		Possible life-threatening effects on neonate
Castor oil	Avoid if taking diuretics	Nausea, abdominal cramps, diarrhoea
Ricinus communis	Do not chew castor oil seeds	Fluid, electrolyte loss
	Maximum single dose of 60ml	Meconium-stained liquor, fetal distress with excessive use

Name	Contraindications, precautions, side effects	Side effects
Clary sage *Salvia sclarea*	See Table 7.1	
Evening primrose oil *Oenothera biennis*	Avoid with anti-epilepsy medication. Avoid with anticoagulants, anti-platelets, aspirin. Discontinue at least two weeks prior to elective Caesarean section	Delayed membrane rupture. Increased need for oxytocin, instrumental delivery. Possible petechiae in neonate
Pineapple *Ananas comosus* Also papaya, mango	Avoid if allergic to these fruit, wheat, celery, carrot, fennel or flowers from Compositae family, e.g. daisies. Avoid if vaginal bleeding. Avoid with anticoagulants	Allergic reactions, anaphylaxis. Bruising, bleeding with excessive use. Diarrhoea
Raspberry leaf *Rubus ideus*	Not to be used for self-induction of labour – intended as a *preparation* for birth. See Chapter 8	

Homeopathic remedies

There is virtually no research to be found on the use of homeopathic remedies to encourage the onset of labour. A systematic Cochrane review (Smith 2010) found two placebo-controlled, double-blinded studies on homeopathic remedies for labour induction but suggested that they were of poor calibre. The primary difficulty with any homeopathy study is the need to individualise the prescription of a relevant remedy; thus randomised trials in which a single remedy is used, such as caulophyllum, are unlikely to produce statistically significant results, since caulophyllum will not be appropriate for all women in the trial.

Professional homeopaths often prescribe remedies to help women keen to avoid medical induction but this is dependent on an individualised clinical consultation.

There are, however, many websites, aimed both at consumers and professional homeopaths, advocating certain specific remedies. Many suggest that women could use both cimicifuga and caulophyllum in homeopathic doses, yet this advice is wrong on several counts. These two remedies are certainly effective, separately, for some women but may be inappropriate for others. In UK homeopathic practice it is normal to prescribe a single remedy that most closely fits with the woman's individual symptom picture. Some websites were found to advise taking three tablets four times daily, yet there is no need to take more than one tablet at a time: one dose is *one episode* of ingestion regardless of the number of tablets taken. It is also of concern to note that some websites suggest taking the remedies for at least a week (and sometimes considerably longer) prior to term, a practice more likely to cause a reverse proving (see Chapter 2) and significantly disrupt the polarity of the uterus.

Table 7.3 summarises three of the commonly used homeopathic remedies that may be suitable for women wanting to self-medicate in order to avoid medical induction of labour. However, there are many more remedies that could be suitable, and women should be advised that it is best to consult a qualified homeopath for the correct prescription unless they are very familiar with the concept of homeopathic prescribing.

Table 7.3 Homeopathic remedies commonly used for post-dates pregnancy

Remedy	Features – physical	Features – emotional	Improves with	Deteriorates with
Caulophyllum	False labour/ excessive Braxton Hicks contractions Exhausted, thirsty, feels hot, nausea Rigid cervical os	Distressed, irritable, fretful	Being out in cool fresh air Having back pressed hard	Being cold NB Do not give routinely – may cause hypertonia or protracted labour
Cimicifuga	Twitching, weak, ineffectual contractions that cease entirely if warm Mild contractions tearing, flying around abdomen Uterine inertia	Fears delivery, dying in labour, going insane Talks incessantly	Being cool	Noise, pain
Pulsatilla	False labour – short, weak, distressing contractions that stop suddenly Backache, spasm in back that appears suddenly, eases gradually	Apologetic, keeps changing mind Erratic behaviour, laughing, weeping Wants sympathy	Being with people Being in fresh air Walking about	Being alone Being too warm/indoors Inactivity

Acupuncture and acupressure

Acupuncture, acupressure and shiatsu (see Chapter 2) are coming under considerable scrutiny as offering alternative ways of initiating labour. There have been many studies, in China and increasingly in western countries, to determine whether stimulation of specific acupoints, either by needling or with thumb and finger pressure, can be effective. Several specific acupoints are considered to be "forbidden points" for pregnancy as they are thought to trigger uterine contractions (Betts and Budd 2011). Although this has been disputed by Cummings (2011), it is these same acupoints which have been investigated in trials on women with post-dates pregnancy, suggesting that the general consensus of opinion remains the same and that most acupuncturists will avoid working on these points until term.

Unfortunately, the research is fairly inconclusive, with many studies reporting results which are not statistically significant. NICE (2008: CG70) states that the available evidence does not support the use of acupuncture as a means of natural induction of labour. There is, perhaps, some truth in this assumption, particularly as the methodology is inconsistent, although many demonstrate success in stimulating contractions. Researchers use different acupoints or different combinations of points, although the commonest points used tend to be Spleen 6 and Large Intestine 4 (Gregson *et al.* 2015; Mollart, Adam and Foureur 2015). Other acupoints include Gall Bladder 21, Bladder 31, Bladder 32 and Bladder 67 (Ajori, Azhari and Eliaspour 2013; Harper *et al.* 2006). In practice, acupuncturists may also incorporate relaxation acupoints into the overall treatment, which further confuses the evidence picture, since it could be argued that the relaxation factor was instrumental in reducing cortisol and increasing oxytocin.

The timing and aims of treatment also varies. Gaudernack, Forbord and Hole (2006) explored the impact of acupuncture on the initiation of contractions following term pre-labour rupture of the membranes, and found a decreased need for oxytocin augmentation. Conversely, Selmer-Olsen, Lydersen and Mørkved (2007) showed no significant difference in the need for intervention between the study group and a control group with pre-labour membrane rupture. Electro-acupuncture has also been used to aid cervical ripening, and compared to the use of misoprostol, with an increase in the number of vaginal births in the trial group (Gribel, Coca-Velarde and Moreira de Sá 2011). In another study, laser acupuncture was used with apparent success and with no adverse effects on fetal wellbeing (Alsharnoubi, Khattab and Elnoury 2015).

Studies with the specific objective of encouraging cervical ripening, inducing labour and/or reducing the need for medical induction commenced acupoint stimulation three or four weeks prior to the EDD (Asher *et al.* 2009); others only commenced treatment at or after 40, or even 41, weeks gestation (Gregson *et al.* 2015; Modlock, Nielsen and Uldbjerg 2010). Smith *et al.* (2013) conducted a prospective randomised controlled trial in which women were given two sessions of acupuncture two days prior to the day they were due to have labour induced, but with little success. Their justification for this regime may have been influenced by organisational limitations, but this particular programme of treatment is not one that is commonly used in professional acupuncture practice.

Most studies include a control group of women who receive only standard maternity care. However, Asher *et al.* (2009) compared acupuncture to both a control group (standard care) and to a group of women who received sham acupuncture, using a traditional Chinese medicine approach, but found no statistically significant differences between the groups.

Treatment may be done weekly or on alternate days (Neri *et al.* 2014). Some trials use acupuncture, whilst others focus on acupressure, sometimes performed by appropriately trained professionals, including midwives. Others teach parents how to apply thumb and finger pressure to the relevant acupoints at home, although it is known that compliance can be an issue in these cases (Gregson *et al.* 2015). Others examine the effectiveness of acupuncture or electro-acupuncture on cervical ripening (Gribel *et al.* 2011; Rabl *et al.* 2001) rather than the initiation of contractions.

Amir *et al.* (2015) explored the effectiveness of Chinese acupressure and acupuncture with conventional methods of labour induction, both singly and in combination. They found favourable results suggesting that acupoint stimulation offered an inexpensive method which appeared to be safe. Some researchers compare acupoint stimulation with membrane sweeping (Andersen *et al.* 2013); others use sham acupuncture (Ajori *et al.* 2013; Asher *et al.* 2009). The timing of treatment is also variable, although treatment performed on alternate days from the EDD to onset of labour is a common regime (Ingram, Domagala and Yates 2005; Neri *et al.* 2014), whereas Modlock *et al.* (2010) treated twice on a single day only. Despite considerable success with acupuncture on the number of women with a post-dates pregnancy who commenced labour (94.7%), a correspondingly high success rate in the control group (89.2%) led Ajori *et al.* (2013) to conclude that acupuncture was ineffective in initiating labour.

A large controlled study of over 400 women by Andersen *et al.* (2013) found that acupuncture appeared to be less successful in reducing the need for medical induction than membrane sweeping, when performed from 41 weeks gestation. Studies by both Asher *et al.* (2009) and Ajori *et al.* (2013) found no significant difference between true and sham acupuncture, although the latter showed a 94 per cent success rate in onset of labour for acupuncture from 38 weeks of pregnancy. Gaudet *et al.* (2008) undertook a small study of just 16 women and demonstrated a significant 62-hour difference in the treatment-to-labour-onset interval between primigravidae who received acupuncture and those who did not. Other researchers have found a reduction in labour duration following acupuncture or acupressure to stimulate contractions (Gaudernack *et al.* 2006). Conversely, Torkzahrani *et al.* (2017) randomised 162 women to receive acupressure, sham acupressure or standard care, but found no statistically significant differences between the three groups in the initiation of labour.

These inconsistent variables and inconclusive results thus lead to ambiguous, imprecise or uncertain conclusions and it is difficult to extrapolate from the evidence whether or not acupressure and acupuncture offer reliable methods of non-medical induction of labour. However, they do appear to be more medically acceptable and probably more effective than supportive therapies such as aromatherapy or reflexology, and there is growing interest in the value of acupuncture for post-dates pregnancy.

Systematic reviews, as always, tend to conclude that there is a need for more research but give tentative backing for the use of acupuncture (Lim *et al.* 2009). There do not appear to be any major adverse effects on either maternal or fetal wellbeing when acupuncture is used professionally, either alone or in combination with oxytocin (Liu *et al.* 2008). It is also possible that, even when treatment success is not statistically significant, maternal satisfaction improves, perhaps because they perceive that non-conventional action is being taken to trigger labour, especially after spontaneous membrane rupture (Selmer-Olsen *et al.* 2007). Acupuncture or acupressure for induction of labour for post-dates pregnancy is generally well tolerated by women, provides a degree of psychological support in the early stages of labour onset and may reduce the incidence of iatrogenic problems associated with induction (Harper *et al.* 2006). Table 7.4 provides a summary of some of the acupuncture/acupressure research for post-dates pregnancy.

Table 7.4 Summary of some acupuncture/acupressure research for post-dates pregnancy

Authors/date	Outcome measures	Gestation (weeks)	Method	Acupoints used	Conclusion
Andersen et al. 2013	Reduction in need for induction		Acupuncture, acupuncture with sweep, sweep, control (4 groups)	General	Not effective, membrane sweep more effective
Ajori et al. 2013	Reduction in need for induction	From 38	RCT double-blind Acupuncture vs sham acupuncture	Large Intestine 4 Spleen 6 Bladder 67	Not effective (despite 94% and 87% success in labour onset)
Asher et al. 2009	Acupuncture for induction, primigravidae	From 38	Acupuncture vs sham acupuncture vs control, usual care	Large Intestine 4, Spleen 6, Bladder 32, Bladder 54	Not effective
Gregson et al. 2015	Acupressure for induction, primi-gravidae, post-dates	From 41	Acupressure taught to mothers for use on alternate days until onset of labour, no control	Large Intestine 4 Spleen 6	Not statistically significantly effective
Gribel et al. 2011	Cervical ripening in women with Bishop score 7+	Variable, based on Bishops score	Electro-acupuncture vs misoprostol	General	Electro-acupuncture cervical ripening similar to misoprostol
Modlock et al. 2010	Acupuncture for induction, post-dates	41+6	Acupuncture vs sham acupuncture, same points, twice on same day	Governing Vessel 20, Bladder 67 Large Intestine 4, Spleen 6	Not effective
Neri et al. 2014	Acupuncture for induction, post-dates	40+2 until 40+6	Acupuncture alternate days for one week, control – no treatment		Not effective
Torkzahrani et al. 2015	Acupressure for cervical ripening	Term	Acupressure for 20 minutes for 1–5 days; group 1, administered by researcher, group 2, self-administered, group 3, control, standard care	Spleen 6	Effective

Professional use of complementary therapies and natural remedies for women with post-dates pregnancy

There is a definite place for maternity caregivers to consider complementary therapy strategies for women with a post-dates pregnancy, although the issue of pre-birth preparation remains contentious. "Pre-birth" treatments involve the use of therapy techniques or natural remedies normally used to stimulate uterine contractions, from about 37 weeks gestation, usually administered weekly by a practitioner such as an acupuncturist; acupressure points may be taught to the expectant parents to self-administer at home or women may be advised about the home use of natural remedies such as aromatherapy essential oils. It is, however, generally shown from the research, and from anecdotal evidence, that pre-birth treatments, especially those incorporating relaxation in the form of therapies such as massage, aromatherapy or reflexology, facilitate the physiological onset of labour. They also enhance satisfaction by offering women opportunities for continuing face-to-face consultations with a birth professional so that they can discuss any worries. This in itself may contribute to spontaneous onset of labour by relaxing women and helping them to appreciate the benefits of allowing labour to commence physiologically rather than risking inappropriate interventions, either complementary or conventional.

Several midwives have established special clinics for women with post-dates pregnancy, or are in the process of doing so (personal communications). These initiatives can be financially advantageous, reducing admissions for medical induction and the use of further interventions such as epidural anaesthesia and operative delivery. The option to try "natural induction" does not preclude women from having a conventional induction of labour when necessary, but in the event of having received apparently unsuccessful complementary treatment, prior use of complementary therapies may aid a medically induced onset.

Weston and Grabowska (2013) established a post-dates pregnancy clinic at the West Middlesex Hospital in west London, which runs two days per week. Midwives were trained to use a package of treatment incorporating acupressure point stimulation, reflex zone therapy and aromatherapy massage with oils that are appropriate for labour contractions. The 2014 and 2015 audit results indicate a consistent success rate (spontaneous onset of labour after the "post-dates" treatment package) of between 67 and 76 per cent in primigravidae and 70 and 82 per cent in multiparae.

Of the women who declined membrane sweep and had the complementary post-dates pregnancy treatment, the average rate of spontaneous labour was 74 per cent in nulliparae and around 76 per cent for multiparae (Weston, personal communication on audit).

Pauley and Percival (2014) also set up a clinic in Hinchingbrooke, Cambridgeshire, offering a similar package of treatment. They reduced the number of inductions of labour for post-dates pregnancy by 5 per cent within six months. In this unit, with approximately 2400 births per year, 5 per cent represents a reduction in the need for induction of approximately 120 women. Given that the cost of a prostin pessary is around £13 and the Propess® intravaginal gel system is £30 (British National Formulary 2017), the cost of induction drugs alone could be between £1560 and £3600 per year, even without the on-costs of additional staff time, in-patient stay and the likelihood of further intervention. Facilitating women to start labour spontaneously may contribute to a more normal first stage labour, potentially reducing the need for Caesarean section, with a cost saving of at least £1000 per birth.

Midwives in these and many other maternity units have been taught by this author to use a "package" of care that includes the use of acupressure (Spleen 6, Gall Bladder 21 and Large Intestine 4), combined with aromatherapy massage using essential oils known to promote uterine action, and occasionally incorporating reflex zone therapy.

Spleen 6 (Sanyinjiao) is an acupuncture point at which several meridians intersect, namely the Spleen, Liver and Kidney meridians. It is said to strengthen the Spleen, encourage blood flow and tonify the Kidney, which is closely linked with the uterus (see also Chapter 2 and Chapter 6 on moxibustion for breech presentation). It is particularly effective for triggering labour onset and can be used to treat retained placenta. It is also good for pain relief in labour and is instrumental in helping with various disorders of the reproductive system, in women and men. This acupoint is located four finger-breadths up from the inner ankle (according to the woman's own finger width) – see Figure 7.1.

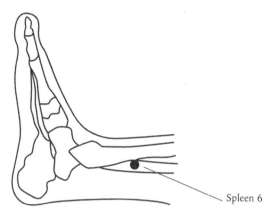

Spleen 6

Figure 7.1 Location of the Spleen 6 acupoint

Gall Bladder 21 (Jian jing) on the top of the shoulders is an acupoint that has a specific function in encouraging downwards movement (see Figure 7.2). This is why it is a contraindicated point in pregnancy, to avoid downwards movement (i.e. expulsion) of the fetus prior to term. It would also be contraindicated in an older woman with a uterine prolapse. Conversely, this point is good for relieving problems such as tense shoulders, as it encourages downwards movement of the local muscles.

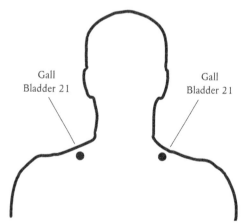

Gall
Bladder 21

Gall
Bladder 21

Figure 7.2 Location of the Gall Bladder 21 accupoint

Large Intestine 4 (Hegu) on the hands (see Figure 8.1 in Chapter 8) is vital in digestion and bowel function but also impacts on psychological wellbeing, by tonifying the Blood and qi. It is effective in relieving headache (but not in pregnancy) and is good for many problems in the face, neck and head because of its action in reducing stagnation and encouraging movement. It is, however, very powerful and is therefore contraindicated in pregnancy to avoid excessive movement of the fetus before it is ready. This point is another that is useful for encouraging the onset of labour, aiding progress and dealing with retained placenta (see Chapter 8).

These three pairs of acupoints can easily be learned by midwives to incorporate into a post-dates pregnancy treatment, and women can also be shown how to locate and stimulate them at home.

If aromatherapy is added to the "package" offered to women, essential oils such as clary sage (*Salvia sclarea*), jasmine (*Jasminum officinalis*), rose (*Rosa centifolia*) or lavender (*Lavandula angustifolia*) may be effective in stimulating contractions, combined with other, gentler oils to provide a pleasant and relaxing blend. In a clinic setting, it may be cost effective and time efficient to blend up the oils beforehand to reduce the time spent choosing and blending oils. However, there must be at least two different blends to offer women, since they may not like the aroma of one particular blend. More importantly, women may react adversely to one of the oils within the blend. For example, those with an allergy to citrus fruit will not be able to have a blend with a citrus oil such as bergamot (*Citrus bergamia*) in it; those with asthma or hayfever may respond adversely to oils from plants that trigger their respiratory symptoms, such as lavender. See Tiran (2016a) for more information on aromatherapy.

Logistically, for an NHS maternity unit to benefit from a specialist complementary therapy post-dates pregnancy clinic, it is important to offer the service to as many women as possible. A service offering specific treatments with added time for relaxation may be popular but is unlikely – and, therefore, unethical – to be equitable in a large unit. Similarly, offering treatments to women prior to 40 weeks gestation is not cost effective unless it is offered as a service for which, perhaps, a fee is charged, since the time could be better spent in offering treatments to more women who are technically "overdue". Conversely, for those working in private practice, offering courses of treatment from 36 or 37 weeks gestation may help women through the last few weeks of their pregnancies and enable ongoing discussion about the appropriateness of self-administered natural techniques and remedies.

Conclusion

Post-dates pregnancy could be considered to be a major issue in maternity care, causing distress to women who want to start labour naturally in order to avoid medical induction. Midwives and doulas are often caught in the "cross-fire" between women and obstetricians and, while they may want to act as the women's advocates, they are usually constrained by local or national policies which may conflict with their own personal views. It is, however, vital that maternity care providers are able to advise women on the safety of the many strategies and remedies that they may wish to self-administer, in order to avoid stimulating contractions at an inappropriate stage of the pregnancy or triggering excessively strong contractions at term, which in itself may lead to a "cascade" of intervention.

However, midwives with comprehensive knowledge and appropriate skills can play a part in helping women with post-dates pregnancy by offering specialist treatments aimed at relaxing them, facilitating cervical ripening and the onset of contractions. This will also have a positive impact on the maternity services by potentially reducing the number of medical inductions of labour and the instrumental and operative deliveries which often follow the procedure.

CHAPTER 8

Complementary Therapies for Labour

Labour is a time when women benefit enormously from human touch, emotional support and other strategies that can help to relax them. A sense of relaxation reduces stress hormones, particularly cortisol, and enables labour hormones, notably oxytocin, to work efficiently. More than at any other time in the childbearing year, complementary therapies can be invaluable tools to help women through their labours. However, women are sometimes so keen to expedite labour that they self-administer natural remedies and apply pressure point techniques inappropriately.

This chapter explores the complementary options for preparing for birth, therapies for pain relief and alternative means of aiding progress in labour, including discussion on the following aspects:

- introduction
- preparation for birth
- pain relief in labour
- progress in labour
- retained placenta

- combining complementary therapies for labour care
- conclusion.

Introduction

Most women spend time during their pregnancies exploring options for the birth, including seeking out antenatal classes and considering ways in which they can prepare their bodies for labour. This appears to be a universal activity amongst women of all races and cultures as they turn inward-looking and concentrate on their ultimate function as a woman.

Many women actively seek out independent complementary practitioners for treatment of specific antenatal conditions such as backache or sickness, or for general relaxation, particularly as they near term. Group sessions such as "hypnobirthing" to help women prepare mentally and emotionally for labour, are now commonly offered, both in the conventional maternity services and by private practitioners. Exercise classes, including water-based sessions, Pilates, yoga or mindfulness training, are also popular. As labour approaches, women start to explore ways to ease the anticipated pain, and it is known that women who are relaxed as they approach term will be likely to experience less pain during the labour. Many want to avoid unnecessary interventions such as induction of labour and search for natural ways of starting labour, as well as exploring their options for after the birth, including healing the perineum in the event of stitches and establishing breastfeeding.

In years gone by, women may not have worked, or were able to stop working in the early third trimester. Decades ago, women were content to defer to the decisions of midwives and doctors but are now prepared to challenge professional expertise in order to achieve the birth they want. Some women even choose actively to decline professional help and opt for unassisted or "free-birthing". However, the plethora of information now available to pregnant women, from other mothers, in magazines, on pregnancy Internet websites and particularly on social media, has contributed to an overload of information, much of which is either incorrect or incomplete. Nowhere is this more true than with the huge subject of complementary therapies and natural remedies for childbirth. The sheer extent of the information available can be confusing for women and sometimes dangerously misinterpreted. It also potentially causes conflict and concern for midwives when women wish to use selected remedies or complementary techniques, particularly in conjunction with conventional drugs.

On the other hand, childbirth is the time when complementary therapies seem to find their natural place in the maternity continuum, providing alternative methods of pain relief, aiding progress and easing anxiety. The nature of caring for a labouring woman is such that touch and physical contact can contribute to a much more satisfying experience, reducing stress hormones and facilitating oxytocin production to encourage as natural a birth as possible. Midwives and doulas are increasingly incorporating aspects of complementary therapies and natural remedies into their care, and many maternity units now offer aromatherapy, massage, acupuncture and occasionally reflexology. Further, although not a complementary therapy in the true sense of the word, many units also offer "hypnobirthing" classes. For women unfamiliar with complementary therapies, the notion of incorporating them into labour care can be introduced during pregnancy and may contribute to enhanced parental knowledge and more realistic expectations, reduced stress and anxiety and consequently a reduction in interventions in labour (Levett *et al.* 2016a, 2016b).

Midwives enjoy being able to be "with woman", returning to the nurturing which is so much a part of supporting a woman during arguably the most significant time in their lives. This generates an attitude which embraces the physical, emotional and spiritual aspects of birth, and has been shown, in units where complementary therapies are provided by midwives, to increase midwifery recruitment and retention (Burns *et al.* 2000). It is also well known that the support of a doula or birth companion contributes to a more relaxed mother and improved outcomes (Kozhimannil *et al.* 2013). Indeed, a study by Akbarzadeh *et al.* (2015) showed that doula care, combined with the application of a single acupressure point, significantly reduced maternal anxiety and duration of labour. The team also surmised that doula support and acupressure facilitated improved fetal oxygenation.

Incorporating complementary therapies into midwifery practice does not have to mean increasing the workload; indeed, it may actually reduce it if women achieve a normal labour without induction, epidural anaesthesia or Caesarean section, which also, of course, saves money (Donnelly 2016). Midwives integrating complementary therapies into their care learn how to use their time differently to engender a greater sense of satisfaction in both the women for whom they care and for themselves. Also, since so many women are now interested in complementary therapies and natural remedies in labour, offering them as part of normal maternity care fosters a greater attention to safe and appropriate use. When these "alternatives" become complementary to conventional labour care, midwives are better able to determine how they interact with mainstream medications and procedures, and to take any necessary steps to minimise risk. Midwives and doulas need to be able to advise women on appropriate ways of preparing for birth and to offer intrapartum care that includes basic complementary therapy strategies that enhance the overall experience of the mother. From a cost-saving perspective, the difference in cost between a normal birth and a Caesarean in the UK is over £1700; reducing the Caesarean section rate within a 6000-birth maternity unit from 25 per cent to 20 per cent could save 300 operative deliveries at an annual cost of over £510,000.

When searching the literature for research evidence, it can be difficult to separate studies on birth preparation, pain relief and the onset and progress of labour since the three aspects are so closely intertwined. Women who are well prepared, physically and mentally, for labour may have a different perception of the pain and discomfort caused by the uterine contractions, with lower stress levels and improved oxytocin levels. It will therefore be seen from the following discussion that many studies measure both *pain* – or a reduction in the need for conventional analgesia – and *progress* in labour – or the reduced use of oxytocics to augment contractions.

Preparation for birth

Antenatal classes

The provision of antenatal classes to prepare women and their partners for birth and parenthood has hitherto been part of mainstream maternity services in the UK. The original intention of "parentcraft classes" which commenced in the 1960s was to introduce the women to the place where they would give birth, to provide suggestions to help them prepare for labour and motherhood and to offer the opportunity for a regular "relaxation and breathing" session that introduced techniques for use in the first stage. The emphasis was on physical preparation of the mother's body to cope with the physical demands of labour. Nowadays there is greater acknowledgement of the psycho-emotional aspects of pregnancy, birth and early parenthood, and birth preparation needs to encompass this as well as preparation of the body.

Unfortunately, contemporary service demands and staff and financial shortages have impacted gravely on the provision of antenatal classes and often focus solely on preparation for the birth, with emphasis on physiology, pain relief and the environment. Many maternity units limit the number of sessions which are usually over-subscribed, and there is little individualisation (Gavin-Jones 2016). Sadly, even the traditional labour ward visit has commonly been replaced by an online "virtual tour" which may suit some women but limits the opportunities for others to obtain answers to their myriad questions about labour. Indeed, it could be argued that, for those women with acute fear of birth or hospitals, online viewing of the environment in which most will give birth could exacerbate their anxieties. Conversely, accessibility to online information (however correct or otherwise) enables women to investigate topics of interest to them and to ignore those about which they already have an understanding or which are not relevant to them.

Many women now choose alternative types of group activities, which provide them with opportunities to meet other like-minded women/ couples and to develop relationships which often last many years. It is possible that antenatal education will be removed completely from the mainstream maternity services and become an independent service which offers women a variety of options. Young (2008) found that women desire a range of classes with some being available earlier in pregnancy, as well as after delivery in the form of "birth after-thoughts" sessions. Classes need to be offered in a variety of settings, including the workplace, so that those who continue working for most of the pregnancy have an opportunity to attend. Classes for women with or without their partners should be available, and for specialist client groups, for example teenagers, women whose first language is not English or those with particular needs such as women expecting more than one baby.

In Australia, Levett et al. (2016a) developed a programme of antenatal classes in which couples were taught how to use massage, simple acupressure techniques, breathing, yoga positions and visualisation. This "Complementary Therapies for Labour and Birth" study demonstrated that women and their partners appreciated the opportunity to learn various coping strategies and enhanced their knowledge and understanding of normal birth. The team concluded that new ways of offering antenatal classes could incorporate some of these techniques and could potentially revolutionise current preparation for birth education.

"Hypnobirthing"

"Hypnobirthing" is one of the most popular forms of group activity in which pregnant women engage, and has enjoyed a real growth since the Duchess of Cambridge effectively gave it royal patronage. "Hypnobirthing" is not, in itself, a complementary therapy but a guided form of deep relaxation using some of the principles of hypnosis, but it differs considerably from clinical hypnotherapy. See Chapter 2 for information on the differences between hypnotherapy and "hypnobirthing".

Antenatal "hypnobirthing" is often described as a calm, focused state of consciousness similar to day-dreaming, with the aim of reducing stress hormones. It also provides a group environment in which women can practise relaxation techniques and which equips them to use them during labour to ease pain. In some respects, "hypnobirthing" is similar to the relaxation sessions included in the original parentcraft classes of the 1960s and 1970s, although additional visualisations are generally included now, with less overt muscle relaxation techniques. In addition to learning how to induce a sense of deep relaxation, the classes also offer couples an opportunity to learn about birth, with the emphasis on physiological labour.

When compared to contemporary conventional antenatal classes, "hypnobirthing" appears to produce a more positive mental outlook in women and an improved expectation of childbirth (Streibert et al. 2015). An Australian study concluded that the women most likely to use "hypnobirthing", or self-hypnosis in labour, tend to be those who are familiar with other complementary modalities and who generally opt to give birth in a birthing centre or at home (Steel et al. 2016). Women who practise more, especially in conjunction with their intended birthing companions, generally cope better with labour pain than those who do not practise or who expect only to start self-hypnosis as they approach term. Learning self-hypnosis is useful for women from all types of background, including adolescent mothers, one particular study demonstrating reduced complications and length of in-patient stay in this client group (Martin et al. 2001).

When using "hypnobirthing" during labour, there is often an emphasis on the use of "appropriate" language (as determined by the teacher), with practitioners expected to avoid the use of words such as "pain" and "contraction" (the latter being referred to as "surges") and on enabling the mother to labour as she wishes without being touched. Using hypnosis principles to encourage women to feel "pressure" instead of "pain" increases their self-confidence in their ability to birth their babies, and is thought to enhance maternal satisfaction and decrease fear (Abbasi et al. 2009). However, this emphasis on the use of "correct" language may, on occasions, cause difficulty for midwives who are unfamiliar with the concepts of "hypnobirthing", especially when classes are not offered by midwives in the local area. McAllister *et al.* (2017) surveyed 129 midwives, obstetricians and anaesthetists to determine their knowledge and attitudes to the use of "self-hypnosis" in labour. They found that midwives' apparent knowledge was higher than doctors' and that those who would personally use hypnosis in childbirth were both more amenable to and better informed about its use. However, this study failed adequately to differentiate between "hypnobirthing" and true clinical hypnosis and perpetuates the confusion that is rife amongst maternity professionals.

There are, in fact, several different types of what is now generically termed "hypnobirthing", a word that implies a system specifically aimed at preparing for birth. Most birth preparation methods available in the UK are fairly similar, the names often being commercially trademarked. The Mongan method, devised by the American hypnotherapist Marie Mongan, claims to be the first style to use the term *HypnoBirthing*™. The Mongan method has, however, been accused of being too rigid in its format and is often adapted by midwives in the UK to make it more appropriate for the culture in which it is used. *KG Hypnobirthing* is the method adapted by Katharine Graves, another hypnotherapist, and classes for expectant parents also include simple massage techniques for use in labour. Maggie Howell, a hypnotherapist who offers *Natal Hypnotherapy* classes for birth preparation as well as individualised hypnotherapy sessions for women with particular antenatal problems, uses a flexible individualised approach that is more closely aligned to clinical hypnosis than standardised birth preparation self-hypnosis classes. Most types of "hypnobirthing" aim to relax and calm women, providing "birth affirmations" to be practised during pregnancy and used in labour, as well as encouraging them to develop more confidence in the potential of their bodies to give birth to their babies without perceptions of excessive pain and in as normal a way as possible.

There are still relatively few studies assessing the use of "hypnosis" for labour and childbirth, a strategy which warrants further investigation (Beebe 2014). Most trials evaluate the effects of "hypnobirthing" used in labour by couples who have learned it antenatally, rather than intrapartum clinical hypnosis delivered by a practitioner in which individualised therapeutic cues are used. A systematic review by Madden *et al.* (2016) found that self-hypnosis may reduce the overall use of inhalational and intramuscular analgesia during labour, although an earlier review (Cyna *et al.* 2013) disputed this. Furthermore, Werner *et al.* (2013) and Downe *et al.* (2015) did not demonstrate any significant difference in the use of epidural anaesthesia between hypnosis and control groups. Conversely, a review of 13 controlled studies by Landolt and Milling (2011) concluded that both self-hypnosis learned during pregnancy, and intrapartum hypnosis guided by a practitioner, was effective in easing labour pain and potentially reduced the length of the first stage and improved infant Apgar scores at birth.

The largest contemporary study into self-hypnosis in pregnancy, the SHIP trial (Downe et al. 2015), aimed to establish the impact of self-hypnosis, taught to groups of primigravidae, on their use of epidural anaesthesia. This randomised controlled study was undertaken across three maternity services in the UK and involved 680 women. Women were self-selected to enter the trial and randomised to either the self-hypnosis or control group in the third trimester. Two 90-minute sessions to teach self-hypnosis to women in the intervention group were undertaken between 32 and 35 weeks gestation and women were then expected to continue at home by listening to an audio self-hypnosis disc. The primary outcome was the use of epidural anaesthesia in labour; other outcome measures included the incidence of hypertension, labour onset, interventions and outcomes, duration of first and second stage labour, Apgar scores, admissions to the neonatal unit, infant feeding method at six weeks postpartum and stillbirths. The study also explored maternal satisfaction with the birth experience and early parenting. A cost analysis was undertaken as well but was not the focus of this paper (Finlayson et al. 2015). Although there was a slight reduction in epidural use in the trial group, this was not statistically significant, neither was there any real difference in secondary clinical outcomes. There was, however, a marked reporting of improved psychological factors, with women identifying a reduction in fear and anxiety in labour compared to that anticipated before labour.

Although the authors acknowledge that other factors could have impacted on this finding, the results are similar to a Danish study by Werner et al. (2013). One of the problems for the SHIP trial (Downe et al. 2015) was that around 10 per cent of the control group reported using self-hypnosis in labour, having been trained to use it outside the trial protocol, a problem encountered by other researchers (Cyna et al. 2013; Werner et al. 2013). Further, only two sessions were allocated to teach women how to trigger the self-hypnotic state, when it is more common to offer a longer course of preparatory sessions.

The Cochrane review (Madden et al. 2016) found no clear evidence that "hypnosis" is significantly better than standard childbirth preparation. It must however be concluded that, when taught antenatally, self-hypnosis is generally appreciated by women and can be effective when used in labour for pain relief (Finlayson *et al.* 2015). Certainly, there appears to be a greater satisfaction amongst women who use self-hypnosis, with increased relaxation and reduced stress and anxiety (Kenyon 2013). It is empowering for women who can harness a heightened state of relaxation, enabling them to distance themselves mentally from the physiological discomfort of uterine muscular contractions and to focus on the impending birth of the baby.

Mindfulness

Mindfulness training is also gaining in popularity and may be especially useful for women with tocophobia. Mindfulness is a way of processing thoughts so that individuals can see more clearly what is happening in their lives and learn to focus on ways to deal with their pressures. It is a psychological way of learning to live in the moment without regret for the past or worry about the future, and to develop a better understanding of themselves and the ways they cope with stress. It may incorporate breathing, meditation, visualisations and exercise such as yoga or tai chi. Although the neurological effects of mindfulness remains unclear, preliminary results suggest that it may impact on gene expression and reverse the physiological effects of chronic stress (Buric *et al.* 2017). When set in the context of the client group, mindfulness training can be more effective than applying general principles (Aslami *et al.* 2017).

It is known that fear of childbirth contributes to greater pain perception (Alehagen, Wijma and Wijma 2001) and increased intervention (Laursen, Johansen and Hedegaard 2009). The pilot Prenatal Education About Reducing Labour Stress (PEARLS) study (Duncan *et al.* 2017) offered a weekend workshop to primigravidae approaching term and compared the study participants to a control group that received a standard childbirth preparation course. Mindfulness training was designed to address fear and anxiety regarding labour. Women in the trial group required less intrapartum analgesia and improved mental wellbeing and reduced the impact of hormonal changes in the puerperium, with less postnatal depression. Mindfulness may also enhance women's readiness for birth and motherhood (Korukcu and Kukulu 2017).

EMDR

A single-blinded study currently in progress in the Netherlands at the time of writing, the OptiMUM study (Baas *et al.* 2017), aims to address tocophobia amongst women with post-traumatic stress following a previous delivery, using eye movement desensitisation and reprocessing (EMDR). EMDR was developed in the 1980s by the psychologist Shapiro, who recognised that eye movements can reduce the intensity of traumatic thoughts. He began to treat victims of trauma with a system which appears to change the way the brain processes information. The therapy is designed to release the images, sounds and feelings from previous traumatic events so that normal brain processing is resumed and the person can view previous events in a less distressing way; this is similar in principle to mindfulness, although the practice differs. It is thought to be physiologically akin to brain activity during rapid eye movement (REM) sleep and dreaming and may involve changes in noradrenaline (Littel *et al.* 2017). Most research has focused on post-traumatic stress disorder (Boterhoven de Haan *et al.* 2017; Mevissen *et al.* 2017; Moreno-Alcázar *et al.* 2017; Schäfer *et al.* 2017), but there is sufficient evidence to apply the findings to fear of birth, especially in women with a previous poor obstetric experience.

Exercise classes

Exercise classes specifically designed for expectant mothers offer an alternative form of group activity with the intention of maintaining health and fitness in preparation for birth. They do not usually incorporate discussion on what actually happens in labour. Pilates and yoga are especially popular. However, the opportunity for women to learn postures, visualisation and breathing techniques in a safe, women-only group allowing for the sharing of worries and experiences can have a profound effect on those who attend (Campbell and Nolan 2016), especially when classes are facilitated by midwives.

Pilates

Pilates has been shown to improve flexibility, potentially aiding pelvic capacity at birth, to ease discomforts such as musculoskeletal issues and to increase maternal self-confidence in birthing and mothering abilities (Uppal *et al.* 2016). It can also help to strengthen the pelvic floor (Balogh 2005; Gomes *et al.* 2017; Hagen *et al.* 2017), although Bø and Herbert (2013) dispute this. Pregnant women who regularly practise Pilates are empowered to take control of their bodies, with reduced stress and increased mindfulness (Caldwell *et al.* 2013).

Yoga

Yoga can be pleasurable, providing a supportive environment for women preparing for birth, especially when combined with discussion and storytelling (Doran and Hornibrook 2013). However, the style of yoga should be such that the activity is largely sedentary rather than the excessive exercise of some types, such as "hot" yoga which would raise the woman's temperature excessively (Peters and Schlaff 2016), although Polis *et al.* (2015) found no adverse maternal or fetal effects in women who practised Bikram yoga. In general, yoga can have a positive physical and mental effect, reducing stress in pregnancy, which contributes to a positive approach to labour (Kusaka *et al.* 2016) and may reduce depression in some women (Battle *et al.* 2015; Davis *et al.* 2015). Yoga may contribute to decreased interventions, reduce first stage duration and alter women's perception of pain in labour so that they require less pharmacological pain relief (Jahdi *et al.* 2017). This may result from a generalised impact on stress and biomarkers such as cortisol, salivary amylase and immunoglobulins (Kusaka *et al.* 2016).

Sophrology

Sophrology involves learning a combination of dynamic physical and mental exercises that help to relax the body and calm the mind. It is commonly offered to pregnant women in France and Italy and is gradually gaining popularity in the UK. In essence, sophrology is a combination of yoga and other gentle exercise methods, breathing exercises and hypnotic suggestions. Very few research papers could be accessed, although some abstracts of French studies were found postulating that sophrology can ease anxiety and regulate breathing (Besnier 2016; Diehr 2016). A Japanese study of 220 pregnant women who practised sophrology incorporating yoga exercise, deep inspiratory and expiratory breathing, music and guided imagery revealed a reduction in stress biomarkers compared with a control group (Suzuki *et al.* 2012).

Autogenic training

Autogenic training also focuses on relaxation through the use of suggestions. It is similar to hypnosis and sophrology in its overall concept, but autogenic training is less well known. Autogenic training involves the induction of an altered state of consciousness similar to hypnosis, often incorporating progressive muscle relaxation and guided imagery. Treatment leads to a marked reduction in cortisol levels (Kiba *et al.* 2017) and may be a mechanism for reducing pain perception (Kanji 2000).

Tai chi

Field *et al.* (2013) investigated the impact of a 12-week course of combined Tai chi and yoga on a group of women with antenatal depression and achieved good results, but the effect on labour was not specifically elucidated. Tai chi may also positively impact on glucose levels in diabetic women, offering an effective system of pregnancy relaxation (Yamamoto *et al.* 2016).

Guided imagery

Guided imagery, a form of relaxation that encourages a focus on positive images, has been shown to be effective in reducing antenatal stress in pregnant teenagers (Flynn, Jones and Ausderau 2016), African American women (Jallo *et al.* 2015) and women at risk of preterm birth (Chuang *et al.* 2015). A Cochrane review (Marc *et al.* 2011) found some evidence to demonstrate that mind-body interventions such as autogenic training, biofeedback, hypnotherapy, guided imagery, meditation, prayer, tai chi and yoga may relieve stress and anxiety in late pregnancy, contributing to a more relaxed approach to labour, but there was no significant body of evidence for any one modality.

Antenatal exercises in water

Antenatal exercises in water may improve quality of life during pregnancy (Vallim *et al.* 2011). Exercising in water reduces the impact on joints and ligaments that can occur during land-based exercise, easing backache and other skeletal problems, while the hydrostatic pressure may ease oedema and enhances respiratory and gastrointestinal functioning (ACPWH 2010). It is important that the water temperature remains between 28 and 32 degrees Celsius. Very little evidence on the use of water-based exercise could be found, but two studies appear to be currently in progress, one at the University of York (Bgeginski *et al.* 2016) and the other, a more general exercise study, at the University of Swansea (the Exercise in Pregnancy Evaluative Controlled Trial – EXPECT – headed by Professor Lewis[1]).

---

1   See www.bbc.co.uk/news/uk-wales-south-west-wales-20982641

Raspberry leaf

In the UK and other developed countries, red raspberry leaf (*Rubus idaeus*) is probably one of the most commonly used self-help remedies to prepare for childbirth. Some studies have shown that up to 58 per cent of pregnant women use it (Holst, Haavik and Nordeng 2009; Nordeng *et al.* 2011). However, clinical experience and discussions of this author with numerous midwives and mothers suggest that the number of women in the UK now taking raspberry leaf in pregnancy is considerably higher, although no definitive survey has been conducted in recent years. This prevalence may be due in part to dissemination of consumer information and experience via the Internet, although most of this is insufficient to ensure safe self-administration, and sometimes it is dangerously incorrect.

Raspberry leaf is a traditional herbal remedy that was first recorded as a therapeutic agent in 1597 (Bamford, Percival and Tothill 1970), although some authorities believe it to have been used as early as the 6th century (Nordeng, Saboni and Samuelsen 2014). Raspberry leaf has long been a popular remedy for gynaecological issues such as dysmenorrhoea and menorrhagia and it has a reputation as a versatile herbal medicine for preventing miscarriage or easing pregnancy sickness (under the direction of a qualified medical herbalist) and for facilitating labour and birth. It is said to aid diuresis, enhance the immune system, stimulate bile production and purify the blood, act as an anti-ageing agent (Tito *et al.* 2015) and, due to its effect on lipid metabolism, may also aid weight loss (Morimoto *et al.* 2005).

There are several misconceptions about raspberry leaf which need clarifying. This raises the issue of whether midwives and doulas should initiate discussions with women about the use of such a popular herbal remedy. Indeed, the NMC (2009) states that midwives, at the point of registration, should be able to advise on over-the-counter herbal remedies such as raspberry leaf, yet very few students receive adequate information during training to enable them to do this. Lack of professional knowledge thus leads midwives either to decline to advise women on the subject, or to attempt to offer what they believe is correct information, but which is often wrong or, more frequently, incomplete. Given that so many women now choose to take raspberry leaf in the UK, there is an urgent need to ensure that midwives and doulas have sufficient knowledge to help them appropriately.

Many women and maternity caregivers erroneously believe that raspberry leaf is a remedy for starting labour (see Chapter 7), and it is of grave concern that over 50 per cent of midwives may be advising women to use raspberry leaf at term to avoid induction of labour (Mollart *et al.* 2017). However, it is intended as a *preparation* for birth to be taken during the third trimester. It is thought to tone smooth muscle, thus having an effect on the myometrium, ostensibly shortening pregnancy and enhancing uterine efficiency so that labour starts spontaneously and progresses normally. However, there is no direct research to support this claim, or the belief that it may also reduce pain in labour. Unless prescribed by a qualified medical herbalist, raspberry leaf should not be self-administered prior to the third trimester, nor should it be delayed until term with the intention of initiating contractions.

Raspberry leaf is oestrogenic (Eagon *et al.* 2000), rich in iron, antioxidants and antithrombotic agents (Han *et al.* 2012). However, studies on the uterine-contracting effects of raspberry leaf are inconclusive (Parsons, Simpson and Ponton 1999). Holst *et al.* (2009) elicited conflicting results and questioned its routine use by women. Reviews of animal studies by Johnson *et al.* (2009) and Zheng *et al.* (2010) suggest a dose-dependent effect, with *increased* duration of pregnancy and first stage labour with ingestion of larger doses, and at least two chemical constituents have been shown to have muscle *relaxation* effects (Rojas-Vera, Patel and Dacke 2002). Further, a study on rats by Makaji *et al.* (2011) found long-term alterations in cytochrome activity in female offspring, suggesting a possible lifelong effect on the individual's ability to metabolise toxic substances.

The question of whether raspberry leaf should be professionally promoted as a birth preparation is contentious. Women's bodies are physiologically designed to be pregnant and to labour spontaneously, but stresses of modern daily life conspire to convince women that they should try everything they can to encourage labour. This psychological pressure adds to the physical stresses of pregnancy, contributing to higher cortisol levels and adversely affecting the natural process of labour. However, as with any pharmacologically active remedy, there are certain women who should refrain from taking raspberry leaf, and women who choose to take it should be assessed to ensure that there are no contraindications or precautions. Box 8.1 summarises the contraindications and precautions.

BOX 8.1

Contraindications to the use of raspberry leaf in pregnancy

- avoid in early pregnancy unless prescribed by a qualified medical herbalist

- *not* to be used as a means of labour induction at term/post-term

- previous Caesarean section, or other uterine surgery; elective Caesarean section planned

- excessive or painful Braxton Hicks contractions (reduce dose)

- multiple pregnancy

- abnormal presentation or lie – breech, transverse, oblique, unstable lie

- placenta praevia or low-lying placenta

- antepartum haemorrhage, whether placenta praevia, abruption or incidental causes

- epilepsy, irrespective of need for medication

- hypertension, pre-eclampsia, history in previous pregnancy

- current or previous varicosities, thrombophlebitis, deep vein thrombosis

- threatened preterm labour, or history of preterm labour in previous pregnancy

- history of precipitate labour in previous pregnancy

- on anticoagulants/other drugs with anticoagulant action, or history of coagulation disorder

- any pre-existing or gestational medical condition requiring medication

- irritable bowel syndrome, Crohn's disease

- hormone-sensitive cancer – ovarian, uterine, cervical

- endometriosis, fibroids

- anaemia (dependent on cause, may affect absorption)

- diabetes mellitus.

Many ill-informed midwives and doulas, who seek to protect women from the possible risk of preterm labour, advise that raspberry leaf should not be commenced until 37 weeks gestation, but over-use at this late stage without having slowly increased the dose in the previous few weeks can lead to hypertonia. The remedy is best commenced at around 32 weeks gestation. The normal dose is between 300 and 400mg, equating to one cup of the tea or one commercially prepared tablet or capsule daily from around 32 weeks of pregnancy, increasing to two a day and then three, spread throughout the day, over the next couple of weeks. The dose should be maintained at three cups/tablets per day until term, unless there is a reason to reduce or discontinue it. It is generally considered that drinking the tea made from the fresh or dried leaves is more effective than tablets, since digestion of the coating of some products may interfere with absorption of the active ingredients. However, the duration of steeping the leaves will obviously affect the strength of the tea. It can be taken during labour if contractions are inefficient but should be avoided if prescribed oxytocics are administered. During the puerperium it may aid uterine involution but, rather than discontinuing abruptly, a gradual reduction in dose may be wise, to avoid a reactionary smooth muscle relaxation.

Possible side effects include excessively strong Braxton Hicks contractions, in which case women should be advised to reduce the dose, or discontinue it if preterm labour is threatened. If a woman is admitted to the maternity unit in preterm labour for which no direct cause can be found, she should be asked if she has taken raspberry leaf (or any other natural remedies) and, if so, advised to discontinue or reduce it. Headaches can occur in some women due to vasoconstriction in the cerebral vessels, although this is not common. Raspberry leaf may cause hypoglycaemia and affect insulin requirements in women with diabetes mellitus (Cheang et al. 2016). Excessive consumption during labour once contractions are well established may theoretically lead to hypertonic uterine action. Postnatal mothers with significant retained products of conception should avoid taking large quantities: although raspberry leaf may assist in emptying of the uterus, it may in this case lead to torrential secondary postpartum haemorrhage. Conversely, those who experienced primary postpartum haemorrhage may benefit from taking raspberry leaf for its iron content.

Pain relief in labour

Women across the world universally appear to accept that childbirth is painful, and seek various means of dealing with it, including folk remedies, massage and other manual techniques. The use of natural remedies and complementary techniques, often classified erroneously as "non-pharmacological" methods, can offer women choices, empower them and provide psychological and physiological benefits, without adverse materno-fetal effects (when used correctly) (Chaillet *et al.* 2014). Lindholm and Hildingsson's study (2015) examined women's pain relief preferences and found, unsurprisingly, that the most popular methods were those most commonly available to women, including relaxation and breathing, massage, warm water, inhalational analgesia and epidural anaesthesia. Epidural anaesthesia was associated with a less positive birth experience, irrespective of whether this had been the first choice for pain relief. However, Jones *et al.* (2012) reach variable conclusions about the effectiveness of different strategies, suggesting that water, relaxation, acupuncture and massage may work, but citing insufficient evidence for the use of hypnosis, aromatherapy and TENS. Despite this, it is interesting to see how, in developed countries, modern maternity care is moving away from pharmacological analgesia and turning to a whole range of traditional and natural remedies which offer simple and relatively safe methods of supporting women at this time.

The birthing environment

Irrespective of whether women choose to give birth at home, in a birth centre or a main obstetric maternity unit, the birthing environment can influence their experiences of pain in labour. The calm, peaceful atmosphere generated in the mother's own home or in many of the midwife-led birthing centres contributes to relaxation and a consequent lowering of cortisol and other stress hormones. Jenkinson, Josey and Kruske (2014) provide a very comprehensive and evidence-based guide to designing an optimum birth environment, considering the room, its windows, doors, furniture, bathroom facilities and privacy, and ways to provide a safe and comfortable place in which the woman can birth her baby.

A room in which the lighting can be dimmed is invaluable and makes the room appear less clinical, as can the avoidance of walls painted white or cream (Newburn and Singh 2003; Stenglin and Foureur 2013). Using the principles of colour therapy, blues, purples, pinks or greens, in a variety of shades, are considered to be the most relaxing colours, and the use of visually attractive artworks and wall murals acts as a distraction (Dalke *et al.* 2006 cited by Jenkinson *et al.* 2014). In colour therapy (chromotherapy), the energy relating to each of the seven spectrum colours of red, orange, yellow, green, blue, indigo and violet is said to resonate with the energy of each of the seven main *chakras* or energy centres of the body. Colour is absorbed by the eyes, skin and skull, impacting on our magnetic energy field and influencing our physical, emotional and spiritual wellbeing. Colour therapists believe that babies first experience colour in the intrauterine environment, being enveloped in a nurturing and comforting field of pink; in later life, associations with different colours may be positive or negative and colour therapy assists in rebalancing the individual's relationship with the colours around us in everyday life. Yousuf Azeemi and Mohsin Raza (2005) provide an interesting analysis of chromotherapy, its scientific evolution and its application to clinical practice.

The safe, private place of birth should also encourage closeness between the labouring woman and her chosen birth companion, and helps to engage the partner in the birthing experience. Couples who view childbirth as a sexual experience should be able, if they so wish, to engage in intimate activities. For some, childbirth is not only a bio-psycho-social experience but also the ultimate sexual experience and orgasm can have a profound effect, both on pain perception and progress in labour, not least through the release of oxytocin (Mayberry and Daniel 2016). Others may wish to have their children present, and this should be considered when arranging a suitable birth setting.

Simple, inexpensive strategies such as listening to music may aid relaxation, decrease fear and anxiety and ease pain, reducing the need for pharmacological analgesia, both during labour and postnatally (Liu, Chang and Chen 2010; Simavli *et al.* 2014). Laopaiboon *et al.* (2009) also suggest that playing music for women having Caesarean section under regional anaesthesia may enhance the maternal experience and aid wellbeing. Using music in a therapeutic way during labour has also been shown to reduce postnatal pain, anxiety and depression and enhance maternal satisfaction with the overall childbearing experience (Simavli *et al.* 2014).

Although some authorities advocate the provision of a complete sensory approach to care in labour (Gutteridge 2014), the use of aromatherapy oils is more controversial. Respiratory reactions can occur in susceptible people exposed to the chemicals in the aromas, potentially causing sensory irritation in the nasal passages or, more severely, bronchial hyper-reactivity which is characterised by reflex bronchospasm, dyspnoea and air hunger. Some essential oils may also cause sensory hyper-reactivity in those with asthma or hay fever, due to an association with the aromas of plants that act as triggers. It is difficult to determine which essential oils are most likely to cause respiratory reactions or to identify which women (or others exposed to the aromas such as the partner or caregivers) could be sensitive to the oils. This means that the intrapartum use of diffusers or vaporisers is inappropriate, unethical and may be acutely dangerous in some circumstances. Aromatic diffusion should *never* be undertaken in public areas such as corridors, communal patient sitting rooms or staff areas. See Tiran (2016a).

Use of water

Labouring in water is internationally popular and a well-researched subject (Nutter *et al.* 2014). It has become almost standard in many maternity units, and structured professional development has helped to enhance midwives' knowledge and skills in working with women requesting pool labour and/or birth (Russell *et al.* 2014). However, water birth is a specialist aspect of midwifery care in its own right and it is not the intention of this book to discuss the subject in any detail. Interested readers are referred to Garland (2017) for further information.

The use of hot or cold water compresses applied to the abdominal fundus, suprapubic or lumbosacral region is also popular and can be useful for some women. Warm heat packs, or intermittent heat and cold applied to the sacrum, may be equally effective (Behmanesh, Pasha and Zeinalzadeh 2009; Ganji *et al.* 2013). Other researchers have investigated the use of heat applied to the sacrum and to the perineum during active labour, finding beneficial effects on both labour pain and maternal satisfaction (Taavoni, Abdolahian and Haghani 2013). Conversely, ice applied to a specific acupuncture point may have some benefit (Can and Saruhan 2015). Dehcheshmeh and Rafiei (2015) also used ice massage on an acupuncture point, but in this study it was compared to the use of music and to standard care. Although both ice and music proved more effective than standard care in reducing pain perception, music was slightly more effective than ice massage. However, ice application may be more long-lasting than simple thumb and finger acupressure applied to the same points (see also acupuncture, below) (Abd El Fadeel Abd el Hamid Afefy 2015; Hajiamini *et al.* 2012).

Injections of sterile water into sacral points that relate to the uterine nerve pathways may be useful for some women (Hutton *et al.* 2009), although NICE (2017b) does not recommend them. This technique claims to have an instantaneous effect with no change in maternal consciousness and no adverse effects on fetal wellbeing. It does not limit mobility and has no apparent impact on labour progress. The sacral points used are the same location as for the transducer pads for TENS. These same points relate to specific acupuncture points known to ease labour pain via the gate control mechanism of pain relief, particularly when there is an occipito-posterior fetal position. An early study by Labrecque *et al.* (1999) demonstrated that sterile water injections are more effective at relieving back pain in labour than TENS, whilst Lundberg (2008) found them to be more effective than acupuncture. Similarly, although acupuncture can be very effective (see below), water injections are often preferred by women (Mårtensson, Stener-Victorin and Wallin 2008). However, Mello, Nóbrega and Lemos (2011) and Derry *et al.* (2012) dispute the efficacy of sterile water injections in alleviating labour pain.

Movement and posture

It has long been known that adopting various postures and being ambulant in labour can help the woman progress through her labour. The incorporation of dance-like movements, including pelvic tilting and hip rocking and rotating, may ease pain and increase maternal satisfaction (Abdolahian *et al.* 2014). Yoga postures can also be effective in easing pain, as well as facilitating fetal progress through the pelvis during birth as a result of movements that impact on pelvic joints and ligaments. Unfortunately, the NICE intrapartum guideline (2017b) does not recommend the use of yoga in labour, due to perceived lack of robust evidence. Surely, however, the mother should be facilitated to engage in whatever activity suits her at the time?

Many dance movements and yoga postures incorporated into first stage labour are similar to those achieved with the rebozo technique used by South American birth attendants, although midwives more commonly use rebozo for fetal malposition such as occipito-posterior than primarily for pain relief (Iversen *et al.* 2017). A rebozo is a shawl used to aid the birth process by acting as a support for the abdomen. Rebozo is becoming increasingly popular in western midwifery (Cohen and Thomas 2015). A retrospective Danish study conducted telephone interviews with postnatal mothers who had used rebozo in labour. It found that women were generally satisfied with having used rebozo; they reported less pain and valued the close relationship between themselves and their midwives. Similarly, the use of a birthing ball can aid fetal positioning and comfort (Taavoni *et al.* 2016), especially when women have been introduced to the concept as part of antenatal preparation for birth (Miquelutti, Cecatti and Makuch 2013).

The use of touch

Massage is a traditional childbirth technique used in all cultures of the world (Anarado *et al.* 2015; McCauley, Stewart and Kebede 2017; Zeng *et al.* 2014). It is especially valuable in labour, facilitating a close physical and emotional bond with the person providing the massage and enabling the application of firm pressure to areas of tension and pain. It is relaxing and may contribute to a shortening of the first and second stages of labour (Bolbol-Haghighi *et al.* 2016) and may reduce epidural use (Janssen, Shroff and Jaspar 2012). Massage is easily learned and can be taught to partners and birth companions in pregnancy. Many women prefer back massage, especially lumbosacral techniques if there is an occipito-posterior position, whilst others enjoy massage of the neck and shoulders, limbs or head. In some cultures abdominal massage is often performed by traditional birth attendants in rural areas to encourage fetal descent (Wanyua *et al.* 2014), although such firm pressure is not generally encouraged in western countries. Gentle clockwise effleurage (stroking) of the abdomen can, however, be pleasant for some women, although abdominal massage should be avoided if the placenta is situated on the anterior uterine wall, as over-zealous stimulation could theoretically cause placental separation.

Unfortunately, the NICE intrapartum guidelines (2017b) condescendingly sanction the use of massage in labour when performed by birth companions who have been taught how to use it, but advise that massage should not be offered by midwives as a form of pain relief in the latent phase or in established labour as there is, apparently, a paucity of evidence to support its use. This is an example of arbitrary dependence on randomised controlled trials when massage is a universally popular strategy which women often find satisfying and effective, irrespective of the availability of formal evidence. Massage performed by trained professionals would surely be potentially safer and more appropriate to the woman's condition, and there is absolutely no logic to the statement permitting partners to use massage whilst discouraging caregivers from using it. This is somewhat confusing, since NICE bases its recommendations on currently available evidence, much of which the working party seems not to have accessed. Either massage is safe, irrespective of whoever performs it, or it is not. Given that midwives have incorporated massage and touch into their care of women for centuries, to good effect and without any known major adverse reactions, it seems to be a retrograde step to discourage its use now.

McNabb *et al.* (2006) developed a programme to teach couples antenatally how to perform massage in labour. They found significantly lower intrapartum pain, although cortisol levels, assessed immediately post-birth, were similar to those for women who had not received massage during the first stage of labour. Chang, Wang and Chen (2002) conducted a randomised controlled study in Taiwan to assess pain and anxiety levels during labour in women who received massage compared to those who did not. Whilst there was, as expected, a steady increase in pain in both groups as labour progressed, the massage group showed significantly lower pain scores in the latent, active and transitional stages of labour, although there was less effect on anxiety levels.

When compared to music or standard care, massage appears to offer a simple, low-cost option for labouring women (Kimber *et al.* 2008; Taghinejad, Delpisheh and Suhrabi 2010). Kamalifard *et al.* (2012) compared first stage massage to breathing techniques, demonstrating reduced pain from both strategies and an apparent reduction in Caesarean sections. However, as there was no control group receiving standard care alone, it is difficult to interpret these results with any certainty. One variation between the two groups was that massage appeared to be most effective at around 4–5cm of cervical dilatation, whereas breathing techniques had a more consistent effect across all phases of the first stage of labour.

Whilst massage can be performed with any medium that prevents the friction of direct skin-to-skin contact, including carrier oils (e.g. grapeseed, sweet almond), talcum powder or even soap, many women and midwives now like to receive massage enhanced with aromatherapy essential oils (see Chapter 2 for precautions). The use of aromatherapy is increasingly widespread in labour, the chemicals in the essential oils, together with the effect of administering them via massage, potentially contributing to reducing pain, aiding progress and normalising birth. Suitable analgesic oils include black pepper (*Piper nigrum*) and common lavender (*Lavandula angustifolia*), whilst those which are mood-enhancing can contribute to an improved sense of wellbeing and a perceived reduction in pain. Sweet orange (*Citrus aurantium*), geranium (*Pelargonium graveolens*) and lavender oils have been shown to reduce anxiety in labour, thereby altering pain perception (Rashidi-Fakari, Tabatabaeichehr, Kamali *et al.* 2015; Rashidi-Fakari, Tabatabaeichehr and Mortazavi 2015; Vakilian and Keramat 2013; Zahra and Leila 2013). In these studies, the mode of delivery of the oils was, however, not via massage but through respiratory administration with individualised doses of the oils via an individually administered taper or on a swab or similar.

Burns *et al.* (2000) conducted a large evaluative study of 8085 women who received intrapartum aromatherapy over an eight-year period, in Oxford, UK. Midwives trained to use 12 essential oils offered aromatherapy, with or without massage, to labouring women who fitted the inclusion criteria. Women enjoyed the relaxation effects of the aromatherapy treatment – and midwives enjoyed giving the treatments, which also had an unexpected effect in improving the recruitment and retention of midwives. There were very few maternal side effects to the oils, all of which were relatively minor, such as nausea, headache or itching skin. There were no fetal/neonatal adverse reactions. Although this was not a randomised controlled trial and has not therefore been included in the NICE guideline on intrapartum care, the sheer size of the study gives credence to the results. Two essential oils, chamomile (*Chamomilla reticulata*) and clary sage (*Salvia sclarea*), appeared to be particularly effective at relieving pain. This analgesic effect on the uterus has also been shown in non-pregnant women with dysmenorrhoea (Hur *et al.* 2012; Ou *et al.* 2012). See also Chapter 7 on post-dates pregnancy.

However, clary sage should be used with care once contractions are well established as over-use can lead to uterine hypertonia and consequent fetal distress. Whilst the evidence that aromatherapy reduced the need for other analgesia was not statistically significant, the overall use of systemic opioids in the unit decreased from 6 per cent to less than 1 per cent over a six-year period. It is difficult to state, however, whether this was due to the pharmacology of the essential oils, the analgesic effects of massage, the change in women's relationships with their midwives, or a combination of factors.

Unfortunately, this large study was not a randomised controlled trial (RCT), so it is not acknowledged in the NICE intrapartum guidelines (2017b), despite being the largest ever study on aromatherapy and childbirth. However, a later study (Burns *et al.* 2007) investigated whether it was possible to use RCT methodology to study aromatherapy use in labour. There appeared to be a greater reduction in pain in the intervention group, and more babies of women in the control group were transferred to the neonatal unit, but the authors acknowledged that the study was underpowered. Despite this, these two studies provide some useful information on aromatherapy for pain relief in labour.

However, careful interpretation of research results is necessary to avoid making assumptions about the use of aromatherapy in labour.

More importantly, although there is a trend to demonstrate that "aromatherapy" as a concept has some value in relieving labour pain, some recent studies have used essential oils that are considered unsafe in pregnancy and labour. For example, Kaviani *et al.* (2014) used jasmine (*Jasminum officinale*) and common sage (*Salvia officinale*) oils, the latter being completely contraindicated in maternity work due to its high content of potentially harmful chemicals, including the very real risk of antepartum or postpartum haemorrhage with large doses. Overall, despite a phenomenal interest amongst mothers and midwives in the use of aromatherapy for pain relief in labour, evidence of good calibre is lacking, leading the Cochrane review (Smith *et al.* 2011a) to conclude that there is insufficient evidence to support its use in labour and NICE (2017b) to recommend that it should not "be offered or advised" for women in either the latent or active phases of labour. This is not helpful given the number of UK maternity units now offering aromatherapy, but it is true that more research on the use of specific essential oils in labour is required, and greater attention by midwives to understanding the chemistry underpinning the mechanism of action is vital.

Research on the use of reflexology in labour suggests that it may have a beneficial effect on women's perceptions of pain. Several Middle Eastern studies appear to offer similar treatments, with control groups receiving standard care. Dolation *et al.* (2011) provided women entering the active phase of labour with a 40-minute session of reflexology, emotional support or standard care. Pain severity was assessed via a visual analogue scale at 4–5cm, 6–7cm and 8–10cm of cervical dilatation and shown to be statistically significantly lower in the reflexology group compared to the emotional support and standard care groups. There also appeared to be a slight decrease in the duration of the first stage, which may have been due to a reduction in cortisol from the relaxing effects of the reflexology. Moghimi-Hanjani *et al.* (2015) and Dolatian *et al.* (2011) also conducted controlled reflexology studies on labouring women. The studies produced similar results, with reflexology appearing to decrease pain intensity, anxiety and duration of the first stage; Dolatian *et al.* claimed an effect not only on the duration of the first stage, but also the second and third stages of labour. Another Middle Eastern study (Valiani *et al.* 2010) compared general care with specific reflexology techniques in the active phase of labour and found reduced reported pain in the women who received reflexology; there was also a corresponding decrease in first stage duration.

However, all of these studies were undertaken in countries where labour care involves frequent examinations per vaginam and other routine medical interventions, a factor which may contribute to women's perception of greater discomfort. It is possible that the reflexology could have been simply a placebo effect, especially as the numbers of participants in the studies were generally fairly small. Further, no detailed description of the nature of the reflexology treatment was given in any of the papers, nor was the specific style of reflexology identified. The short duration of treatment was not justified in clinical terms and appears arbitrary. Although researchers in each of these studies described the interventions as "reflexology", it may have been simply an adapted foot massage rather than the appropriate stimulation or sedation of specific reflex points for individual clinical indications (see Tiran 2010b).

In the UK, midwives providing reflexology during labour are more likely to perform short repeated sessions, responding to the woman's needs, position and mobility. Ten-minute specific reflexology techniques may be adapted according to whether the woman is in pain, anxious, nauseous or needing treatment to aid progress. It is unlikely that a single session of reflexology would be sufficient to facilitate a woman's progress throughout labour, although it may act as a means of relaxation and easing anxiety on admission to the birth centre or delivery suite. Despite the lack of good quality research, however, reflexology can be helpful in labour. Specific reflex zone therapy techniques can be employed to loosen pelvic joints and ligaments and to relieve pelvic congestion, particularly in a prolonged labour. Women seem to enjoy the hands-on approach, although it is unclear how intrapartum reflexology differs from massage, with or without essential oils.

Stimulation of acupuncture points

TENS has been used to good effect for pain relief following both normal birth and Caesarean section (Kayman-Kose et al. 2014). This works by stimulating the sacral foramen points in the lower back, intercepting neural pathways to the uterus and relieving pain via the gate control theory (Melzack and Wall 1965). These points also correspond to certain acupuncture points used for pain relief and labour progress (see below).

A systematic review of TENS in labour (Mello, Nóbrega and Lemos 2011) found nine studies in which women in the first stage had used TENS, but there was no statistically different reported pain relief, use of other analgesia or other outcome measures. The NICE intrapartum guidelines (2017b) recommend that TENS is not offered to women in labour since there does not appear to be sufficient evidence to support its use.

Conversely, Santana *et al.* (2016) conducted a randomised trial of TENS commenced at the beginning of the active phase of labour. The study demonstrated that, although there was no change in the location or distribution of pain, there was a statistically significant variation between the experimental and control groups in terms of pain reduction and the time between the intervention and the need for pharmacological analgesia. In practice, as there is little evidence of any risks of using TENS in term labour, women should be supported if they wish to use it. TENS offers an inexpensive but potentially effective means of pain relief that may avoid the need for more expensive and risky analgesia such as epidural anaesthesia.

NB TENS should not be used prior to term as there is a small possibility that it may trigger labour contractions because the transducers are positioned over acupuncture points used to stimulate contractions (see below).

The increasing interest in acupuncture has led to many authorities exploring its use for pain relief in labour, either as needling or via thumb and finger stimulation (acupressure). Stimulation of specific acupoints appears to raise maternal satisfaction and reduce pain and the need for pharmacological analgesia including epidural anaesthesia (Smith *et al.* 2011b). Midwives in Germany, Austria, Iceland and other countries often train in maternity acupuncture so they can include it in routine midwifery care in labour, and UK midwives are starting to follow this trend.[2]

When compared to pethidine, acupuncture appears to have a greater analgesic effect within 30 minutes of administration during the first stage but is understandably less effective in the transition phase (Allameh, Tehrani and Ghasemi 2015). Other researchers have concluded that, whilst acupuncture can offer good pain relief, and may have an impact on the duration of labour, it does not appear to reduce the likelihood of Caesarean section (Mafetoni and Shimo 2015).

Ozgoli *et al.* (2016) conducted a randomised controlled study of 105 primigravidae in established labour to assess whether acupressure stimulation had an effect on perceived pain levels. The women were randomly allocated to receive standard labour care only, or to one of two groups to receive acupressure. Of these, one group received acupressure to the Large Intestine 4 point on the hand and the other group received stimulation to the Bladder 32 acupressure point in the lumbar area. Acupressure was given during contractions when the cervix was assessed as being 4–5 cm, 6–7 cm and 8–10 cm dilated. Acupressure was found to be more pain-relieving

---

2   See www.expectancy.co.uk/acupuncture

than standard care, but there were some interesting variations between the two acupressure points. Stimulation of the Bladder 32 acupoint was more effective at relieving pain in earlier labour when there was less cervical dilatation, but no significant difference was found between the Bladder 32 and Large Intestine 4 acupoints as women approached the transition stage. Acupoints Bladder 2 and Spleen 6 were stimulated with electro-acupuncture in a randomised controlled study by Dong *et al.* (2015). In clinical practice it would be normal practice to use a combination of both these and other acupuncture points, altering them according to the stage of labour and the woman's individual needs.

Other studies have also investigated the use of thumb and finger pressure (acupressure) to the Large Intestine 4 and Bladder 32 acupoints, although Large Intestine 4 seems to be the point of choice, perhaps as it is more easily located and can be stimulated by the caregiver or the labouring woman herself (see Figure 8.1). In India, Sebastian (2014) compared Large Intestine 4 stimulation with conventional care, also concluding that acupressure is an effective analgesic. Dabiri and Shahi (2014) randomised 149 women to receive either acupressure to the Large Intestine 4 acupoint or general touch; both were compared to a matched group of women who received no complementary or conventional pain relief at all. Acupressure or general touch was applied during contractions for a period of 30 minutes during the active first stage of labour. Although acupressure had no significant effect on the duration of labour, there was a statistically significant difference in the use of acupressure for pain relief. Whilst it is understandable in research terms that a short period of treatment would be assessed, it would be preferable for acupressure to be used intermittently throughout the first stage, irrespective of duration.

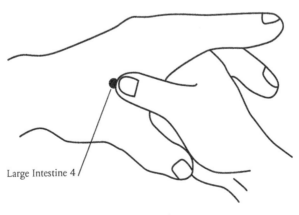

Figure 8.1 Location of the Large Intestine 4 acupoint

Vixner, Mårtensson and Schytt (2015) undertook a long-term follow-up to an earlier study (Vixner *et al.* 2014) which had demonstrated that neither manual nor electro-acupuncture significantly affected pain levels, although it did reduce the need for other methods of pain relief, including epidural anaesthesia. This secondary analysis explored the data from the previous RCT to assess women's recollections of labour pain, comparing manual acupuncture, electro-acupuncture and standard care. The 303 women in the original study were asked to complete questionnaires on the day following the birth and, again, two months later. There was considerable difference between the groups in the perception of pain immediately following delivery, but at two months postpartum, women in both groups retrospectively evaluated their labour pain as having been similar, despite those in the acupuncture groups having required less conventional analgesia. See also Chapter 7 for more on the specific acupoints used to stimulate contractions.

Homeopathic remedies

Women who are familiar with homeopathic remedies may wish to use them in labour, although there is very little research evidence to support efficacy or safety. In one study in Pakistan, chamomilla, popularly used by traditional birth attendants, was compared to pentazocine and to placebo (Zafar *et al.* 2016). Although both interventions were better at relieving pain than placebo, there was no statistical difference between the homeopathic remedy and the pharmacological drug, neither being found in this study to offer substantial intrapartum pain relief. Whilst searching the literature, several Internet references were found to an old French double-blinded study on the use of homeopathy in labour but the full text was unavailable (Dorfman, Arnal-Lassiere and Tetau 1986). This study apparently demonstrated that homeopathy helped to reduce duration of labour, but the remedies used were not specified in the abstract.

In general clinical practice there are, however, several homeopathic remedies that may prove useful for pain relief in labour, although the overall symptom picture must be taken into account. For example, the nature, duration and location of the contractions may differ from one woman to the next, thus requiring different remedies. Table 8.1 gives a few examples of homeopathic remedies for pain relief, although this list is not exhaustive and specific remedies would be prescribed according to the woman's individual situation.

Table 8.1 Homeopathic remedies for pain relief in labour

	Caulophyllum	Chamomilla	Cimicifuga	Nux vomica	Pulsatilla	Sepia
Features	Short distressing spasmodic contractions, sharp cramps in pelvic ligaments, flying in all directions, fever, thirsty, faint, nausea Exhausted	Contractions unbearable, tear round abdomen, shooting down inner legs, back pain, protracted labour, hot perspiration, nausea, thirsty	Contractions come if woman is cool, stop when hot, tearing, flying around abdomen, cramp in hip, twitching, chilly, faint	Severe irregular contractions, spasmodic, drawing sensation in back and thighs, cramps in hands and legs, urge to pass urine, defaecate, headache, faintness, exhaustion, possibly in preterm labour	Distressing, irregular, ineffective contractions, cutting, pressing in back, appear suddenly, ease gradually; pale face, thirstless, dry mouth, faintness, nausea, vomiting	Severe spasmodic shooting contractions, extend upwards, felt in back, sensation of weight in anus; cold extremities with heat flushes, faintness
Emotionally	Fretful, irritable	"I can't bear it", rude, nervous, moaning, over-sensitive to noise and pain	Talks incessantly even during contractions, hysterical, complaining, restless, says she will go crazy	Over-sensitive, especially to touch, irritable, nervous	Changeable, apologetic, wants sympathy, distressed	Snappy, irritable, indifferent, says she has had enough
Better for	Cool fresh air	Cool fresh air			Fresh air	Crossing legs
Worse for	Cold	Noise and pain	Noise and pain		Movement of fetus	

Unfortunately, the politics affecting homeopathy credibility in the UK means that it is less prominent in the choices for analgesia in childbirth, even by women who are very familiar with complementary therapies. Conversely, in Germany, Austria, Switzerland and eastern European countries, midwives frequently administer homeopathic medicines alongside conventional drugs for pain relief, with reported good effects (Hrgovic *et al.* 2010; Münstedt, Brenken and Kalder 2009).

Progress in labour

It must be remembered that labour is a normal physiological process for which, normally, no intervention should be necessary, either to initiate or accelerate contractions. Injudicious augmentation with natural remedies can be detrimental to the overall progress of the labour, but the selective use of complementary therapies can be helpful, especially for a long latent phase of labour or in the event of previously good contractions slowing down. In this latter case it is important to utilise one's midwifery skills first to assess the woman's condition and to eliminate or deal with factors that may be adversely affecting contractions, such as a full bladder, hypoglycaemia, nausea, fear, pain or obstructed labour. Many aspects of complementary therapy can be employed to reduce fear, anxiety and pain before resorting to those that aim specifically to accelerate uterine contractions.

Clary sage (*Salvia sclarea*) is an essential oil of particular concern. Women seem to be aware that clary sage can be helpful in aiding progress in labour, but often they erroneously use it prior to term, perhaps in an attempt to prepare for labour, rather than to trigger contractions (for detailed information on clary sage, see Chapter 7). Lack of understanding, however, means that some women continue using it in labour, even when pharmacological oxytocics are administered. Online support groups for pregnant women are awash with comments about using clary sage before and during labour, with almost all being unsafe and inappropriate suggestions. Midwives frequently report issues arising due to excessive use of clary sage, both in terms of hypertonia and fetal distress and adverse effects on themselves and others present at the labour. Midwives attempting to conceive or those who are pregnant, as well as caregivers who may be menstruating, should avoid inhaling the vapours of clary sage and other oils known to be uterotonic (e.g. jasmine, rose). Clary sage does not only have an impact on the uterus but also acts as a relaxant, sometimes causing drowsiness, which can be a problem for those needing to make clinical decisions in an emergency, or to drive. It is now a priority to educate women about the possible dangers of inadvertent over-use of clary sage.

In practice, it is important to examine the whole picture rather than considering pain relief and progress in labour as two separate entities, since the one may impact on the other. As is seen with homeopathic prescribing, viewing the woman as a whole, including her personality and the way in which she deals with her labour and the factors that exacerbate or improve her wellbeing, assists in choosing the most appropriate strategy to help her. Many of the remedies used for pain relief in labour are also those appropriate for aiding progress, since the prescription is made for the *woman*, not for the *condition*.

As with natural induction for post-dates pregnancy, acupuncture and acupressure can be an effective, simple and non-invasive method of stimulating uterine contractions that is relatively well evidenced, compared to other complementary therapies. Midwives can be taught selected acupressure points and the method of stimulation and incorporate these into normal intrapartum care without the risk of any major problems. Many acupuncture and acupressure studies simultaneously address pain relief needs and duration of labour (see below), and the points used are often the same as those for induction of labour (see Chapter 7). Mollart *et al.* (2015) conducted a systematic review of seven trials investigating acupressure on the onset and duration of labour as well as pain relief. The most commonly used acupoints were Spleen 6 and Large Intestine 4, both of which appeared to contribute to reduction in the first stage of labour.

In Turkey, Mucuk and Baser (2014) compared the Large Intestine 4 acupoint to stimulation of the Spleen 6 acupoint on the leg, and both were compared with a control group. Acupoint stimulation in this study was not by thumb or finger pressure but with the use of a transcutaneous electrical nerve stimulator "pen". Labour pain visual analogue scores and duration of labour were lower in the acupoint stimulation group and, although the difference was not statistically significant, it was concluded that this technique could offer an easily implemented method of easing pain in the first stage of labour. The team (Mucuk, Baser and Ozkan 2013) had previously shown that this method of pain relief reduced serum cortisol and adrenocorticotrophic hormone levels, suggesting, at the very least, that reducing stress hormones facilitates women's coping strategies, altering their perception of contraction pain and indirectly aiding progress in labour. However, the acupoints used in both studies are used primarily to aid onset and progress of contractions, and use for pain relief in established labour could theoretically increase the risk of hypertonic uterine action. See Chapter 7 for more debate on these points.

Women's inappropriate use of pharmacologically active herbal medicines to augment labour is of concern as very little scientific work has been undertaken on their potential risks, or even on their possible therapeutic benefits. In particular, women seem to select plant remedies aimed at enhancing contractions in order to shorten labour duration. Black cohosh (*Cimicifuga racemosa*) and blue cohosh (*Caulophyllum thalictroides*) are two herbal remedies commonly used by American nurse-midwives, but more usually to induce than to augment labour (see Chapter 7). Crampbark (*Viburnum opulus*), skullcap (*Scutellaria lateriflora*), motherwort (*Leonarus cardiaca*) and other herbs are also used, both for pain relief and for induction or acceleration of labour. Midwives and doulas should enquire of women whether they are using any herbal medicines in order to be alert to their potential to disturb uterine polarity or interact with prescribed medications.

Retained placenta

The third stage of labour is usually considered to be the most potentially hazardous for the mother in terms of possible haemorrhage. Thus, the use of complementary therapies and natural remedies for retained placenta should only be undertaken by midwives with a thorough understanding of the third stage of labour, an appreciation of the individual mother's specific condition and a precise knowledge of the physiological effects of the chosen modality. For example, it would be inappropriate to use an essential oil thought to cause smooth muscle contraction if it was thought that the placenta had separated and was situated within the cervix; in this case, treatment would require a remedy or technique to *relax* the cervix to facilitate expulsion of the placenta. Similarly, employing an acupuncture or acupressure technique with the aim of encouraging downwards movement (of the placenta) may be inappropriate if the placenta is morbidly adherent, as this could theoretically lead to uterine inversion.

However, there have been some case reports and small studies included in the literature on the use of complementary therapies and natural remedies to aid placental separation and expulsion. A retrospective case note review of women with retained placenta in a Danish hospital was undertaken by

Chauhan, Gasser and Chauhan (1998). Of these, 45 had needed manual placental removal while 30 received acupuncture, 25 of whom expelled the placenta without further complications within 20 minutes; of the remaining five women, four were later found to have placenta accreta. The incidence of haemorrhage following placental expulsion was 13 per cent in the acupuncture group compared to 47 per cent in the manual removal group. In a more recent review, Djakovic et al. (2015) suggested that first and second stage acupuncture may reduce delay in the third stage by facilitating placental separation. López-Garrido et al. (2015) undertook a randomised controlled study in Spain of 76 women in the third stage of labour, administering either true acupuncture to the relevant acupoints or sham acupuncture, and found statistically significant differences in the time from birth of the baby to expulsion of the placenta and membranes. The true acupuncture group had a third stage of around five minutes, whilst the sham acupuncture group had an average time of over 15 minutes.

Combining complementary therapies for labour care

The current trends in relation to the use of complementary therapies and natural remedies during labour focus primarily on easing pain and aiding progress. However, all practitioners, whether midwives, doulas or independent complementary therapists, must be able to apply a working knowledge of the mechanism of the individual therapies to the practice of those therapies in intrapartum care, based on a comprehensive understanding of labour physiology and how over-zealous use of "natural" therapies could potentially interfere with normal uterine action or interact with prescribed medication. Further, whilst an experienced midwife trained in a range of complementary therapies may be able to justify using a combination of strategies at this time, others need to be mindful of the effects of one therapy on another. For example, if a woman wishes to administer homeopathic remedies, aromatherapy oils should not be used on or near the woman as these will inactivate the chemically fragile homeopathic medicines. Table 8.2 outlines precautions relevant to therapies that are popularly used in labour (see also Chapter 2).

Table 8.2 Precautions to the use of complementary therapies and natural remedies commonly used in labour

Acupuncture	• check all needles are accounted for and disposed correctly • normal infection control precautions • do not use acupuncture points on the back with epidural *in situ*
Aromatherapy	• do not use clary sage, jasmine or rose oils with oxytocics • avoid hypotensive oils with epidural anaesthesia • essential oils should not be added to the birthing pool water • in the obstetric unit, keep one or two labour rooms completely aromatherapy-free for women with high-risk pregnancies/labours • do not use in anaesthetic room or theatre • pregnant midwives should not be exposed to uterotonic oils
Herbal medicine	• women should be advised to inform midwife if they wish to self-administer herbal remedies, herbal teas, aromatherapy oils • do not use herbal medicines/teas aimed at increasing contractions once labour is well established • avoid all herbal remedies with prescribed medication in labour, particularly oxytocics • avoid all herbal remedies if Caesarean section is required, or if woman has coagulation disorder or haemorrhage
Homeopathy	• use only one remedy at a time • careful prescribing according to the woman's precise symptom picture, to avoid reverse proving from use of incorrect remedy • should not be used with aromatherapy oils or herbal teas such as peppermint – will be inactivated
Hypnosis/ "hypnobirthing"	• observe woman for state of consciousness throughout labour
Massage	• avoid abdominal massage if placenta is situated on anterior wall of uterus • avoid over-stimulation of acupressure points that aid contractions particularly if labour is well established
Reflexology	• avoid direct stimulation of reflex zone for pituitary gland unless there is a specific indication to stimulate, e.g. contractions, retained placenta • NEVER stimulate or sedate the reflex zone for the uterus – theoretically may cause placental separation • only stimulate reflex zone for the pituitary if contractions need to be augmented prior to oxytocics, but care once syntocinon in progress

Conclusion

Labour and birth are the time when a woman is potentially at her most vulnerable. Preparation for birth is key to a satisfying experience and midwives and doulas are best placed to provide care, advice and information to help her. Many women are now interested in using "alternatives" or "natural" means of maintaining their physical and emotional health and wellbeing during pregnancy and in preparing for the rigours of labour and the beginnings of parenthood.

There are several ways in which complementary therapies and natural remedies can be utilised for this process, and to facilitate as normal and satisfying a labour experience as possible. However, as with other stages of the childbearing period, it is vital that the therapies, techniques and remedies are used appropriately and safely. With regards to natural remedies such as herbal medicines, homeopathic preparations and aromatherapy oils, women should be helped to understand that these are powerful substances that should be treated like drugs. If an expectant mother wishes to consult a complementary practitioner, she should ensure that the therapist is trained and insured to treat women, especially in relation to encouraging the onset of labour, which is possibly the most common reason for choosing complementary therapies at and around term.

Women wishing to use natural remedies during the first stage of labour should be facilitated in their decisions, but professionals have a responsibility to ensure that labour continues to progress normally and that, in the event of any deviation from the norm, advice to discontinue any alternatives may need to be given. Conversely, midwives and doulas who have trained in the application of one or more therapies for labour have much to offer as alternatives to conventional pain relief and augmentation and for helping to keep the woman relaxed and in control. Incorporating complementary therapies into mainstream labour care enhances the woman's experience, encourages normal birth and reduces interventions that may have long-term sequelae, for the mother, the baby, the midwife and the maternity services.

Complementary Therapies for the Postnatal Period

Although many women appear to use complementary therapies less in the early days of the puerperium than during pregnancy and birth, there are some issues for which natural remedies and alternative techniques can be effective. Women who do consider complementary therapies at this time tend to resort to them primarily to help with lactation and to aid wound healing, especially after episiotomy. Women also sometimes ask professionals about using complementary therapies and natural remedies for their babies. Whilst there are some ways in which natural therapies can be of help, it is important to be much more cautious if considering their use for infants, especially those below three months of age. It is not the intention of this book to cover in detail the use of complementary therapies for neonates, but a general introduction to their benefits and risks is included at the end of this chapter.

This chapter includes:

- introduction

- recovery from birth

- lactation issues

- perineal wound healing

- mental health

- complementary therapies for the neonate

- conclusion.

Introduction

Becoming a mother, especially for the first time, is a period of psycho-emotional, social and physical adaptation which can be fraught with anxieties and worries. Social expectations to conform to being the "perfect parent", changes in family dynamics and issues around whether or not to return to work bring additional pressures to bear. Physical recovery from the birth takes time – up to a year in the case of the musculoskeletal system – and extra stress can delay a full return to normal.

Whilst some women will turn to complementary therapies or self-administer natural remedies, some of these strategies can also easily be included in standard postnatal care. They offer options for easing pain and discomfort, aiding recovery from the birth and facilitating adaptation from pregnancy to motherhood. Relaxation therapies reduce stress hormones, aiding breast milk production, improving sleep patterns and enhancing the immune system, thus promoting wound healing and preventing infection.

Research on the value of using complementary therapies in the puerperium appears to be confined largely to lactation issues and wound healing, although some studies address stress reduction. However, there appears to be a wider gap between the use of complementary therapies in the postnatal period and the available evidence to support its professional incorporation into mainstream maternity care than with some aspects of antenatal and intrapartum care. This may be because, once a mother and her baby are discharged from the midwife's care, there is less contact with the health services and perhaps less inclination to investigate ongoing family use of complementary therapies (except aspects such as infant massage, which is well researched).

Recovery from birth

Most women experience a range of discomforts in the first few days after giving birth. This may be abdominal, perineal, back or neck pain, the severity of discomfort commonly being related to the mode of delivery.

The majority of research studies focus on post-Caesarean section recovery, presumably because symptoms tend to be more severe and operative delivery has a higher risk of complications than normal birth. It is perhaps cynical to postulate also that medical staff attach far less importance to the postnatal period once their role in monitoring pregnancy and delivering the baby has been completed. Midwives and doulas, however, emphasise the bio-psycho-social aspects of care following birth and the adaptation required for the mother, baby and whole family.

For pain relief in the early days following the birth, simple hand and foot massage could be helpful, particularly after instrumental or operative delivery (Abbaspoor, Akbari and Najar 2014). A study by Saatsaz *et al.* (2016) randomly allocated 156 post-Caesarean primiparae to receive hand and foot massage or foot massage alone, or to act as a control. Both massage groups experienced significantly less pain than control subjects for up to 90 minutes post-treatment. Hand and foot bathing has also been found to reduce pain and restore homeostatic balance (Cal *et al.* 2016).

Adding essential oils to the massage oil may be an effective method of providing post-operative analgesia and aiding relaxation, although care must be taken to consider the possible interaction with any prescribed medication or the potentiation of drugs by essential oils with similar actions. Bearing in mind also that neonates must not be exposed to the aromas of essential oils, care must be taken to ensure treatment is given in an area away from the baby (see Chapter 2, Aromatherapy). Lavender oil (*Lavandula angustifolia*) individually administered via a face mask following general surgery (Kim *et al.* 2006; Yu and Seol 2017) or Caesarean section (Olapour *et al.* 2013) may offer a partial analgesic effect, although these studies found no real statistically significant differences when compared with conventional analgesic use. It is interesting to note that no discussion on the possible hypotensive effects of lavender oil was included in any of these research reports, despite evidence suggesting that lavender oil may influence blood pressure (Bikmoradi *et al.* 2015; Lytle, Mwatha and Davis 2014). It is vital that midwives, doulas and other maternity professionals focus not only on the potential benefits but also the possible risks of natural remedies and use them in the context of the clinical setting. Also, the use of a face mask may be inappropriate since this will deliver only minimal amounts of the chemicals from the essential oils and the analgesic effect is less likely to be sustained. Further, it is paramount to ensure no interaction with, or potentiation or inhibition of the oils with, other pharmacological drugs that may still be being administered and to avoid overwhelming the liver with the need to metabolise both the oils and the drugs simultaneously.

Reiki (Therapeutic Touch®) could be offered as a pain-relieving strategy, and may be particularly effective when applied over the surgical incision area (Sagkal Midilli and Ciray Gunduzoglu 2016). Midilli and Eser (2015) conducted a randomised controlled trial in which reiki was administered twice a day for two days post-Caesarean section and demonstrated a positive effect on the study group compared to the control group, with less reported pain and a consequent decrease in the use of pharmacological analgesia. Conversely, a Canadian study in which distant reiki was offered to post-Caesarean mothers proved inconclusive (Vandervaart *et al.* 2011). Listening to music also appears to reduce pain and the need for analgesic medication (Ebneshahidi and Mohseni 2008).

Acupuncture is especially beneficial for holistic recovery from birth. Rather than treating each symptom in isolation (pain, intestinal transit, wound healing, etc.), an assessment of the mother's internal energies aims to determine the points to be stimulated or sedated in order to treat the whole person. Acupuncture is known to reduce stress hormones, stimulate endorphins and enhance the immune system (Kawakita and Okada 2014), effects which all contribute to physical and psychological recovery. Auricular acupuncture has been found, in post-Caesarean mothers, to lower cortisol levels, thereby easing fatigue and promoting sleep, reducing anxiety and regulating blood pressure and heart rate (Kuo *et al.* 2016). This could easily and inexpensively be incorporated into midwifery care for women who have had a normal birth. In another study, auricular and general acupuncture were administered to 22 women after Caesarean section; treatment was well tolerated, pain was considerably lessened and women reported satisfaction with the intervention (Hesse *et al.* 2016). Similarly, TENS may be helpful, especially when applied to the relevant acupuncture points. A study by Kayman-Kose *et al.* (2014) allocated 100 post-Caesarean section mothers to receive either TENS or a placebo, plus 100 women who had achieved a normal birth without episiotomy into two further groups to receive TENS or a placebo. Women in both TENS groups required significantly less analgesia eight hours after delivery than the women in the placebo groups, suggesting that TENS offers a practical method of relieving pain in the postnatal period.

In post-operative bowel care, chewing mint-flavoured gum may help in preventing or treating paralytic ileus following operative delivery (but should not be used if the woman is also using homeopathic medicines as the latter will be inactivated) (Abd-El-Maeboud *et al.* 2009). Acupuncture has also been used successfully for paralytic ileus in general post-operative patients (Jung *et al.* 2017; Ng *et al.* 2013). From a herbal medicine perspective, *daikenchuto* (daikon radish/mooli) is a popular Japanese remedy for intestinal disorders, although large doses can cause gastric irritation. Abstracts of numerous studies on this herbal remedy were found, implying that it may offer an effective solution to sluggish intestinal movement. Constipation is anecdotally reported to respond to acupuncture, and several abstracts of Chinese-language studies using acupuncture for paralytic ileus or irritable bowel syndrome (IBS) were found, but no direct evidence could be located relating specifically to bowel problems in the postnatal period. Abdominal massage also stimulates peristalsis (Turan and Aşt 2016) but should be avoided until the uterine fundus has involuted below the level of the pelvic brim, particularly if the woman has retained products of conception; women who have had a Caesarean section will be unable to tolerate the pressure required from abdominal massage for this to be a realistic option. Reflexology incorporating clockwise massage of the arches of the feet, the reflex zones for the intestines, may be more comfortable and more effective (Tiran 2010b), although a single-blinded study on patients with IBS did not demonstrate that reflexology relieved the constipation (Tovey 2002).

Lactation issues

Breastfeeding women will normally achieve optimum milk supply by encouraging physiological baby-led feeding. However, when milk supply does not meet demand, galactogoguic (milk-stimulating) herbal remedies or homeopathic medicines may be used by some new mothers to improve lactation. Commonly used pharmacologically active herbal galactogogues include fenugreek, milk thistle and others (Zuppa *et al.* 2010), whilst the application of cabbage leaves to the breasts is popular to relieve engorgement. There are, however, relatively few studies on the use of herbs during breastfeeding, mostly with small sample sizes, sometimes using multi-herbal preparations and often with variable breastfeeding practices between subjects (Bazzano *et al.* 2016; Mortel and Mehta 2013).

Sim *et al.* (2013) found that almost 60 per cent of breastfeeding women used herbal remedies, with fenugreek (*Trigonella foenum-graecum*) being one of the most popular (18%). There is some evidence, mainly anecdotal, for the ingestion of fenugreek seed tea specifically to encourage lactation

(Forinash *et al.* 2012), although this is disputed by Reeder, Legrand and O'Connor-Von (2013). Fenugreek possibly works through the stimulation of dopamine receptors that stimulate prolactin production (Gabay 2002). It may increase the antioxidant properties of breast milk, offering protection to the baby from oxidative stress (Kavurt *et al.* 2013). Fenugreek may contribute indirectly to infant weight gain (Ghasemi, Kheirkhah and Vahedi 2015; Turkyılmaz *et al.* 2011), presumably due to the increase in available breast milk. However, adverse reactions can occur with maternal ingestion of fenugreek. The babies of women who consume fenugreek tea, either in late pregnancy or during breastfeeding, may develop an unusual body odour similar to that of maple syrup urine disease (Korman, Cohen and Preminger 2001; Sewell, Mosandl and Böhles 1999), and it is important to differentiate this side effect from clinical manifestation of the disease. One report also highlighted the case of a woman who took fenugreek for four weeks prior to delivery and developed toxic epidermal necrolysis, an unpleasant skin reaction (Bentele-Jaberg *et al.* 2015).

Cabbage leaves have long been used to relieve the discomfort of engorged breasts, and many midwives, doulas and lactation consultants advise their use (Lee 2010). However, as with other traditional remedies, information given to new mothers about cabbage leaves needs to be accurate, comprehensive and, where possible, based on contemporary evidence (Schaffir and Czapla 2012). A recent Cochrane review found that there are some promising findings to support the application of cabbage leaves to the breasts to relieve engorgement (Mangesi and Zakarija-Grkovic 2016); Boi, Koh and Gail (2012) and Saini and Saini (2014) agreed, but concur that more studies are needed.

The mechanism of action when cabbage leaves are applied to the skin of the breasts is unclear, although any effects are local rather than systemic since the active chemical constituents do not appear to be absorbed into the circulation. Many midwives believe cabbage leaves work because of the presence of an enzyme, but equally effective relief can be obtained from using lettuce, geranium or even rhubarb leaves which contain different chemical constituents, suggesting that some other mechanism may be at work. (NB Rhubarb is poisonous; the breasts must be washed before putting the baby to feed and it is probably wise to refrain from using rhubarb at all.) An abstract of an Iranian study was found in which even hollyhock leaves (*Althaea officinalis L*) were used to good effect (Khosravan *et al.* 2017).

It has also been suggested that the action of cabbage is due to the chlorophyll in the leaves, suggesting that the darker green cabbages could be more effective, but since white cabbage or pale lettuce also appear to work, this may also not be the complete mechanism by which cabbage leaves work. Even red cabbage can be used but tends to stain the skin.

Cabbage (*Brassica oleracea*) contains the amino acid methionine, which may increase vasodilatation to reduce engorgement and inflammation, but it is difficult to elucidate from searching the literature the difference between oral consumption and dermal application. It is also possible that the excess fluid is drawn from the breasts through a process of osmosis. If this is so, the fresh, raw cabbage leaves should not be washed prior to use as contact with water will trigger the osmotic action, nor should they be chilled in the freezer, since thawing will cause them to wilt and become wet, again nullifying their potential therapeutic effect. Nikodem *et al.* (1993) found that women who used cabbage leaves to relieve engorgement in the early puerperium were more likely than controls to be breastfeeding exclusively at six weeks postpartum, but the researchers were unable to clarify the mechanism of action and postulated that the consequent reassurance, reduced discomfort and increased self-confidence in breastfeeding may have contributed to the effects. Most women appear to prefer cold leaves, but there appears to be little difference in clinical effectiveness between chilled or room temperature leaves (Arora, Vatsa and Dadhwal 2008; Roberts, Reiter and Schuster 1995).

The outer leaves should be discarded and any field dirt removed by wiping. It may be necessary to remove the fibrous central stalk of larger leaves to enable them to be wrapped around the breast inside the brassiere. They are left in place until they become wet – they smell like cooked cabbage – and typically takes about 20 minutes but can be as soon as five minutes after application. The leaves are replaced with fresh ones and the process is repeated as many times as necessary until the mother feels some relief. Although the evidence base is limited, there appear to be no risks associated with the practice of using cabbage leaves to relieve engorgement, and it offers an inexpensive, safe and possibly effective method of easing a common discomfort of the puerperium. However, women who are allergic to cabbage and other plants in the brassica family should avoid using the leaves for engorgement.

Other herbal remedies may be used in certain cultures. Meng *et al.* (2015) found that breast massage, combined with a cactus and aloe vera preparation, relieved pain and swelling in women with engorgement and helped to re-stimulate lactation, although it is difficult to determine whether the breast massage alone would have helped. It is worth noting that aloe vera (*Aloe barbadensis*) also has a reputation as an effective wound healing agent (Nimma *et al.* 2017) and is often advocated as a remedy for sore nipples (Eshgizade *et al.* 2015; Tafazoli *et al.* 2010). However, care should be taken to wash the breasts prior to feeding, because the baby may react adversely, especially with long-term use. Common unfavourable effects to ingestion of aloe gel include diarrhoea, abdominal cramping and allergic reactions. Over time, the mother may also experience side effects of the topical application, including skin irritation and a burning sensation.

Non-pharmacological homeopathic remedies, including a combination remedy of apis and bryonia, may assist in stimulating or suppressing lactation or easing engorgement (Berrebi *et al.* 2001). There is extremely limited evidence on homeopathy for lactation issues, but a study on cows (in which there is no placebo effect) showed that various remedies, given in combination, were effective in treating mastitis (Varshney and Naresh 2005). Practitioners of homeopathy may prescribe phytolacca, bryonia, chamomilla, belladonna, pulsatilla or other remedies, according to the precise symptoms (see Chapter 2, Homeopathy).

Acupuncture may also help with lactation issues. Numerous Chinese-language abstracts were found when searching the literature on this subject; additional studies published in English-language journals indicate that acupuncture may sustain exclusive breastfeeding when compared to a control group (Neri *et al.* 2011) and regulate milk supply, preventing engorgement (Wei *et al.* 2008; Zhou *et al.* 2009). A Swedish randomised, non-blinded trial (Kvist *et al.* 2007) suggested that acupuncture may be a preferable treatment option for women with poor lactation than the use of nasal oxytocin sprays and other conventional strategies. It is interesting to note that acupuncture treatment in non-parturient patients may cause galactorrhoea, probably due to an iatrogenic increase in prolactin (Campbell and Macglashan 2005; Jenner and Filshie 2002), suggesting a mechanism of action for the increase in milk production in new mothers.

There is some evidence for the use of mindfulness strategies to improve milk supply. Laughter therapy improves the immune response and appears to have a positive effect on lactation (Perez-Blasco, Viguer and Rodrigo 2013; Ryu, Shin and Yang 2015). An abstract was found of a Croatian study by Vidas *et al.* (2011) in which autogenic training combined with breastfeeding support was offered to women in a counselling centre. Women in the study group were significantly more likely to be still exclusively breastfeeding their babies at six months than those in the control group and reported an improved relationship with their babies. However, as with other studies, it is difficult to determine whether the results could have been skewed by the fact that breastfeeding advice was also offered to these women, when perhaps normal practices in some countries do not give women so much individualised attention. Sobrinho (2003) demonstrated the link between raised cortisol levels and reduced prolactin, suggesting that any therapy aimed at relaxing the mother will facilitate lactation. Clinical hypnosis has been shown to be particularly effective in increasing breast milk production (Sobrinho *et al.* 2003), which is likely to be due to the increase in oxytocin that occurs as cortisol is reduced (Uvnäs-Moberg 1998).

Chiropractors believe that breastfeeding difficulties associated with fixing the baby on the breast may develop as a result of neonatal spinal subluxations (misalignments) sustained during the birth, especially with instrumental delivery. A systematic review by Alcantara, Alcantara and Alcantara (2015) concluded that misalignments of the fetal neck, cranium and mandible from traumatic delivery contributes to intracranial strain and jaw tension in the infant, making it difficult for the baby to attach to the nipple adequately to draw milk. In this case, chiropractic treatment of the baby may be the best solution to continuing breastfeeding. Indeed, the establishment of a joint midwifery and chiropractic clinic has been shown to achieve exclusive breastfeeding in almost 90 per cent of women who attended (Miller *et al.* 2016).

Perineal wound healing

Perineal pain following delivery, either from lacerations or an episiotomy, is one of the most common discomforts for women in the early puerperium, yet one for which conventional care has limited options. Prevention of perineal trauma is preferable to dealing with the consequences of tears or episiotomy. Haavik *et al.* (2016) suggest that chiropractic spinal manipulation during the second trimester of pregnancy may prepare the musculature of the pelvic floor for the birth and result in less perineal trauma at delivery. The practice of perineal massage may also contribute to fewer severe lacerations, reduce the need for episiotomy and lessen the severity of postpartum perineal pain (Beckmann and Stock 2013; Hastings-Tolsma 2014; Seehusen and Raleigh 2014).

Some authorities advocate perineal massage being performed during the last few weeks of pregnancy, whilst others suggest that it can be done in labour, although the NICE guideline on intrapartum care recommends that it is not performed during the second stage (NICE 2017b). Aasheim *et al.*'s

Cochrane review (2011) indicated that warm compresses or perineal massage applied during labour appear to be safe and effective for reducing perineal trauma, although Mei-dan *et al.*'s review (2008) proved inconclusive. Interestingly, an earlier study by Hastings-Tolsma *et al.* (2007) found an *increase* in the incidence of lacerations following the use of oils or lubricants. On a physical level, antenatal perineal massage appears, anecdotally, to have some benefits in reducing trauma at delivery. On a psychological level it may help the expectant mother to adjust to the idea of preparing this area of her body for the birth of her baby.

Several Middle Eastern studies support the use of intrapartum perineal massage, and a systematic analysis by Karaçam, Ekmen and Calişir (2012) concurred. However, the choice of medium used in some of these studies is concerning. It is generally thought that a light, non-greasy vegetable oil such as grapeseed should be used for perineal massage. A study by Harlev *et al.* (2013) attempted to determine the most appropriate oil, but this trial is flawed because the two oils used in the study are not suitable for all women. The oils used were jojoba liquid wax, which is not necessarily the best consistency, and a combination of olive oil with sweet almond oil, the latter of which potentially causes allergic reactions in some people. Demirel and Golbasi (2015) used glycerol during the first and second stages of labour, and Geranmayeh *et al.* (2012) used Vaseline™, which is intended for external use only. Using petroleum jelly on moist mucous membranes tends to linger and can encourage an increase in bacteria, leading to infection (Brown *et al.* 2013). Many of these Middle Eastern studies appeared to demonstrate a reduction in the need for episiotomy compared to control groups. On the other hand, episiotomy is performed routinely in many of these countries, and positive results may simply have been due to the lack of standard surgical intervention in the study group, irrespective of the use of perineal massage.

In the UK, a case is known to this author of a woman who self-administered a commercial steroid-based cream to massage the perineum during pregnancy in the belief that it would thin the perineum and encourage stretching at delivery. Unfortunately, the cream caused complete breakdown of the perineal tissues in labour when the presenting part exerted pressure on the pelvic floor. Essential oils (aromatherapy) should not be used for perineal massage during pregnancy or labour. Many chemical constituents in essential oils potentially cause irritation in this delicate mucosal area and it is unsafe for the baby to come into contact with the oils at birth.

There are however several essential oils thought to help with post-delivery wound healing, easing discomfort and reducing the incidence of infection. These include common lavender (*Lavandula angustifolia*) and tea tree (*Melaleuca alternifolia*) (Chin and Cordell 2013; Mori *et al.* 2016). However, whilst there is an increasing amount of literature in the professional press regarding the possible effectiveness of "lavender oil", the studies are very variable, both in terms of the robustness of the research methodology but also, more importantly, the ways in which the lavender is administered. Like all essential oils, lavender essential oil is antibacterial (Sienkiewicz *et al.* 2014) and contains large amounts of a particular chemical group called terpenes, which are known to be analgesic (Giovannini *et al.* 2016). However, its direct wound healing capacity is questionable. Two UK midwives, Dale and Cornwell (1994), conducted a randomised controlled trial of 635 postnatal women divided into three groups to receive either pure *Lavandula angustifolia* essential oil or a synthetic lavender product or a placebo inert substance, added to the bath water for ten consecutive days following delivery. There were no statistically significant differences between the groups in terms of wound healing, although reported maternal pain was lower in the natural lavender group, particularly after the third postnatal day. It was surmised that the analgesic effect enabled women to cope better with the discomfort of perineal sutures and that any perceived improvement in wound healing may be due more to the anti-infective properties of the lavender oil in preventing infection and wound breakdown than to a direct impact on incision aggregation and healing. It is also possible that the linalyl acetate content of lavender, which is thought to relax smooth muscle, could have a vasodilatory effect, thus improving blood supply to the wound area (Koto *et al.* 2006).

In countries such as Iran and Turkey, where perineal wound care remains embedded in traditional medical practices long since discontinued in western countries, such as the routine use of povidone-iodine or betadine applications directly to the perineum, the enthusiasm for natural, plant-based remedies has produced a plethora of studies investigating natural alternatives. However, the substances used are not necessarily the same as those used by midwives in the west. For example, Marzouk *et al.* (2015) conducted a single-blinded, placebo-controlled study of 60 primiparae in which *lavender-thymol* was applied topically to the perineal wound area. There appeared to be a statistically significant improvement in redness, oedema and wound cohesion in those who received lavender-thymol and a greater reduction in dyspareunia by the end of the puerperium. This led the researchers to conclude that lavender-thymol is an effective and safe strategy to treat perineal wounds when compared to those who received normal care. However, this study did not use lavender in isolation and the safety of thymol following childbirth has not been clarified. Thymol is a crystalline compound derived from *Thymus vulgaris*, from thyme and other plants; it has an aromatic similarity to the culinary herb thyme, and is strongly anti-infective, possibly reducing the resistance of bacteria to penicillin (Palaniappan and Holley 2010).

Another Iranian study (Sheikhan *et al.* 2012) compared lavender *essence* to normal care (betadine), and although the results were less conclusive, the team considered that "lavender" was a preferable treatment. However, essential oils are the extracted volatile oils from plants, whereas the definition of essences is more indistinct and often refers to fragrant oils, which may be synthetic, or used as flavourings in foods. Similarly, Vakilian *et al.* (2011) compared lavender oil with povidone iodine, demonstrating reduced erythema and oedema. However, topically applied povidone-iodine, in itself, can cause skin and mucosal irritation and sensitisation in susceptible women and, again, any improvements may have arisen from the omission of standard care rather than the inclusion of a natural oil treatment.

Midwives and doulas advocating the use of lavender or other essential oils for perineal healing must apply a comprehensive knowledge of aromatherapy to clinical practice, both in terms of standard practice and wound management. For example, whilst adding a few drops of essential oil to the bath water is a simple means of administering the oil, it is important that the correct lavender essential oil (*Lavandula angustifolia*) is used, diluted in a small amount of a suitable carrier oil such as grapeseed and given in an appropriate dose (maximum six drops). The carrier oil prevents the neat essential oil from floating on the surface of the bath water and coming into direct contact with the mother's skin which may cause irritation. Sufficient information must be given to the mother to enable her to make an informed decision about its use. As with all drugs (i.e. chemicals) the midwife must take responsibility for administering the oil by physically adding it to the bath water, particularly in a hospital setting. The bath must be cleaned afterwards, both for hygiene and for safety reasons to avoid other mothers slipping in the bath on any remaining oil. In the absence of a suitable vegetable oil carrier, it is permissible to use milk but this must be *full-fat* milk (not semi-skimmed or skimmed) so that the fatty globules can facilitate dilution of the essential oils in the water. Mineral-based baby oil is not appropriate as it impairs absorption of the oil via the skin. Once the mother has exited the bath, the wound area should be dried thoroughly in accordance with contemporary wound management practice.

Several inappropriate practices in relation to the use of lavender for perineal healing have come to the notice of this author in recent years. Some midwives are known to advocate adding neat drops of lavender essential oil to a sanitary pad, in a line equivalent to the suture line, or making a lavender spray in a water bottle for the mother to spray onto the perineal wound. These are both inappropriate methods. In the first example, essential oils should rarely be used neat but, in any case, adding them to a sanitary pad is an expensive waste of money since the pad is specifically designed to draw fluid away from the skin. In the second example, mixtures of essential oil in water will chemically last only 24 hours before oxidation alters the chemical composition. The bottle should therefore be labelled with a use-by time and date. Further, the use of a plastic bottle is inappropriate because the organic oil chemicals interact with the synthetic chemicals in the plastic, causing further oxidation (deterioration) of the essential oil, thus changing the original chemicals to others which may be more hazardous, possibly causing irritation.

Tea tree essential oil has also been used in the bath, either alone or in combination with lavender oil. Tea tree (*Melaleuca alternifolia*) is particularly valuable as an anti-infective agent and has been researched extensively since the 1970s in relation to many different pathogens. There is some evidence to suggest it can be useful for wound healing (Chin and Cordell 2013; Edmondson *et al.* 2011), but whether this is due to a direct effect on granulation or an indirect effect through the prevention of wound infection is not clear. However, tea tree oil can cause serious skin or mucosal irritation in some women and should therefore be used or advised with caution, ensuring good dilution and low doses. It is possible to obtain tea tree oil rich in terpinen 4-ol, which is thought to reduce the incidence of irritation, but this is more expensive and there does not appear to be any evidence to support its use for wound healing above the use of standard tea tree oil.

Homeopathic arnica is well known as a remedy for shock, trauma and bruising and is often used by newly birthed mothers to ease pain and reduce bruising to the perineum and buttocks following episiotomy or lacerations. It can also be used after operative or instrumental delivery and is particularly effective for wounds with pain, swelling and tissue bruising. A localised patch containing arnica can also be used for small wounds such as needle puncture or epidural cannula bruising (Barkey and Kaszkin-Bettag 2012), although this would not be appropriate for perineal healing.

Arnica is produced from the plant *Arnica Montana*, also known as Leopard's bane, and women should be careful to obtain the homeopathically prepared version (which has been diluted and succussed; see Chapter 2) and to avoid the pharmacologically active herbal form or the essential oil. Following a normal birth the dose would be the 30C strength, one tablet taken three times daily for three days, then discontinued to avoid a reverse proving. If the mother has had more severe trauma or a more complicated delivery, the dose for self-administration is increased to one 30C strength tablet, taken every hour on day one (whilst awake), every two hours on day two and every three hours on day three, then discontinued. When prescribed by a qualified homeopath following Caesarean section, professional-strength tablets, such as 1M, may be used but are given less frequently. Arnica is also available in cream or ointment form, but this must not be applied to broken skin or the sutured wound nor should it be used for a prolonged period, because it can cause further inflammation, blistering, eczema and other skin problems. If a woman is known to be sensitive to the actual plant, even homeopathic arnica cream should be avoided. Homeopathic arnica and lavender or tea tree essential oil baths should not be used concomitantly as the aromatic oils inactivate the homeopathic remedies.

The evidence for effectiveness of arnica is varied. Some studies lack robust methodology, and randomised controlled trials are often inconclusive or produce negative results. This has led to sceptics of homeopathy disparaging its use and claiming that its effect (like other homeopathic medicines) is nothing more than a placebo. Several studies have investigated the use of arnica following surgery and found beneficial effects on bruising, trauma and oedema (Chaiet and Marcus 2016; Iannitti *et al.* 2016; Robertson, Suryanarayanan and Banerjee 2007), although the effects may not be immediate (Pumpa *et al.* 2014) and may, occasionally, exacerbate the symptoms (Adkison, Bauer and Chang 2010).

Excessive consumption of homeopathic remedies can trigger a reverse proving, in which the symptoms intended to be treated can worsen. The impact of arnica on the control of haemorrhage has been demonstrated (Sorrentino *et al.* 2017), but this suggests that if excessive doses are ingested the reverse may occur and the woman may experience increased bleeding. Cases are known to this author of women who have taken prolonged prophylactic doses of arnica prior to delivery or excessively frequent doses in the first 24 to 48 hours following delivery and have subsequently suffered postpartum haemorrhage, either primary or secondary. This reinforces the principle that homeopathic remedies should not be commenced until the "problem", in this case perineal trauma, has actually occurred and that prophylactic administration is inappropriate, especially over such a prolonged period of time. One abstract was found in the literature of a case in which toxic optic neuropathy occurred following inadvertently excessive consumption of arnica (Venkatramani *et al.* 2013).

Other studies use arnica in combination with other homeopathic, herbal or synthetic substances. For example, Castro *et al.* (2012) studied the effect on rats of arnica compared to homeopathic hypericum and in combination with microcurrent stimulation, finding that the use of a microcurrent enhanced the benefits of both homeopathic remedies. Simsek *et al.* (2016) used a cream containing arnica and an anti-inflammatory analgesic, which was found to reduce oedema and bruising after rhinoplasty. Conversely, van Exsel *et al.* (2016) found no statistically different reduction in bruising or swelling following blepharoplasty compared to a placebo cream, and a systematic review by Ho, Jagdeo and Waldorf (2016) concluded that there is insufficient evidence to support the use of topical arnica or bromelain (see below) for post-operative oedema.

Other natural remedies which researchers have attempted to evaluate include bromelain, a chemical constituent of pineapple (*Ananas comosus*). Bromelain is a traditional remedy used for pain, wound healing and musculoskeletal issues (see also Chapter 7 in relation to using pineapple for post-dates pregnancy). In a double-blinded placebo-controlled study by Golezar (2016), women were given oral tablets of bromelain three times a day for six days that appeared to reduce pain and promote wound healing more quickly than the placebo. However, the bromelain was isolated from the pineapple and produced as oral tablets, which may have a different impact and produce a greater risk of side effects than from using it as part of the whole plant in context with its other chemical constituents. Moreover, it appears to possess anticoagulant and antiplatelet activities, with a possibility of bleeding (Gläser and Hilberg 2006). This implies the need for caution in women with excessively heavy lochia; therapeutic doses should be avoided in women taking anticoagulants.

Various other topical herbal ointments have been trialled with varying results, including horsetail (*Equisetum arvense*), cinnamon (*Cinnamomum verum*) and an ointment containing calendula (marigold, *Calendula officinalis*) and aloe vera (*Aloe barbadensis*) (Asgharikhatooni *et al.* 2015; Eghdampour *et al.* 2013; Mohammadi *et al.* 2014). Witch hazel water (*Hamamelis virginiana*) is also sometimes used for its astringent and anti-inflammatory effects (Thring, Hili and Naughton 2011).

Acupuncture can be an effective analgesic when compared to normal pharmacological methods of relieving perineal pain, and the immunostimulant effect of acupuncture may contribute to wound healing. The precise acupoints used may vary between women when assessed individually, although Marra *et al.* (2011) used wrist and ankle points to good effect. Working along similar principles, TENS has also been used to good effect in reducing pain following both episiotomy and post-Caesarean section (de Sousa, Gomes-Sponholz and Nakano 2014; Dionisi and Senatori 2011; Kayman-Kose *et al.* 2014; Pitangui *et al.* 2014).

A single-blinded study of biofeedback taught by physiotherapists to mothers for home self-administration showed no real benefit, but the researchers postulated that the mothers find it difficult to allocate sufficient time to perform the technique (Peirce *et al.* 2013). A Cochrane review of localised cooling (East *et al.* 2012) found limited evidence of analgesia, wound repair and oedema compared to other natural and conventional clinical strategies, although many women report satisfaction.

Mental health

Stress, anxiety and lack of confidence are common emotions amongst newly birthed mothers, which can predispose them to more significant postnatal "blues" which, for some, may develop into clinical depression. Lack of sleep often exacerbates symptoms in susceptible women, while those who experience emotional trauma during pregnancy, as well as those with pre-existing depression, are much more likely to develop postnatal mental health problems because of the hugely fluctuating hormone levels and the immense social changes wrought by having a new baby. Several aspects of complementary medicine have been explored, both for the prevention and treatment of depression, with some being more acceptable than others. It must be stressed however that complementary therapies cannot replace conventional medical care when women are severely clinically depressed and caution must be employed when advising women at risk of depression or with a pre-existing mental health condition on natural remedies or aspects of other modalities.

Placentophagy

Placentophagy – eating the placenta – has become popular in recent years as a means of preventing depression, although the practice is comparatively rare in humans across all cultures (Young and Benyshek 2010). Most women wanting to consume the placenta have the placental tissue encapsulated to make it easier and more palatable to ingest, but others eat it raw or cooked. There is a belief that eating the placental tissue provides hormones to prevent postnatal depression, as well as iron to replace that lost during pregnancy and birth. It is also thought to reduce post-delivery pain, boost energy levels, aid lactation, promote skin elasticity and enhance maternal bonding with the baby. Women generally report perceived positive effects, particularly for subjective symptoms, but there is little evidence to support these claims (Selander *et al.* 2013).

In an American study, Schuette *et al.* (2017) investigated women's and professionals' attitudes to, and knowledge of, placentophagy. Approximately two thirds of women and almost 90 per cent of midwives and doctors had heard of the practice but most knew very little about its benefits and risks. Gryder *et al.* (2017) conducted a randomised placebo-controlled trial to investigate the claim that encapsulated placenta is a rich source of iron for women who are iron deficient. Whilst encapsulated placenta contained significantly more iron than a placebo (beef), it was not sufficient to meet the recommended daily amounts for lactating mothers, and the authors expressed concern that women whose only source of iron came from the placenta may not receive a sufficient amount. Abstracts of some very old papers were found online and claimed variously that placentophagy increased breast milk production (Hammett 1918) and the protein and lactose content of breast milk (McNeile and Lyle 1918) and eased pain (in rats) following birth (DiPirro and Kristal 2004). No studies appear to have been undertaken on the possible risks of eating the placenta, although Hayes (2016) suggests that infection, thromboembolism from oestrogenic tissue and accumulation of environmental toxins are possible.

Touch therapies

Touch therapies such as massage, aromatherapy and reflexology may be helpful in aiding relaxation and facilitating sleep in women with postnatal "blues". However, touch therapies should be used with caution for mothers with clinical depression, whether pre-existing or antenatally or postnatally manifested. This is because deep relaxation may be inappropriate for some women, perhaps precipitating a serious emotional release, a fact that reinforces the need for counselling and listening skills in professionals who provide massage.

Massage has been shown to aid sleep in the early postpartum period (Ko and Lee 2014) and to ease anxiety in mothers of babies in the neonatal intensive care unit (Feijó *et al.* 2006), whilst teaching depressed mothers how to massage their babies may improve the maternal-infant relationship (Onozawa *et al.* 2001). Women with pre-existing antenatal depression have been shown to benefit from regular massage throughout pregnancy, administered by their partners, with a reduction in postnatal depression and cortisol levels (Field *et al.* 2009).

It is also possible to combine the massage with essential oils. Imura, Misao and Ushijima (2006) offered women a single 30-minute aromatherapy massage on the second postpartum day and found improved anxiety and depression scores compared to a control group. However, this may have been due more to the interaction with caregivers, or a positive reaction to the massage, than specifically related to the essential oils. Conrad and Adams (2012) provided a more realistic programme of 15-minute treatments with rose (*Rosa centifolia*) and lavender (*Lavandula angustifolia*) oils, administered either by inhalation or via a hand massage. The Edinburgh Postnatal Depression score and Generalized Anxiety Disorder scale evaluations were significantly improved in both the trial groups compared to a control group.

In another study (Kianpour *et al.* 2016) anxiety, stress and depression were significantly lower in the postpartum women who received lavender inhalation, even up to three months after delivery. The methodology involved women inhaling three drops of lavender essential oil from the palms of their hands, eight-hourly for four weeks. However, as with many other Iranian trials, the lavender was specifically prepared at a local laboratory and the research paper does not specify the type of lavender. Further, no mention was made of any woman experiencing skin irritation from the dermal application or respiratory adverse effects from the inhalation, although one woman withdrew from the study because she did not like the aroma of the lavender. It is interesting to note that a systematic review by Perry *et al.* (2012) found that, despite limited evidence for *Lavandula angustifolia* as an anxiolytic, oral consumption of a tea made from lavender (i.e. as a herbal remedy rather than as an aromatherapy treatment) may have some value in reducing anxiety.

One abstract of a Korean trial using "reflexology" for women with postnatal depression was found (Choi and Lee 2015) and appeared to show reduced fatigue and lowered cortisol levels, leading the researchers to conclude that "foot reflexology massage" may be a useful intervention for women with fatigue, stress and depression in the postnatal period.

However, although it is not possible to state categorically without viewing the paper, as with many other reflexology studies, it is likely that the treatment was more akin to a foot massage than based on specific reflex zone techniques aimed at alleviating the condition. Conversely, the quality of sleep in Taiwanese women who received a 30-minute reflexology treatment each evening for five days was shown to be better than in women in the control group (Li *et al.* 2011).

Mindfulness

Mindfulness techniques such as guided imagery impact positively on the mood, and help to reduce stress (Beattie *et al.* 2017), particularly that experienced by mothers whose babies are in the neonatal intensive care unit (Howland *et al.* 2017). Learning mindfulness techniques during pregnancy can be especially effective in the postnatal period (Roy Malis, Meyer and Gross 2017), and women explicitly at risk of mental health disorders may benefit from mindfulness yoga before and after delivery (Muzik *et al.* 2012). Group sessions can help some women, although the logistics of arranging these and gathering newly birthed mothers together must be considered. A study by Buttner *et al.* (2015) found that when depressed new mothers participated in yoga sessions, with 16 treatments over eight weeks, there were improved depression and anxiety scores and enhanced quality of life for 78 per cent of the trial group. It is however difficult to elucidate whether the yoga was the primary means of improvement or the fact that women were in a dedicated group setting, presumably allowing for interactions between participants.

Ko *et al.* (2013) initiated an exercise programme, based on yoga and Pilates principles, to help new mothers to lose weight, ease fatigue and prevent or reduce depression. A course of 12 one-hour weekly sessions was provided. Fatigue levels pre- and post-course were not significantly different, but there were noticeable reductions in body weight, fat mass and basic metabolic rate. When measured in terms of women's quality of life there was considerable improvement. Although the primary aim of the study was to investigate exercise for postnatal weight loss, it was concluded that improved body image contributed to enhanced emotional states and that group exercise programmes could contribute to a reduction in postnatal depression.

St John's wort

St John's wort (SJW) (*Hypericum perforatum*) has long been known as an herbal remedy for treating mild to moderate depression and may be one of the most commonly used remedies in the postnatal period (Budzynska *et al.* 2012). It is often used orally for mood disturbances, including premenstrual syndrome, menopausal symptoms, seasonal affective disorder and other mental health issues, whilst topical application aids wound healing. SJW has been found in numerous clinical trials to be more effective than placebo in reducing depressive symptoms and is at least as effective as tricyclic antidepressants and selective serotonin reuptake inhibitors (SSRIs) including sertraline, fluoxetine and paroxetine (Apaydin *et al.* 2016; Linde, Berner and Kriston 2008; Rahimi, Nikfar and Abdollahi 2009). Short-term use seems to be particularly effective (Linde and Knüppel 2005), the active constituents being hypericin and related chemicals, which appear to regulate serotonin, noradrenaline and dopamine and reduce cortisol (Schüle *et al.* 2001).

General side effects to SJW include gastrointestinal disturbance, insomnia, headaches, photosensitivity and skin rashes. More serious adverse reactions include manic episodes and suicidal tendencies, as well as serotonin syndrome if administration is discontinued abruptly. SJW should not be taken concurrently with antidepressants with similar actions and may inhibit the use of the contraceptive Pill, anticoagulants and certain drugs used in cancer and HIV treatments (Jiang *et al.* 2006; Murphy *et al.* 2005). It may also possibly induce psychotic episodes in women who take it injudiciously (Ferrara, Mungai and Starace 2017).

The safety of SJW in pregnancy and breastfeeding is still under discussion. Although researchers and medical professionals were of the opinion in the late 20th and early 21st centuries that SJW should be completely avoided in the preconception, antenatal and breastfeeding periods, cautious approval has been forthcoming in recent years (Dugoua, Mills *et al.* 2006; Moretti *et al.* 2009) with apparently little neonatal risk (Klier *et al.* 2006). However, women should be advised to seek medical advice before changing from prescribed antidepressants to SJW and that any change should be gradual and preferably under medical or herbalist supervision to avoid the risk of side effects. Similarly, withdrawal from SJW should also be gradual. As a point of interest for post-puerperal use, concomitant use of SJW with the contraceptive Pill can trigger breakthrough bleeding and reduced contraceptive efficacy (Berry-Bibee *et al.* 2016).

Complementary therapies for the neonate

Minor conditions affecting the baby may be helped with complementary therapies or natural remedies, although parents should be advised to use all home-administered remedies and techniques with caution. Aromatherapy is completely contraindicated in the neonate (see Chapter 2).

Babies with colic respond well to gentle abdominal massage, which has been found to be more effective than the traditional shoulder-rocking action performed by many mothers (Nahidi et al. 2017; Sheidaei et al. 2016). Chiropractic and cranial osteopathy (see Chapter 2, Chiropractic) also have a reputation for being beneficial in treating crying babies with colic (Miller, Newell and Bolton 2012). Dobson et al. (2012) undertook a meta-analysis of randomised controlled studies in which chiropractic, osteopathy and craniosacral therapy were used to treat infant colic. Most studies were small, but a theme across many was a statistically significant reduction in infant crying following treatment. Miller and Phillips's study (2009) also found chiropractic to be successful, particularly in older children who demonstrated less behavioural issues such as temper tantrums, and the authors suggest that chiropractic may offer a long-term solution to colic. However, Wiberg and Wiberg (2010) undertook a retrospective study in Denmark in which 276 babies under three months of age were treated with chiropractic but, despite some resolution in slightly older infants, the treatment was not found to be a statistically significant option for colic in newborns. Similarly, Johnson, Cocker and Chang (2015) found little evidence to support the use of osteopathy, chiropractic or massage and suggested that giving the infant a probiotic supplement (lactobacillus) and encouraging the mother to reduce dietary allergens was more effective. They also raised the issue of safety, which has not been well researched in chiropractic studies. One case report was found of an infant who sustained posterior rib fractures following chiropractic for colic (Wilson, Greiner and Duma 2012), although the authors acknowledged the need to eliminate genetic bone fragility and non-accidental injury.

Acupuncture may also be helpful for neonates. A large multicentre, randomised controlled, blinded trial compared standardised western acupuncture, individualised acupuncture according to Chinese medicine principles and conventional care for colic in 147 infants (Landgren and Hallström 2017). The study demonstrated significant reduction in crying of the babies in both acupuncture groups compared to standard care and the authors concluded that acupuncture offers a safe, effective option to parents.

However, a study in Sweden by Skjeie *et al.* (2013) found no clinically relevant changes in crying of babies treated with acupuncture and went so far as to suggest that acupuncture for infant colic should be confined to clinical research trials only. This recommendation was supported by Raith, Urlesberger and Schmölzer (2013) who found no justification for treating infants with acupuncture. In addition, they suggest that clinical trials should only be undertaken by senior acupuncturists with considerable experience of treating babies and children.

In respect of herbal remedies, some commercially produced remedies for infant colic contain a mixture of therapeutic agents, such as chamomile, fennel and melissa, which was shown in a randomised controlled trial by Savino *et al.* (2005) to reduce infant crying from colic within one week of administration. Sweet fennel (*Foeniculum vulgare*) is well known as a possible solution to colic. The seeds of the plant, made into an emulsion, appear to be at least more effective than a placebo (Alexandrovich *et al.* 2003), and giving the baby a small amount of fennel tea may also be helpful (Weizman *et al.* 1993). Perry, Hunt and Ernst (2011) suggested from their systematic review that there may be some encouraging results for fennel for infant colic but concluded that there was little real evidence to support its use at that time. One case report was found of two women who drank fennel tea as a galactogogue; it appeared to cause toxic effects in their babies (Rosti *et al.* 1994), and although there has hitherto been a suggestion that the anethole content of fennel may be carcinogenic, this theory now seems to be disputed (Gori *et al.* 2012). The essential oil of sweet fennel is contraindicated in newborns, although small amounts of fennel tea are safe enough (see Chapter 2).

Infant massage has long been shown to be very beneficial, for both babies and mothers. In preterm babies it is relaxing, reduces cortisol and promotes growth and wellbeing (Asadollahi *et al.* 2016; Badr, Abdallah and Kahale 2015; Diego, Field and Hernandez-Reif 2014; Field, Diego and Hernandez-Reif 2011). It can also aid neurological development (Lai *et al.* 2016) and reduce pain in babies undergoing venepuncture (Chik, Ip and Choi 2017). The use of a lotion to avoid the friction of direct skin-to-skin contact appears to aid the onset and duration of sleep (Field *et al.* 2016) and promote weight gain in preterm and small babies (Jabraeile *et al.* 2016). However, this latter study used olive oil, which is contraindicated in neonates because it may cause eczema, as does sunflower oil (Cooke *et al.* 2016). There is some suggestion that baby massage may improve jaundice (Basiri-Moghadam *et al.* 2015; Dalili *et al.* 2016), although Seyyedrasooli *et al.* (2014) dispute this. Massaging the baby also acts as a relaxant for the mother, reducing anxiety (Afand *et al.* 2017) and postnatal depression scores (Field 2010). It also appears to enhance the relationship of both parents with the baby (Gnazzo *et al.* 2015).[1]

Conclusion

Complementary therapies and natural remedies may have a part to play in helping women to recover from the birth, especially in reducing pain, aiding lactation and promoting wound healing. The relaxation effects of many therapies can contribute to adaptation to motherhood, improved sleep and possibly reducing the effects of anxiety and stress. Although self-administration of natural remedies appears to be much less in the puerperium than during pregnancy or labour, encouraging women to receive regular relaxation therapy from a professional gives them some time for themselves which is often sorely lacking in the early weeks and months after the birth of a baby. In the longer term, complementary therapies may prevent or reduce the severity of mild depression, and assist parents to develop a close relationship with their babies. However, apart from massage, the use of complementary therapies for infants should be under the direction of a qualified practitioner who is experienced in treating babies and children.

---

[1]   See also the Touch Research Institute, Miami, at www6.miami.edu/touch-research for more research and information.

References

Aasheim V, Nilsen AB, Lukasse M, Reinar LM (2011) Perineal techniques during the second stage of labour for reducing perineal trauma. Cochrane Database of Systematic Reviews. (12):CD006672.

Abbasi M, Ghazi F, Barlow-Harrison A, Sheikhvatan M, Mohammadyari F (2009) The effect of hypnosis on pain relief during labor and childbirth in Iranian pregnant women. International Journal of Clinical and Experimental Hypnosis. 257(2):174–83.

Abbaspoor Z, Akbari M, Najar S (2014) Effect of foot and hand massage in post-cesarean section pain control: a randomized control trial. Pain Management Nursing. 15(1):132–6.

Abbassi J (2017) Amid reports of infant deaths, FTC cracks down on homeopathy while FDA investigates. JAMA network, 28 February 2017. Viewed online 13/09/2017 at http://jamanetwork.com/journals/jama/article-abstract/2602995

AbdEl Fadeel Abd el Hamid Afefy N (2015) Effect of ice cold massage and acupressure on labor pain and labor duration: a randomized controlled trial. Journal of Natural Sciences Research, ISSN 2224-3186 (paper), ISSN 2225-0921 (online). Vol.5, 137.

Abd-El-Maeboud KH, Ibrahim MI, Shalaby DA, Fikry MF (2009) Gum chewing stimulates early return of bowel motility after caesarean section. BJOG. 116(10):1334–9.

Abdolahian S, Ghavi F, Abdollahifard S, Sheikhan F (2014) Effect of dance labor on the management of active phase labor pain and clients' satisfaction: a randomized controlled trial study. Global Journal of Health Science. 6(3):219–26.

Abdulrazzaq YM, Al Kendi A, Nagelkerke N (2009) Soothing methods used to calm a baby in an Arab country. Acta Paediatrica. 98(2):392–6.

Abebe W (2002) Herbal medication: potential for adverse interactions with analgesic drugs. Journal of Clinical Pharmacy and Therapeutics. 27(6):391–401.

ACOG (American College of Obstetrics and Gynecology) (2004) Practice bulletin: nausea and vomiting of pregnancy. Obstetrics & Gynecology. 103(4):803–14.

ACPWH (2010) Aquanatal guidelines: guidance on antenatal and postnatal exercises in water. Viewed online 13/09/2017 at www.csp.org.uk/sites/files/csp/secure/acpwh-aquanatal_copy.pdf

Adams J (2006) An exploratory study of complementary and alternative medicine in hospital midwifery: models of care and professional struggle. Complementary Therapies in Clinical Practice. 12(1):40–7.

Adams J, Frawley J, Steel A, Broom A, Sibbritt D (2015) Use of pharmacological and non-pharmacological labour pain management techniques and their relationship to maternal and infant birth outcomes: examination of a nationally representative sample of 1835 pregnant women. Midwifery. 31(4):458–63.

Adams J, Lui CW, Sibbritt D, Broom A, Wardle J, Homer C (2011) Attitudes and referral practices of maternity care professionals with regard to complementary and alternative medicine: an integrative review. Journal of Advanced Nursing. 67(3):472–83.

Adkison JD, Bauer DW, Chang T (2010) The effect of topical arnica on muscle pain. Annals of Pharmacotherapy. 44(10):1579–84.

Afand N, Keshavarz M, Fatemi NS, Montazeri A (2017) Effects of infant massage on state anxiety in mothers of preterm infants prior to hospital discharge. Journal of Clinical Nursing. 26(13–14):1887–92 (Abstract).

Ajori L, Nazari L, Eliaspour D (2013) Effects of acupuncture for initiation of labor: a double-blind randomized sham-controlled trial. Archives of Gynecology and Obstetrics. 287(5):887–91.

Akbarzadeh M, Ghaemmaghami M, Yazdanpanahi Z, Zare N, Azizi A, Mohagheghzadeh A (2014) The effect of dry cupping therapy at acupoint BL23 on the intensity of postpartum low back pain in primiparous women based on two types of questionnaires: a randomized clinical trial. International Journal of Community Based Nursing and Midwifery. 2(2):112–20.

Akbarzadeh M, Masoudi Z, Zare N, Vaziri F (2015) Comparison of the effects of doula supportive care and acupressure at the BL32 point on the mother's anxiety level and delivery outcome. Iranian Journal of Nursing and Midwifery Research. 20(2):239–46.

Akdogan M, Gultekin F, Yontem M (2004) Effect of Mentha piperita (Labiatae) and Mentha spicata (Labiatae) on iron absorption in rats. Toxicology and Industrial Health. 20(6–10):119–22.

Akmeşe ZB, Oran NT (2014) Effects of progressive muscle relaxation exercises accompanied by music on low back pain and quality of life during pregnancy. Journal of Midwifery and Women's Health. 59(5):503–9.

Alaniz VI, Liss J, Metz TD, Stickrath E (2015) Cannabinoid hyperemesis syndrome: a cause of refractory nausea and vomiting in pregnancy. Obstetrics & Gynecology. 125(6):1484–6.

Alcantara J, Alcantara JD, Alcantara J (2015) The chiropractic care of infants with breastfeeding difficulties. Explore (NY). 11(6):468–74.

Aldabe D, Ribeiro DC, Milosavljevic S, Dawn Bussey M (2012) Pregnancy-related pelvic girdle pain and its relationship with relaxin levels during pregnancy: a systematic review. European Spine Journal. 21(9):1769–76.

Alehagen S, Wijma K, Wijma B (2001) Fear during labor. Acta Obstetricia et Gynecologica Scandinavica. 80(4):315–20.

Alexander B, Turnbull D, Cyna A (2009) The effect of pregnancy on hypnotisability. Americal Journal of Clinical Hypnosis. 52(1):13–22.

Alexandrovich I, Rakovitskaya O, Kolmo E, Sidorova T, Shushunov S (2003) The effect of fennel (Foeniculum Vulgare) seed oil emulsion in infantile colic: a randomized, placebo-controlled study. Alternative Therapies in Health and Medicine. 9(4):58–61.

Al-Kuran O, Al-Mehaisen L, Bawadi H, Beitawi S, Amarin Z (2011) The effect of late pregnancy consumption of date fruit on labour and delivery. Journal of Obstetrics and Gynaecology. 31(1):29–31.

Allameh Z, Tehrani HG, Ghasemi M (2015) Comparing the impact of acupuncture and pethidine on reducing labor pain. Advanced Biomedical Research. 4:46.

Almog B, Levin I, Winkler N, Fainaru O *et al.* (2005) The contribution of laminaria placement for cervical ripening in second trimester termination of pregnancy induced by intra-amniotic injection of prostaglandin F(2)alpha followed by concentrated oxytocin infusion. European Journal of Obstetrics & Gynecology and Reproductive Biology. 118(1):32–5.

Alsharnoubi J, Khattab A, Elnoury A (2015) Laser acupuncture effect on fetal well-being during induction of labor. Lasers in Medical Science. 30(1):403–6.

Amir N, Berger R, Grinfeld T, Kaner P, Gabinet Y (2015) Efficacy comparison between Chinese medicine's labor inducement methods and conventional methods customary in hospitals. Harefuah. 154(1):47–51, 67, 66 (Abstract only).

Amorosa JM, Stone JL (2015) Outpatient cervical ripening. Seminars in Perinatology. 39(6):488–94.

Amster E, Tiwary A, Schenker MB (2007) Case report: potential arsenic toxicosis secondary to herbal kelp supplement. Environental Health Perspectives. 115(4):606–8.

Anarado A, Ali E, Nwonu E, Chinweuba A, Ogbolu Y (2015) Knowledge and willingness of prenatal women in Enugu Southeastern Nigeria to use in labour non-pharmacological pain reliefs. African Health Sciences. 15(2):568–75.

Andersen BB, Knudsen B, Lyndrup J, Fælling AE (2013) Acupuncture and/or sweeping of the fetal membranes before induction of labor: a prospective, randomized, controlled trial. Journal of Perinatal Medicine. 41(5):555–60.

Andres C, Chen WC, Ollert M, Mempel M, Darsow U, Ring J (2009) Anaphylactic reaction to camomile tea. Allergology International. 58(1):135–6.

Annagür BB, Kerimoğlu ÖS, Gündüz Ş, Tazegül A (2014) Are there any differences in psychiatric symptoms and eating attitudes between pregnant women with hyperemesis gravidarum and healthy pregnant women? Journal of Obstetrics and Gynaecology Research. 40(4):1009–14.

Anzai A, Vázquez Herrera NE, Tosti A (2015) Airborne allergic contact dermatitis caused by chamomile tea. Contact Dermatitis. 72(4):254–5.

Apaydin EA, Maher AR, Shanman R, Booth MS (2016) A systematic review of St. John's Wort for major depressive disorder. Systematics Review. 5(1):148.

Armstrong N, Ernst E (2001) A randomised double-blind placebo controlled investigation of a Bach flower remedy. Complementary Therapies in Nursing and Midwifery. 7:215–21.

Arnadottir TS, Sigurdardottir AK (2013) Is craniosacral therapy effective for migraine? Tested with HIT-6 Questionnaire. Complementary Therapies in Clinical Practice. 19(1):11–49.

Arora S, Vatsa M, Dadhwal V (2008) A comparison of cabbage leaves vs. hot and cold compresses in the treatment of breast engorgement. Indian Journal of Community Medicine. 33(3):160–2.

Asadi N, Maharlouei N, Khalili A, Darabi Y *et al.* (2015) Effects of LI-4 and SP-6 acupuncture on labor pain, cortisol level and duration of labor. Journal of Acupuncture and Meridian Studies. 8(5):249–5.

Asadollahi M, Jabraeili M, Mahallei M, Asgari Jafarabadi M, Ebrahimi S (2016) Effects of gentle human touch and field massage on urine cortisol level in premature infants: a randomized, controlled clinical trial. Journal of Caring Sciences. 5(3):187–94.

Asgharikhatooni A, Bani S, Hasanpoor S, Mohammad Alizade S, Javadzadeh Y (2015) The effect of equisetum arvense (horse tail) ointment on wound healing and pain intensity after episiotomy: a randomized placebo-controlled trial. Iranian Red Crescent Medical Journal. 17(3):e25637.

Asher GN, Coeytaux RR, Chen W, Reilly AC, Loh YL, Harper TC (2009) Acupuncture to initiate labor (Acumoms 2): a randomized, sham-controlled clinical trial. Journal of Maternal-Fetal and Neonatal Medicine. 22(10):843–8.

Aslami E, Alipour AD, Najib FS, Aghayosefi A (2017) A comparative study of mindfulness efficiency based on islamic-spiritual schemes and group cognitive behavioral therapy on reduction of anxiety and depression in pregnant women. International Journal of Community Based Nursing and Midwifery. 5(2):144–52.

Audi J, Belson M, Patel M, Schier J, Osterloh J (2005) Ricin poisoning: a comprehensive review. JAMA. 294(18):2342–51.

Avis NE, Coeytaux RR, Levine B, Isom S, Morgan T (2016) Trajectories of response to acupuncture for menopausal vasomotor symptoms: The Acupuncture in Menopause study. Menopause. 24(2):171–9.

Awad R, Mallah E, Khawaja BA, Dayyih WA et al. (2016) Pomegranate and licorice juices modulate metformin pharmacokinetics in rats. Neuro Endocrinology Letters. 37(3):202–6.

Aydin Y, Aslan E, Yalcin O (2016) Effect of reflexology to depressive symptoms in women with overactive bladder. Holistic Nursing Practice. 30(5):294–300.

Azhari S, Pirdadeh S, Lotfalizadeh M, Shakeri MT (2006) Evaluation of the effect of castor oil on initiating labor in term pregnancy. Saudi Medical Journal. 27(7):1011–14.

Aziz MA, Adnan M, Begum S, Azizullah A, Nazir R, Iram S (2016) A review on the elemental contents of Pakistani medicinal plants: implications for folk medicines. Journal of Ethnopharmacology. 188:177–92.

Baas MA, Stramrood CA, Dijksman LM, de Jongh A, van Pampus MG (2017) The OptiMUM-study: EMDR therapy in pregnant women with posttraumatic stress disorder after previous childbirth and pregnant women with fear of childbirth: design of a multicentre randomized controlled trial. European Journal of Psychotraumatology. 8(1):1293315.

Babbar S, Hill JB, Williams KB, Pinon M, Chauhan SP, Maulik D (2016) Acute fetal behavioral response to prenatal yoga: a single, blinded, randomized controlled trial (TRY yoga). American Journal of Obstetric Gynecology. 214(3):399.e1–8.

Babbar S, Shyken J. (2016) Yoga in pregnancy. Clinical Obstetrics and Gynecology. 59(3):600–12.

Badr LK, Abdallah B, Kahale L (2015) A meta-analysis of preterm infant massage: an ancient practice with contemporary applications. MCN: The American Journal of Maternal/Child Nursing. 40(6):344–58.

Baillie N, Rasmussen P (1997) Black and blue cohosh in labour. New Zealand Medical Journal. 110:20–1.

Balakrishnan A (2015) Therapeutic uses of peppermint – a review. Journal of Pharmaceutical Sciences and Research. 7(7):474–6.

Baldwin AL, Vitale A, Brownell E, Kryak E, Rand W (2017) Effects of reiki on pain, anxiety, and blood pressure in patients undergoing knee replacement: a pilot study. Holistic Nursing Practice. 31(2):80–9.

Balogh A (2005) Pilates and pregnancy. RCM Midwives. 8(5):220–2.

Bamford DS, Percival RC, Tothill AU (1970) Raspberry leaf tea: a new aspect for an old problem. British Journal of Pharmacology. 40(1):161P–162P.

Bamford JT, Ray S, Musekiwa A, van Gool C, Humphreys R, Ernst E (2013) Oral evening primrose oil and borage oil for eczema. Cochrane Database of Systematic Reviews. (4):CD004416.

Bao C, Zhang J, Liu J, Liu H et al. (2016) Moxibustion treatment for diarrhea-predominant irritable bowel syndrome: study protocol for a randomized controlled trial. BMC Complementary and Alternative Medicine. 16(1):408.

Barkey E, Kaszkin-Bettag M (2012) A homeopathic arnica patch for the relief of cellulitis-derived pain and numbness in the hand. Global Advances in Health and Medicine. 1(2):18–20.

Barratt C (2017) Exploring how mindfulness and self-compassion can enhance compassionate care. Nursing Standard. 31(21):55–63.

Basirat Z, Moghadamnia A, Kashifard M, Sharifi-Razavi A (2009) The effect of ginger biscuit on nausea and vomiting in early pregnancy. Acta Medica Iranica. 47(1):51–6.

Basiri-Moghadam M, Basiri-Moghadam K, Kianmehr M, Jani S (2015) The effect of massage on neonatal jaundice in stable preterm newborn infants: a randomized controlled trial. Journal of the Pakistan Medical Association. 65(6):602–6.

Bastu E, Celik C, Nehir A, Dogan M, Yuksel B, Ergun B (2013) Cervical priming before diagnostic operative hysteroscopy in infertile women: a randomized, double-blind, controlled comparison of 2 vaginal misoprostol doses. International Surgery. 98(2): 140–4.

Battle CL, Uebelacker LA, Magee SR, Sutton KA, Miller IW (2015) Potential for prenatal yoga to serve as an intervention to treat depression during pregnancy. Women's Health Issues. 25(2):134–41.

Bayles B, Usatine R (2009) Evening primrose oil. American Family Physician. 80(12):1405–8.

Bazzano AN, Littrell L, Brandt A, Thibeau S, Thriemer K, Theall KP (2016) Health provider experiences with galactagogues to support breastfeeding: a cross-sectional survey. Journal of Multidisciplinary Healthcare. 9:623–30.

Beattie J, Hall H, Biro MA, East C, Lau R (2017) Effects of mindfulness on maternal stress, depressive symptoms and awareness of present moment experience: a pilot randomised trial. Midwifery. 50:174–83.

Beaumont E, Irons C, Rayner G, Dagnall N (2016) Does compassion-focused therapy training for health care educators and providers increase self-compassion and reduce self-persecution and self-criticism? Journal of Continuing Education in the Health Professions. 36(1):4–10.

Beckmann MM, Stock OM (2013) Antenatal perineal massage for reducing perineal trauma. Cochrane Database of Systematic Reviews. (4):CD005123.

Beebe KR (2014) Hypnotherapy for labor and birth. Nursing for Women's Health. 18(1):48–58.

Beevi Z, Low WY, Hassan J (2015) Successful treatment of ptyalism gravidarum with concomitant hyperemesis using hypnosis. American Journal of Clinical Hypnosis. 58(2):215–23.

Behmanesh F, Pasha H, Zeinalzadeh M (2009) The effect of heat therapy on labor pain severity and delivery outcome in parturient women. Iranian Red Crescent Medical Journal. 11(2):188–92.

Bendich A (2000) The potential for dietry supplements to reduce premenstrual syndrome (PMS) symptoms. Journal of the American College of Nutrition. 19(1):3–12.

Benito P, Rodríguez-Perez R, García F, Juste S, Moneo I, Caballero ML (2014) Occupational allergic rhinoconjunctivitis induced by Matricaria chamomilla with tolerance of chamomile tea. Journal of Investigative Allergology and Clinical Immunology. 24(5):369–70.

Bennett S, Bennett MJ, Chatchawan U, Jenjaiwit P (2016) Acute effects of traditional Thai massage on cortisol levels, arterial blood pressure and stress perception in academic stress condition: a single blind randomised controlled trial. Journal of Bodywork and Movement Therapies. 20(2):286–92.

Bensoussan A, Myers SP, Carlton AL (2000) Risks associated with the practice of traditional Chinese medicine: an Australian study. Archives of Family Medicine. 9(10):1071–8.

Bentele-Jaberg N, Guenova E, Mehra T, Nägeli M et al. (2015) The phytotherapeutic fenugreek as a trigger of toxic epidermal necrolysis. Dermatology. 231(2):99–102.

Bergström C, Persson M, Mogren I (2016) Sick leave and healthcare utilisation in women reporting pregnancy related low back pain and/or pelvic girdle pain at 14 months postpartum. Chiropractic and Manual Therapies. 24:7.

Bernard M, Tuchin P (2016) Chiropractic management of pregnancy-related lumbopelvic pain: a case study. Journal of Chiropractic Medicine. 15(2):129–33.

Berrebi A, Parant O, Ferval F, Thene M *et al.* (2001) Treatment of pain due to unwanted lactation with a homeopathic preparation given in the immediate post-partum period. Journal of Gynecology, Obstetrics and Biological Reproduction (Paris). 30(4):353–7 (Abstract).

Berry-Bibee EN, Kim MJ, Tepper NK, Riley HE, Curtis KM (2016) Co-administration of St. John's wort and hormonal contraceptives: a systematic review. Contraception. 94(6):668–77.

Bertuit J, Van Lint CE, Rooze M, Feipel V (2017) Pregnancy and pelvic girdle pain: analysis of pelvic belt on pain. Journal of Clinical Nursing. 25 May. doi: 10.1111/jocn.13888.

Besnier V (2016) Relaxation, a complementary approach for mental health nurses. [Article in French. Soins Psychiatrie. 37(306):17–22.

Betts D (2006) The Essential Guide to Acupuncture in Pregnancy and Childbirth. Hove, UK: Journal of Chinese Medicine.

Betts D, Budd S (2011) "Forbidden points" in pregnancy: historical wisdom? Acupuncture in Medicine. 29(2):137–9.

Bgeginski R, Ramos JG, Nagpal T, Mottola M (2016) The effects of water-based exercise during pregnancy: a systematic review. PROSPERO 2016:CRD42016039473. Viewed online 18/09/2017 at www.crd.york.ac.uk/PROSPERO/display_record. asp?ID=CRD42016039473

Bikmoradi A, Seifi Z, Poorolajal J, Araghchian M, Safiaryan R, Oshvandi K (2015) Effect of inhalation aromatherapy with lavender essential oil on stress and vital signs in patients undergoing coronary artery bypass surgery: a single-blinded randomized clinical trial. Complementary Therapies in Medicine. 23(3):331–8.

Bishop A, Ogollah R, Bartlam B, Barlas P *et al.* (2016) Evaluating acupuncture and standard care for pregnant women with back pain: the EASE Back pilot randomised controlled trial (ISRCTN49955124). Pilot Feasibility Studies. 2:72.

Bishop FL, Yardley L, Cooper C, Little P, Lewith G (2017) Predicting adherence to acupuncture appointments for low back pain: a prospective observational study. BMC Complementary and Alternative Medicine. 17(1):5.

Bishop JL, Northstone K, Green JR, Thompson EA (2011) The use of complementary and alternative medicine in pregnancy: data from the Avon Longitudinal Study of Parents and Children (ALSPAC). Complementary Therapies in Medicine. 19(6):303–10.

Black FO (2002) Maternal susceptibility to nausea and vomiting of pregnancy: is the vestibular system involved? American Journal of Obstetric Gynecology. 186 (5 Suppl Understanding):S204–9.

Blanchette MA, Stochkendahl MJ, Borges Da Silva R, Boruff J, Harrison P, Bussières A (2016) Effectiveness and economic evaluation of chiropractic care for the treatment of low back pain: a systematic review of pragmatic studies. PLoS One. 11(8):e0160037.

Blitz MJ, Smith-Levitin M, Rochelson B (2016) Severe hyponatremia associated with use of black cohosh during prolonged labor and unsuccessful home birth. American Journal of Perinatology Reports. 6(1):e121–4.

BMA (British Medical Association) (1986) Alternative Therapy: Report of the Board of Science and Education. London: British Medical Association.

BMA (British Medical Association) (1993) Complementary Medicine: New Approaches to Good Practice. Oxford: Oxford University Press.

Bø K, Herbert RD (2013) There is not yet strong evidence that exercise regimens other than pelvic floor muscle training can reduce stress urinary incontinence in women: a systematic review. Journal of Physiotherapy. 59(3):159–68.

Boeira JM, Fenner R, Betti AH, Provensi G *et al.* (2010) Toxicity and genotoxicity evaluation of Passiflora alata Curtis (Passifloraceae). Journal of Ethnopharmacology. 128(2):526–32.

Boel M, Lee S, Rijken M, Paw M *et al.* (2009) Castor oil for induction of labour: not harmful, not helpful. Australian and New Zealand Journal of Obstetrics and Gynaecology. 49(5):499–503.

Boi B, Koh S, Gail D (2012) The effectiveness of cabbage leaf application (treatment) on pain and hardness in breast engorgement and its effect on the duration of breastfeeding. JBI Database of Systematic Reviews and Implementation Reports. 10(20):1185–213.

Boitor M, Martorella G, Arbour C, Michaud C, Gélinas C (2015) Evaluation of the preliminary effectiveness of hand massage therapy on postoperative pain of adults in the intensive care unit after cardiac surgery: a pilot randomized controlled trial. Pain Management Nursing. 16(3):354–66.

Bolbol-Haghighi N, Masoumi SZ, Kazemi F (2016) Effect of massage therapy on duration of labour: a randomized controlled trial. Journal of Clinical and Diagnostic Research. 10(4):QC12–15.

Boltman-Binkowski H (2016) A systematic review: are herbal and homeopathic remedies used during pregnancy safe? Curationis. 39(1):1514.

Bona E, Cantamessa S, Pavan M, Novello G *et al.* (2016) Sensitivity of Candida albicans to essential oils: are they an alternative to antifungal agents? Journal of Applied Microbiology. 121(6):1530–45.

Borgatta L, Barad D (1991) Prolonged retention of laminaria fragments: an unusual complication of laminaria usage. Obstetrics and Gynecology. 78(5 pt 2):988–90.

Borgatta L, Chen AY, Vragovic O, Stubblefield PG, Magloire CA (2005) A randomized clinical trial of the addition of laminaria to misoprostol and hypertonic saline for second-trimester induction abortion. Contraception. 72(5):358–61.

Boterhoven de Haan KL, Lee CW, Fassbinder E, Voncken MJ *et al.* (2017) Imagery rescripting and eye movement desensitisation and reprocessing for treatment of adults with childhood trauma-related post-traumatic stress disorder: IREM study design. BMC Psychiatry. 17(1):165.

Boulvain M, Kelly A, Lohse C, Stan C, Irion O (2001) Mechanical methods for induction of labour. Cochrane Database of Systematic Reviews. (4):CD001233.

Brady LH, Henry K, Luth JF 2nd, Casper-Bruett KK (2001) The effects of shiatsu on lower back pain. Journal of Holistic Nursing. 19(1):57–70.

Brämberg EB, Bergström G, Jensen I, Hagberg J, Kwak L (2017) Effects of yoga, strength training and advice on back pain: a randomized controlled trial. BMC Musculoskeletal Disorders. 18(1):132.

British National Formulary (2017) Dinoprostone: interactions. Viewed online 25/10/2017 at https://bnf.nice.org.uk/drug/dinoprostone.html#interactions

Brookes, K (2004) Chemical investigation of isihlambezo or traditional pregnancy-related medicines. PhD thesis. Viewed online 25/10/2017 at https://www.google.co.uk/search?q=Brookes%2C+K+(2004)+Chemical+investigation+of+isihlambezo+or+traditional+pregnancy-related+medicines&oq=brookes%2C+&aqs=chrome.3.69i57j0-l2j69i59j0l2.5425j0j4&sourceid=chrome&ie=UTF-8

Broussard CS, Louik C, Honein MA, Mitchell AA (2010) Herbal use before and during pregnancy. American Journal of Obstetric Gynecology. 202(5):443.e1–6.

Brown JM, Hess KL, Brown S, Murphy C, Waldman AL, Hezareh M (2013) Intravaginal practices and risk of bacterial vaginosis and candidiasis infection among a cohort of women in the United States. Obstetrics and Gynecology. 121(4):773–80.

Buchanan DT, Landis CA, Hohensee C, Guthrie KA *et al.* (2016) Effects of yoga and aerobic exercise on actigraphic sleep parameters in menopausal women with hot flashes. Journal of Clinical Sleep Medicine. pii: jc-00520-15.

Budzynska K, Gardner ZE, Dugoua JJ, Low Dog T, Gardiner P (2012) Systematic review of breastfeeding and herbs. Breastfeed Medicine. 7(6):489–503.

Budzynska K, Gardner ZE, Low Dog T, Gardiner P (2013) Complementary, holistic, and integrative medicine: advice for clinicians on herbs and breastfeeding. Pediatrics in Review. 34(8):343–52.

Bue L, Lauszus FF (2016) Moxibustion did not have an effect in a randomised clinical trial for version of breech position. Danish Medical Journal. 63(2). pii: A5199.

Bukowski EL, Berardi D (2014) Reiki brief report: using Reiki to reduce stress levels in a nine-year-old child. Explore (NY). 10(4):253–5.

Bulchandani S, Watts E, Sucharitha A, Yates D, Ismail KM (2015) Manual perineal support at the time of childbirth: a systematic review and meta-analysis. BJOG. 122(9):1157–65.

Buric I, Farias M, Jong J, Mee C, Brazil IA (2017) What is the molecular signature of mind-body interventions? A systematic review of gene expression changes induced by meditation and related practices. Frontiers in Immunology. 8:670.

Burns E, Zobbi V, Panzeri D, Oskrochi R, Regalia A (2007) Aromatherapy in childbirth: a pilot randomised controlled trial. BJOG. 114(7):838–44.

Burns EE, Blamey C, Ersser SJ, Barnetson L, Lloyd AJ (2000) An investigation into the use of aromatherapy in intrapartum midwifery practice. Journal of Alternative and Complementary Medicine. 6(2):141–7.

Bush TM, Rayburn KS, Holloway SW, Sanchez-Yamamoto DS et al. (2007) Adverse interactions between herbal and dietary substances and prescription medications: a clinical survey. Alternative Therapies in Health and Medicine. 13(2):30–5.

Butani L, Afshinnik A, Johnson J, Javaheri D et al. (2003) Amelioration of tacrolimus-induced nephrotoxicity in rats using juniper oil. Transplantation. 76(2):306–11.

Butt MS, Pasha I, Sultan MT, Randhawa MA, Saeed F, Ahmed W (2013) Black pepper and health claims: a comprehensive treatise. Critical Reviews in Food Science and Nutrition. 53(9):875–86.

Buttagat V, Narktro T, Onsrira K, Pobsamai C (2016) Short-term effects of traditional Thai massage on electromyogram, muscle tension and pain among patients with upper back pain associated with myofascial trigger points. Complementary Therapies in Medicine. 28:8–12.

Butterworth A (2016) Aromatherapy birth botched by midwives. Scottish Daily Mail, 29 October 2016. Viewed online 25/10/2017 at https://www.pressreader.com/uk/scottish-daily-mail/20161029/282406988899982

Buttner MM, Brock RL, O'Hara MW, Stuart S (2015) Efficacy of yoga for depressed postpartum women: a randomized controlled trial. Complementary Therapies in Clinical Practice. 21(2):94–100.

Buyukkayaci Duman N, Ozcan O, Bostanci MÖ (2015) Hyperemesis gravidarum affects maternal sanity, thyroid hormones and fetal health: a prospective case control study. Archives of Gynecology and Obstetrics. 292(2):307–12.

Cal E, Cakiroglu B, Kurt AN, Hartiningsih SS, Suryani, Dane S (2016) The potential beneficial effects of hand and foot bathing on vital signs in women with caesarean section. Clinical and Investigative Medicine. 39(6):27508.

Caldwell K, Adams M, Quin R, Harrison M, Greeson J (2013) Pilates, mindfulness and somatic education. Journal of Dance and Somatic Practices. 5(2):141–53.

Caliskaner Z, Karaayvaz M, Ozturk S (2004) Misuse of a herb: stinging nettle (Urtica urens) induced severe tongue oedema. Complementary Therapies in Medicine. 12(1):57–8.

Calvert I (2005) Ginger: an essential oil for shortening labour? The Practising Midwife. 8(1):30–4.

Cameron EL (2007) Measures of human olfactory perception during pregnancy. Chemical Senses. 32(8):775–82.

Cameron EL (2014) Pregnancy and olfaction: a review. Frontiers in Psychology. 5:67.

Campbell A, Macglashan J (2005) Acupuncture-induced galactorrhoea: a case report. Acupuncture in Medicine. 23(3):146.

Campbell VR, Nolan M (2016) A qualitative study exploring how the aims, language and actions of yoga for pregnancy teachers may impact upon women's self-efficacy for labour and birth. Women and Birth. 29(1):3–11.

Campion M, Glover L (2016) A qualitative exploration of responses to self-compassion in a non-clinical sample. Health and Social Care in the Community. Viewed online 18/09/2017 at http://self-compassion.org/wp-content/uploads/2017/01/Campion 2016.pdf

Can HO, Saruhan A (2015) Evaluation of the effects of ice massage applied to large intestine 4 (hegu) on postpartum pain during the active phase of labor. Iranian Journal of Nursing and Midwifery Research. 20(1):129–38.

Can Gürkan O, Arslan H (2008) Effect of acupressure on nausea and vomiting during pregnancy. Complementary Therapies in Clinical Practice. 14(1):46–52.

Cant S (2011) The knowledgeable doer: nurse and midwife integration of complementary and alternative medicine in NHS hospitals. Wellcome Trust Conference: Regulation and Professionalisation in Complementary and Alternative Medicine: Historical Perspectives and Contemporary Concerns. May 2011, University of Birmingham.

Cant S, Watts P, Ruston A (2011) Negotiating competency, professionalism and risk: the integration of complementary and alternative medicine by nurses and midwives in NHS hospitals. Social Science and Medicine. 72(4):529–36.

Cappello G, Spezzaferro M, Grossi L, Manzoli L, Marzio L (2007) Peppermint oil (Mintoil) in the treatment of irritable bowel syndrome: a prospective double blind placebo-controlled randomized trial. Digestive and Liver Disease. 39(6):530–6.

Cardini F, Basevi V, Valentini A, Martellato A (1991) Moxibustion and breech presentation: preliminary results. The American Journal of Chinese Medicine. 19(2):105–14.

Cardini F, Lombardo P, Regalia AL, Regaldo G et al. (2005) A randomised controlled trial of moxibustion for breech presentation. BJOG. 112(6):743–7.

Cardini F, Marcolongo A (1993) Moxibustion for correction of breech presentation: a clinical study with retrospective control. The American Journal of Chinese Medicine. 21(2):133–8.

Cardini F, Weixin H (1998) Moxibustion for correction of breech presentation: a randomized controlled trial. JAMA. 280(18):1580–4.

Carneiro ÉM, Barbosa LP, Marson JM, Terra JA Junior et al. (2017) Effectiveness of Spiritist "passe" (Spiritual healing) for anxiety levels, depression, pain, muscle tension, well-being, and physiological parameters in cardiovascular inpatients: a randomized controlled trial. Complementary Therapies in Medicine. 30:73–8.

Carpenter P, Richards K (2011) Olive versus mineral oil. Journal of Community Practice. 84(2):40–2.

Carson CF, Hammer KA, Riley TV (2006) Melaleuca alternifolia (Tea Tree) oil: a review of antimicrobial and other medicinal properties. Clinical Microbiology Reviews. 19(1):50–62.

Castro FC, Magre A, Cherpinski R, Zelante PM et al. (2012) Effects of microcurrent application alone or in combination with topical Hypericum perforatum L. and Arnica montana L. on surgically induced wound healing in Wistar rats. Homeopathy. 101(3):147–53.

Castro-Sánchez AM, Lara-Palomo IC, Matarán-Peñarrocha GA, Saavedra-Hernández M, Pérez-Mármol JM, Aguilar-Ferrándiz ME (2016) Benefits of craniosacral therapy in patients with chronic low back pain: a randomized controlled trial. Journal of Alternative and Complementary Medicine. 22(8):650–7.

Chaiet SR, Marcus BC (2016) Perioperative Arnica montana for reduction of ecchymosis in rhinoplasty surgery. Annals of Plastical Surgery. 76(5):477–82.

Chaillet N, Belaid L, Crochetière C, Roy L et al. (2014) Nonpharmacologic approaches for pain management during labor compared with usual care: a meta-analysis. Birth. 41(2):122–37.

Challoner KR, McCarron MM (1990) Castor bean intoxication. Annals of Emergency Medicine. 19(10):1177–83.

Chang HY, Jensen MP, Lai YH (2015) How do pregnant women manage lumbopelvic pain? Pain management and their perceived effectiveness. Journal of Clinical Nursing. 24(9–10):1338–46.

Chang MY, Wang SY, Chen CH (2002) Effects of massage on pain and anxiety during labour: a randomized controlled trial in Taiwan. Journal of Advanced Nursing. 38(1):68–73.

Chaturvedi A, Nayak G, Nayak AG, Rao A (2016) Comparative assessment of the effects of hatha yoga and physical exercise on biochemical functions in perimenopausal women. Journal of Clinical and Diagnostic Research. 10(8):KC01–4.

Chauhan P, Gasser FJ, Chauhan AM (1998) Clinical investigation on the use of acupuncture for treatment of placental retention. American Journal of Acupuncture. 26(1):19–25.

Cheang KI, Nguyen TT, Karjane NW, Salley KE (2016) Raspberry leaf and hypoglycemia in gestational diabetes mellitus. Obstetrics and Gynecology. 128(6):1421–24.

Chen CW, Chen-Jei Tai, Cheuk-Sing Choy, Chau-Yun Hsu et al. (2013) Wave-induced flow in meridians demonstrated using photoluminescent bioceramic material on acupuncture points. Evidence-Based Complementary and Alternative Medicine. 2013:739293. Viewed online 18/09/2017 at www.ncbi.nlm.nih.gov/pmc/articles/PMC3838801

Chen PJ, Yang L, Chou CC, Li CC, Chang YC, Liaw JJ (2017) Effects of prenatal yoga on women's stress and immune function across pregnancy: a randomized controlled trial. Complementary Therapies in Medicine. 31:109–17.

Chen XW, Serag ES, Sneed KB, Liang J et al. (2011) Clinical herbal interactions with conventional drugs: from molecules to maladies. Current Medicinal Chemistry. 18(31):4836–50.

Cherian T (2000) Effect of papaya latex extract on gravid and non-gravid rat uterine preparations in vitro. Journal of Ethnopharmacology. 70(3):205–12.

Chevalier A (2016) Encyclopaedia of Herbal Medicine, 3rd edition. London: Dorling Kindersley.

Chik YM, Ip WY, Choi KC (2017) The effect of upper limb massage on infants' venipuncture pain. Pain Management Nursing. 18(1):50–7 (Abstract).

Chin KB, Cordell B (2013) The effect of tea tree oil (Melaleuca alternifolia) on wound healing using a dressing model. Journal of Alternative and Complementary Medicine. 19(12):942–5.

Chittumma P, Kaewkiattikun K, Wiriyasiriwach B (2007) Comparison of the effectiveness of ginger and vitamin B6 for treatment of nausea and vomiting in early pregnancy: a randomized double-blind controlled trial. Journal of the Medical Association of Thailand. 90(1):15–20.

Choi JS, Han JY, Ahn HK, Lee SW et al. (2015) Assessment of fetal and neonatal outcomes in the offspring of women who had been treated with dried ginger (Zingiberis rhizoma siccus) for a variety of illnesses during pregnancy. Journal of Obstetrics and Gynaecology. 35(2):125–30.

Choi MS, Lee EJ (2015) Effects of foot-reflexology massage on fatigue, stress and postpartum depression in postpartum women (Article in Korean). Journal of Korean Academy of Nursing. 45(4):587–94. Abstract viewed online 18/09/2017 at www.ncbi.nlm.nih.gov/pubmed/26364533

Choi TY, Lee MS, Kim JI, Zaslawski C (2017) Moxibustion for the treatment of osteoarthritis: an updated systematic review and meta-analysis. Maturitas. 100:33–48.

Chojkier M (2003) Hepatic sinusoidal-obstruction syndrome: toxicity of pyrrolizidine alkaloids. Journal of Hepatology. 39(3):437–46.

Chou FH, Avant KC, Kuo SH, Fetzer SJ (2008) Relationships between nausea and vomiting, perceived stress, social support, pregnancy planning, and psychosocial adaptation in a sample of mothers: a questionnaire survey. International Journal of Nursing Studies. 45(8):1185–91.

Chow EC, Teo M, Ring JA, Chen JW (2008) Liver failure associated with the use of black cohosh for menopausal symptoms. Menopause. 15(4Pt1):628–38.

Christodoulou-Smith J, Gold JI, Romero R, Goodwin TM *et al.* (2011) Posttraumatic stress symptoms following pregnancy complicated by hyperemesis gravidarum. The Journal of Maternal-Fetal and Neonatal Medicine. 24(11):1307–11.

Chu H, Li MH, Huang YC, Lee SY (2013) Simultaneous transcutaneous electrical nerve stimulation mitigates simulator sickness symptoms in healthy adults: a crossover study. BMC Complementary and Alternative Medicine. 13:84.

Chuang CH, Doyle P, Wang JD, Chang PJ, Lai JN, Chen PC (2006) Herbal medicines used during the first trimester and major congenital malformations: an analysis of data from a pregnancy cohort study. Drug Safety. 29(6):537–48.

Chuang LL, Liu SC, Chen YH, Lin LC (2015) Predictors of adherence to relaxation guided imagery during pregnancy in women with preterm labor. Journal of Alternative and Complementary Medicine. 21(9):563–8.

Ciganda C, Laborde A (2003) Herbal infusions used for induced abortion. Journal of Toxicology: Clinical Toxicology. 41(3):235–9.

Close C, Sinclair M, Liddle D, Madden E, McCullough J, Hughes C (2014) A systematic review investigating the effectiveness of Complementary and Alternative Medicine (CAM) for the management of low back and/or pelvic pain (LBPP) in pregnancy. Journal of Advanced Nursing. 70(8):1702–16.

Close C, Sinclair M, Liddle D, McCullough J, Hughes C (2016a) Women's experience of low back and/or pelvic pain (LBPP) during pregnancy. Midwifery. 37:1–8.

Close C, Sinclair M, McCullough J, Liddle D, Hughes C (2016b) A pilot randomised controlled trial (RCT) investigating the effectiveness of reflexology for managing pregnancy low back and/or pelvic pain. Complementary Therapies in Clinical Practice. 23:117–24.

Close C, Sinclair M, McCullough J, Liddle D, Hughes C (2016c) Factors affecting recruitment and attrition in randomised controlled trials of complementary and alternative medicine for pregnancy-related issues. Evidence-Based Complementary and Alternative Medicine. 2016:6495410.

Cochrane S, Smith CA, Possamai-Inesedy A, Bensoussan A (2016) Prior to conception: the role of an acupuncture protocol in improving women's reproductive functioning assessed by a pilot pragmatic randomised controlled trial. Evidence-Based Complementary and Alternative Medicine. 2016:3587569.

Cohen DL, Boudhar S, Bowler A, Townsend RR (2016) Blood pressure effects of yoga, alone or in combination with lifestyle measures: results of the lifestyle modification and blood pressure study (LIMBS). Journal of Clinical Hypertension (Greenwich). 18(8):809–16.

Cohen SM, O'Connor AM, Hart J, Merel NH, Te HS (2004) Autoimmune hepatitis associated with the use of black cohosh: a case study. Menopause. 11(5):575–7.

Cohen SR, Thomas CR (2015) Rebozo technique for fetal malposition in labor. Journal of Midwifery and Women's Health. 60(4):445–51.

Conrad P, Adams C (2012) The effects of clinical aromatherapy for anxiety and depression in the high risk postpartum woman: a pilot study. Complementary Therapies in Clinical Practice. 18(3):164–8.

Cooke A, Cork MJ, Victor S, Campbell M *et al.* (2016) Olive oil, sunflower oil or no oil for baby dry skin or massage: a pilot, assessor-blinded, randomized controlled trial (the Oil in Baby Skincare [OBSeRvE] Study). Acta Dermato-Venereologica. 96(3):323–30.

Cooperative Research Group of Moxibustion Version of Jangxi Province (1984) Further studies on the clinical effects and the mechanism of version by moxibustion. In: Abstracts of the Second National Symposium on Acupuncture, Moxibustion and Acupuncture Anaesthesia. 7–10 August, Beijing, China. Cited by Ewies A, Olah K (2002) Moxibustion in breech version: a descriptive review. Acupuncture in Medicine. 20(1):26–9.

Coulon C, Poleszczuk M, Paty-Montaigne MH, Gascard C *et al.* (2014) Version of breech fetuses by moxibustion with acupuncture: a randomized controlled trial. Obstetrics and Gynecology. 124(1):32–9.

Cramer H, Frawley J, Steel A, Hall H *et al.* (2015) Characteristics of women who practice yoga in different locations during pregnancy. BMJ Open. 5(8):e008641.

Cummings M (2011) "Forbidden points" in pregnancy: no plausible mechanism for risk. Acupuncture in Medicine. 29(2):140–2.

Cuthbert SC (2006) Proposed mechanisms and treatment strategies for motion sickness disorder: a case series. Journal of Chiropractic Medicine. 5(1):22–31.

Cuzzolin L, Francini-Pesenti F, Verlato G, Joppi M, Baldelli P, Benoni G (2010) Use of herbal products among 392 Italian pregnant women: focus on pregnancy outcome. Pharmacoepidemiology and Drug Safety. 19(11):1151–8.

Cyna AM, Crowther CA, Robinson JS, Andrew MI, Antoniou G, Baghurst P (2013) Hypnosis antenatal training for childbirth: a randomised controlled trial. BJOG. 120(10):1248–59; discussion 1256–7.

Dabiri F, Shahi A (2014) The effect of LI4 acupressure on labor pain and duration of labor: a randomized controlled trial. Oman Medical Journal. 29(6):425–9.

Da-Costa-Rocha I, Bonnlaender B, Sievers H, Pischel I, Heinrich M (2014) Hibiscus sabdariffa L.: a phytochemical and pharmacological review. Food Chemistry. 165:424–43.

Dako-Gyeke P, Aikins M, Aryeetey R, McCough L, Adongo PB (2013) The influence of socio-cultural interpretations of pregnancy threats on health-seeking behavior among pregnant women in urban Accra, Ghana. BMC Pregnancy and Childbirth. 13:211.

Dalal K, Elanchezhiyan D, Das R, Dalal D *et al.* (2013) Noninvasive characterisation of foot reflexology areas by swept source-optical coherence tomography in patients with low back pain. Evidence-Based Complementary and Alternative Medicine. 2013:983769.

Dale A, Cornwell S (1994) The role of lavender oil in relieving perineal discomfort following childbirth: a blind randomized clinical trial. Journal of Advanced Nursing. 19(1):89–96.

Dalili H, Sheikhi S, Shariat M, Haghnazarian E (2016) Effects of baby massage on neonatal jaundice in healthy Iranian infants: A pilot study. Infant Behavior and Development. 42:22–6.

Dalke H, Little J, Niemann E, Camgoz N, Steadman G, Hill S, Stott L (2006) Colour and lighting in hospital design. Optics and Laser Technology. 38:343–65.

Darmstadt GL, Mao-Qiang M, Chi E, Saha SK *et al.* (2002) Impact of topical oils on the skin barrier: possible implications for neonatal health in developing countries. Acta Paediatrica. 91(5):546–54.

Darwish AM, Ahmad AM, Mohammad AM (2004) Cervical priming prior to operative hysteroscopy: a randomized comparison of laminaria versus misoprostol. Human Reproduction. 19(10):2391–4.

Datta S, Mahdi F, Ali Z, Jekabsons MB *et al.* (2014) Toxins in botanical dietary supplements: blue cohosh components disrupt cellular respiration and mitochondrial membrane potential. Journal of Natural Products. 77(1):111–17.

Davis K, Goodman SH, Leiferman J, Taylor M, Dimidjian S (2015) A randomized controlled trial of yoga for pregnant women with symptoms of depression and anxiety. Complementary Therapies in Clinical Practice. 21(3):166–72.

Davis L, Hanson B, Gilliam S (2016) Pilot study of the effects of mixed light touch manual therapies on active duty soldiers with chronic post-traumatic stress disorder and injury to the head. Journal of Bodywork and Movement Therapies. 20(1):42–51.

Davis N, Campbell D (2017) "A misuse of scarce funds": NHS to end prescription of homeopathic remedies. The Guardian, 22 July. Viewed online 18/09/2017 at www.theguardian.com/lifeandstyle/2017/jul/21/a-misuse-of-scarce-funds-nhs-to-end-prescription-of-homeopathic-remedies

de Boer H, Cotingting C (2014) Medicinal plants for women's healthcare in southeast Asia: a meta-analysis of their traditional use, chemical constituents, and pharmacology. Journal of Ethnopharmacology. 151(2):747–67.

de Boer H, Lamxay V (2009) Plants used during pregnancy, childbirth and postpartum healthcare in Lao PDR: a comparative study of the Brou, Saek and Kry ethnic groups. Journal of Ethnobiology and Ethnomedicine. 5:25.

de Pascalis V, Varriale V, Cacace I (2015) Pain modulation in waking and hypnosis in women: event-related potentials and sources of cortical activity. PLoS One. 10(6):e0128474.

de Sousa L, Gomes-Sponholz FA, Nakano AM (2014) Transcutaneous electrical nerve stimulation for the relief of post-partum uterine contraction pain during breast-feeding: a randomized clinical trial. Journal of Obstetrics and Gynaecology Research. 40(5):1317–23.

Dean C, Marsden J (2017) Satisfaction for treatment of hyperemesis gravidarum in day case settings compared to hospital admissions. MIDIRS Midwifery Digest. 27(1):11–20.

Dehcheshmeh FS, Rafiei H (2015) Complementary and alternative therapies to relieve labor pain: a comparative study between music therapy and Hoku point ice massage. Complementary Therapies in Clinical Practice. 21(4):229–32.

Del Casale A, Ferracuti S, Rapinesi C, De Rossi P et al. (2015) Hypnosis and pain perception: an activation likelihood estimation (ALE) meta-analysis of functional neuroimaging studies. Journal of Physiology – Paris. 109(4–6):165–72.

Demirel G, Golbasi Z (2015) Effect of perineal massage on the rate of episiotomy and perineal tearing. International Journal of Gynecology and Obstetrics. 131(2):183–6.

Demirel G, Guler H (2015) The effect of uterine and nipple stimulation on induction with oxytocin and the labor process. Worldviews on Evidence-Based Nursing. 12(5):273–80.

Deng H, Shen X (2013) The mechanism of moxibustion: ancient theory and modern research. Evidence-Based Complementary and Alternative Medicine. 2013:379291.

Derry S, Straube S, Moore RA, Hancock H, Collins SL (2012) Intracutaneous or subcutaneous sterile water injection compared with blinded controls for pain management in labour. Cochrane Database of Systematic Reviews. (1):CD009107.

Dhany AL, Mitchell T, Foy C (2012) Aromatherapy and massage intrapartum service impact on use of analgesia and anesthesia in women in labor: a retrospective case note analysis. Journal of Alternative and Complementary Medicine. 18(10):932–8.

Dharmananda S (2004) Moxibustion: practical considerations for modern use of an ancient technique. Viewed online 18/09/2017 at www.itmonline.org/arts/moxibustion.htm

Di Francisco-Donoghue J, Apoznanski T, de Vries K, Jung MK, Mancini J, Yao S (2017) Osteopathic manipulation as a complementary approach to Parkinson's disease: a controlled pilot study. NeuroRehabilitation. 40(1):145–51.

Diego MA, Field T, Hernandez-Reif M (2014) Preterm infant weight gain is increased by massage therapy and exercise via different underlying mechanisms. Early Human Development. 90(3):137–40.

Diehr J (2016) Sophrology and psychiatry. Soins Psychiatrie. 37(306):28–31 (Abstract).

Dionisi B, Senatori R (2011) Effect of transcutaneous electrical nerve stimulation on the postpartum dyspareunia treatment. Journal of Obstetrics and Gynaecology Research. 37(7):750–3.

DiPirro JM, Kristal MB (2004) Placenta ingestion by rats enhances delta- and kappa-opioid antinociception, but suppresses mu-opioid antinociception. Brain Research. 1014(1–2):22–33.

Djakovic I, Djakovic Z, Bilić N, Košec V (2015) Third stage of labor and acupuncture. Medical Acupuncture. 27(1):10–13.

Do CK, Smith CA, Dahlen H, Bisits A, Schmied V (2011) Moxibustion for cephalic version: a feasibility randomised controlled trial. BMC Complementary and Alternative Medicine. 11:81.

Dobson D, Lucassen PL, Miller JJ, Vlieger AM, Prescott P, Lewith G (2012) Manipulative therapies for infantile colic. Cochrane Database of Systematic Reviews. (12):CD004796.

Dochez V, Dimet J, David-Gruselle A, Le Thuaut A, Ducarme G (2016) Validation of specific questionnaires to assess nausea and vomiting of pregnancy in a French population. International Journal of Gynecology and Obstetrics. 134(3):294–8.

Dolatian M, Hasanpour A, Montazeri S, Heshmat R, Alavi Majd H (2011) The effect of reflexology on pain intensity and duration of labor on primiparas. Iranian Red Crescent Medical Journal. 13(7):475–9.

Dong C, Hu L, Liang F, Zhang S (2015) Effects of electro-acupuncture on labor pain management. Archives of Gynecology and Obstetrics. 291(3):531–6.

Donnelly L (2016) NHS is rationing Caesarean births to save money, coroner warns. Daily Mail, 15 April 2016. Viewed online 25/10/2017 at www.telegraph.co.uk/news/2016/04/15/nhs-is-rationing-caesarean-births-to-save-money-coroner-warns

Doran F, Hornibrook J (2013) Women's experiences of participation in a pregnancy and postnatal group incorporating yoga and facilitated group discussion: a qualitative evaluation. Women and Birth. 26(1):82–6.

Dorfman P, Arnal-Lassiere M, Tetau M (1986) Preparation for delivery by homeopathic treatment: double blind vs placebo experimentation. T. Medicine Paris-Ouest. Cited by van Wassenhoven M (2005) Priorities and methods for developing the evidence profile of homeopathy. Recommendations of the ECH General Assembly and XVIII Symposium of GIRI Homeopathy. 94(2):107–24.

Dove D, Johnson P (1999) Oral evening primrose oil: its effect on length of pregnancy and selected intrapartum outcomes in low-risk nulliparous women. Journal of Nurse-Midwifery. 44(3):320–4.

Downe S, Finlayson K, Melvin C, Ali S et al. (2015) Self-hypnosis for intrapartum pain management in nulliparous women: a randomized controlled trial of clinical effectiveness. BJOG. 122(9):1226–34.

Drobnik J, Drobnik E (2016) Timeline and bibliography of early isolations of plant metabolites (1770–1820) and their impact to pharmacy: a critical study. Fitoterapia. 115:155–64.

Dugoua JJ, Mills E, Perri D, Koren G (2006) Safety and efficacy of St. John's wort (hypericum) during pregnancy and lactation. The Canadian Journal of Clinical Pharmacology. 13(3):e268–76.

Dugoua JJ, Perri D, Seely D, Mills E, Koren G (2008) Safety and efficacy of blue cohosh (Caulophyllum thalictroides) during pregnancy and lactation. Canadian Journal of Clinical Pharmacology. 15(1):66–73.

Dugoua JJ, Seely D, Perri D, Koren G, Mills E (2006) Safety and efficacy of black cohosh (Cimicifuga racemosa) during pregnancy and lactation. The Canadian Journal of Clinical Pharmacology. 13(3):e257–61.

Duncan LG, Cohn MA, Chao MT, Cook JG, Riccobono J, Bardacke N (2017) Benefits of preparing for childbirth with mindfulness training: a randomized controlled trial with active comparison. BMC Pregnancy and Childbirth. 17(1):140.

Dundee JW, Chestnutt WN, Ghaly RG, Lynas AG (1986) Traditional Chinese acupuncture: a potentially useful antiemetic? BMJ (Clinical Research Edition). 293(6547):583–4.

Dundee JW, Ghaly RG, Bill KM, Chestnutt WN, Fitzpatrick KT, Lynas AG (1989) Effect of stimulation of the P6 antiemetic point on postoperative nausea and vomiting. British Journal of Anaesthesia. 63(5):612–18.

Dundee JW, Ghaly RG, Fitzpatrick KT, Abram WP, Lynch GA (1989) Acupuncture prophylaxis of cancer chemotherapy-induced sickness. Journal of the Royal Society of Medicine. 82(5):268–71.

Eagon PK, Elm MS, Hunter DS et al. (2000) Medicinal herbs: modulation of estrogen action. Era of Hope Meeting, Dept Defense; Breast Cancer Research Program, Atlanta, GA, 8–11 June.

East CE, Begg L, Henshall NE, Marchant PR, Wallace K (2012) Local cooling for relieving pain from perineal trauma sustained during childbirth. Cochrane Database of Systematic Reviews. (5):CD006304.

Ebneshahidi A, Mohseni M (2008) The effect of patient-selected music on early postoperative pain, anxiety, and hemodynamic profile in cesarean section surgery. Journal of Alternative and Complementary Medicine. 14(7):827–31.

Ebrahimi N, Maltepe C, Bournissen FG, Koren G (2009) Nausea and vomiting of pregnancy: using the 24-hour Pregnancy-Unique Quantification of Emesis (PUQE-24) scale. Journal of Obstetrics and Gynaecology Canada. 31(9):803–7.

Edelman AB, Buckmaster JG, Goetsch MF, Nichols MD, Jensen JT (2006) Cervical preparation using laminaria with adjunctive buccal misoprostol before second-trimester dilation and evacuation procedures: a randomized clinical trial. American Journal of Obstetric Gynecology. 194(2):425–30.

Edgcumbe DP, McAuley D (2008) Hypoglycaemia related to ingestion of a herbal remedy. European Journal of Emergency Medicine. 15(4):236–7.

Edmondson M, Newall N, Carville K, Smith J, Riley TV, Carson CF (2011) Uncontrolled, open-label, pilot study of tea tree (Melaleuca alternifolia) oil solution in the decolonisation of methicillin-resistant Staphylococcus aureus positive wounds and its influence on wound healing. International Wound Journal. 8(4):375–84.

Edmunds J (1999) Blue cohosh and newborn myocardial infarction? Midwifery Today with International Midwife. 52:34–5.

Edwards J, Alcantara J (2014) Successful clinical outcomes confirmed via ultrasound in a patient with placenta previa and breech fetal presentation with chiropractic care. Journal of Pediatric, Maternal and Family Health. 3:3–9.

Eghdampour F, Jahdie F, Kheyrkhah M, Taghizadeh M, Naghizadeh S, Hagani H (2013) The impact of Aloe vera and Calendula on perineal healing after episiotomy in primiparous women: a randomized clinical trial. Journal of Caring Sciences. 2(4):279–86.

Elden H, Ladfors L, Olsen MF, Ostgaard HC, Hagberg H (2005) Effects of acupuncture and stabilising exercises as adjunct to standard treatment in pregnant women with pelvic girdle pain: randomised single blind controlled trial. BMJ. 330(7494):761.

Elden H, Fagevik-Olsen M, Ostgaard HC, Stener-Victorin E, Hagberg H (2008) Acupuncture as an adjunct to standard treatment for pelvic girdle pain in pregnant women: randomised double-blinded controlled trial comparing acupuncture with non-penetrating sham acupuncture. BJOG. 115(13):1655–68.

Elden H, Östgaard HC, Glantz A, Marciniak P, Linnér AC, Olsén MF (2013) Effects of craniosacral therapy as adjunct to standard treatment for pelvic girdle pain in pregnant women: a multicenter, single blind, randomized controlled trial. Acta Obstetricia et Gynecologica Scandinavica. 92(7):775–82.

Eliason BC (1998) Transient hyperthyroidism in a patient taking dietary supplements containing kelp. Journal of the American Board of Family Medicine. 11:478–80.

Engel K, Gerke-Engel G, Gerhard I, Bastert G (1992) Fetomaternal macrotransfusion after successful internal version from breech presentation by moxibustion. Geburtshilfe und Frauenheilkd. 52(4):241–3 (Abstract).

Ensiyeh J, Sakineh MA (2009) Comparing ginger and vitamin B6 for the treatment of nausea and vomiting in pregnancy: a randomised controlled trial. Midwifery. 25(6):649–53.

Erick M (1995) Hyperolfaction and hyperemesis gravidarum: what is the relationship? Nutrition Reviews. 53(10):289–95.

Ernst E (2002) Herbal medicine products during pregnancy: are they safe? BJOG. 109(3):227–35.

Ernst E (2010) Bach flower remedies: a systematic review of randomised clinical trials. Swiss Medical Weekly. 140:w13079.

Eshgizade M, Moghaddam MB, Mohammadzadeh H, Sadat MA, Mina M (2015) A comparison of the efficacy of olive oil, aloe vera extract and breast milk on healing breast fissure in the breastfeeding women. Avicenna Journal of Phytomedicine Supplement. 5:86–7 (Abstract).

Essilfie Appiah G, Hofmeyr GJ (2005) Misoprostol in obstetrics and gynaecology: benefits and risks. South African Journal of Obstetrics and Gynaecology. 11(1):9–10.

Evira Finnish Food Safety Authority (2016) General instructions on safe use of foodstuffs. Viewed online 18/09/2017 at www.evira.fi/globalassets/elintarvikkeet/tietoa-elintarvikkeista/elintarvikevaarat/elintarvikkeiden-kayton-rajoitukset/16.11.evira_taulukko1_eng.pdf

Ewies A, Olah K (2002) Moxibustion in breech version: a descriptive review. Acupuncture in Medicine. 20(1):26–9.

Facchinetti F, Pedrielli G, Benoni G, Joppi M et al. (2012) Herbal supplements in pregnancy: unexpected results from a multicentre study. Human Reproduction. 27(11):3161–7.

Facco E (2017) Meditation and hypnosis: two sides of the same coin? International Journal of Clinical and Experimental Hypnosis. 65(2):169–88.

Facco E, Zanette G, Casiglia E (2014) The role of hypnotherapy in dentistry. International Journal of Clinical and Experimental Hypnosis. 62(2):179–87.

Faramarzi M, Yazdani S, Barat S (2015) A RCT of psychotherapy in women with nausea and vomiting of pregnancy. Human Reproduction. 30(12):2764–73.

Farber K, Wieland LS (2016) Massage for low-back pain. Explore (NY). 12(3):215–17.

Feeney C, Bruns E, LeCompte G, Forati A, Chen T, Matecki A (2017) Acupuncture for pain and nausea in the intensive care unit: a feasibility study in a public safety net hospital. Journal of Alternative and Complementary Medicine. 25 Apr. doi: 10.1089/acm.2016.0323.

Feijen-de Jong EI, Jansen DE, Baarveld F, Spelten E, Schellevis F, Reijneveld SA (2015) Determinants of use of care provided by complementary and alternative health care practitioners to pregnant women in primary midwifery care: a prospective cohort study. BMC Pregnancy and Childbirth. 15:140.

Feijó L, Hernandez-Reif M, Field T, Burns W, Valley-Gray S, Simco E (2006) Mothers' depressed mood and anxiety levels are reduced after massaging their preterm infants. Infant Behaviour and Development. 29(3):476–80.

Fejzo MS, Magtira A, Schoenberg FP, MacGibbon K et al. (2013) Antihistamines and other prognostic factors for adverse outcome in hyperemesis gravidarum. European Journal of Obstetrics & Gynecology and Reproductive Biology. 170(1):71–6.

Fernández LF, Palomino OM, Frutos G (2014) Effectiveness of Roasmarinus officinalis essential oil as anti-hypotensive agent in primary hypotensive patients and its influence on health-related quality of life. Journal of Ethnopharmacology. 151(1):509–16.

Ferrara M, Mungai F, Starace F (2017) St John's wort (Hypericum perforatum) – induced psychosis: a case report. Journal of Medical Case Reports. 11(1):137.

Ferraz GAR, Rodrigues MRK, Lima SAM, Lima MAF *et al.* (2017) Is reiki or prayer effective in relieving pain during hospitalization for cesarean? A systematic review and meta-analysis of randomized controlled trials. Sao Paulo Medical Journal. 135(2):123–32.

Fessler DM (2002) Reproductive immunosuppression and diet: an evolutionary perspective on pregnancy sickness and meat consumption. Current Anthropology. 43(1):19–61.

Field T (2010) Postpartum depression effects on early interactions, parenting, and safety practices: a review. Infant Behaviour and Development. 33(1):1–6.

Field T (2016a) Massage therapy research review. Complementary Therapies in Clinical Practice. 24:19–31.

Field T (2016b) Yoga research review. Complementary Therapies in Clinical Practice. 24:145–61.

Field T, Diego M, Delgado J, Medina L (2013) Tai chi/yoga reduces prenatal depression, anxiety and sleep disturbances. Complementary Therapies in Clinical Practice. 19(1):6–10.

Field T, Diego M, Gonzalez G, Funk CG (2014) Neck arthritis pain is reduced and range of motion is increased by massage therapy. Complementary Therapies in Clinical Practice. 20(4):219–23.

Field T, Diego M, Gonzalez G, Funk CG (2015) Knee arthritis pain is reduced and range of motion is increased following moderate pressure massagetherapy. Complementary Therapies in Clinical Practice. 21(4):233–7.

Field T, Diego M, Hernandez-Reif M (2010a) Moderate pressure is essential for massage therapy effects. International Journal of Neuroscience. 120(5):381–5.

Field T, Diego M, Hernandez-Reif M (2010b) Prenatal depression effects and interventions: a review. Infant Behaviour and Development. 33(4):409–18.

Field T, Diego M, Hernandez-Reif M (2011) Potential underlying mechanisms for greater weight gain in massaged preterm infants. Infant Behaviour and Development. 34(3):383–9.

Field T, Diego M, Hernandez-Reif M, Deeds O, Figueiredo B (2009) Pregnancy massage reduces prematurity, low birthweight and postpartum depression. Infant Behaviour and Development. 32(4):454–60.

Field T, Diego M, Hernandez-Reif M, Medina L, Delgado J, Hernandez A (2012) Yoga and massage therapy reduce prenatal depression and prematurity. Journal of Bodywork and Movement Therapies. 16(2):204–9.

Field T, Gonzalez G, Diego M, Mindell J (2016) Mothers massaging their newborns with lotion versus no lotion enhances mothers' and newborns' sleep. Infant Behaviour and Development. 45(Pt A):31–3.

Fink NS, Urech C, Cavelti M, Alder J (2012) Relaxation during pregnancy: what are the benefits for mother, fetus, and the newborn? A systematic review of the literature. The Journal of Perinatal and Neonatal Nursing. 26(4):296–306.

Finkel RS, Zarlengo KM (2004) Blue cohosh and perinatal stroke. The New England Journal of Medicine. 351:302–3.

Finlayson K, Downe S, Hinder S, Carr H, Spiby H, Whorwell P (2015) Unexpected consequences: women's experiences of a self-hypnosis intervention to help with pain relief during labour. BMC Pregnancy and Childbirth. 15:229.

Firouzbakht M, Nikpour M, Jamali B, Omidvar S (2014) Comparison of ginger with vitamin B6 in relieving nausea and vomiting during pregnancy. AYU. 35(3):289–93.

Fishburn S (2015) Pelvic girdle pain: updating current practice. The Practising Midwife. 18(10):12–15.

Flake ZA, Scalley RD, Bailey AG (2004) Practical selection of antiemetics. American Family Physician. 69(5):1169–74.

Flynn TA, Jones BA, Ausderau KK (2016) Guided imagery and stress in pregnant adolescents. The American Journal of Occupational Therapy. 70(5). doi: 10.5014/ajot.2016.019315.

Forinash AB, Yancey AM, Barnes KN, Myles TD (2012) The use of galactogogues in the breastfeeding mother. Annals of Pharmacotherapy. 46(10):1392–404.

Forster DA, Denning A, Wills G, Bolger M, McCarthy E (2006) Herbal medicine use during pregnancy in a group of Australian women. BMC Pregnancy and Childbirth. 6:21.

Foster NE, Bishop A, Bartlam B, Ogollah R et al. (2016) Evaluating Acupuncture and Standard carE for pregnant women with Back pain (EASE Back): a feasibility study and pilot randomised trial. Health Technology Assessment. 20(33):1–236.

Fraser D (ed.) (2009) Myles' Textbook for Midwives, 15th edition. Edinburgh: Churchill Livingstone.

Frawley J, Adams J, Steel A, Broom A, Gallois C, Sibbritt D (2015) Women's use and self-prescription of herbal medicine during pregnancy: an examination of 1,835 pregnant women. Women's Health Issues. 25(4):396–402.

Frawley J, Sibbritt D, Broom A, Gallois C, Steel A (2016) Complementary and alternative medicine practitioner use prior to pregnancy predicts use during pregnancy. Journal of Women's Health. 56(8):926–39.

Frawley J, Sundberg T, Steel A, Sibbritt D, Broom A, Adams J (2016) Prevalence and characteristics of women who consult with osteopathic practitioners during pregnancy: a report from the Australian Longitudinal Study on Women's Health (ALSWH). Journal of Bodywork and Movement Therapies. 20(1):168–72.

Freeman RM, Macaulay AJ, Eve L, Chamberlain GV, Bhat AV (1986) Randomised trial of self hypnosis for analgesia in labour. BMJ. 292:657–8.

Gabay MP (2002) Galactogogues: medications that induce lactation. Journal of Human Lactation. 18(3):274–9.

Gammie N, Key S (2014) Time's up! Women's experience of induction of labour. The Practicing Midwife. 17(4):15–18.

Ganji Z, Shirvani MA, Rezaei-Abhari F, Danesh M (2013) The effect of intermittent local heat and cold on labor pain and child birth outcome. Iranian Journal of Nursing and Midwifery Research. 18(4):298–303.

García-Mochón L, Martín JJ, Aranda-Regules JM, Rivas-Ruiz F, Vas J (2015) Cost effectiveness of using moxibustion to correct non-vertex presentation. Acupuncture in Medicine. 33(2):136–41.

Garland D (2017) Revisiting Waterbirth: An Attitude to Care, 2nd edition. London: Palgrave.

Garry D, Figueroa R, Guillaume J, Cucco V (2000) Use of castor oil in pregnancies at term. Alternative Therapies in Health and Medicine. 6(1):77–9.

Garshasbi A, Faghih Zadeh S (2005) The effect of exercise on the intensity of low back pain in pregnant women. International Journal of Gynecology and Obstetrics. 88(3):271–5.

Gartoulla P, Davis SR, Worsley R, Bell RJ (2015) Use of complementary and alternative medicines for menopausal symptoms in Australian women aged 40–65 years. Medical Journal of Australia. 203(3):146.

Gatward H, Simpson M, Woodhart L, Stainton MC (2010) Women's experiences of being induced for post date pregnancy. Women and Birth. 23(1):3–9.

Gaudernack LC, Forbord S, Hole E (2006) Acupuncture administered after spontaneous rupture of membranes at term significantly reduces the length of birth and use of oxytocin: a randomized controlled trial. Acta Obstetricia et Gynecologica Scandinavica. 85(11):1348–53.

Gaudet LM, Dyzak R, Aung SK, Smith GN (2008) Effectiveness of acupuncture for the initiation of labour at term: a pilot randomized controlled trial. Journal of Obstetrics and Gynaecology Canada. 30(12):1118–23.

Gavin-Jones T (2016) Hypnobirth within the NHS: time to ditch the parent craft? The Practising Midwife. 19(5):16, 18–19.

George JW, Skaggs CD, Thompson PA, Nelson DM, Gavard JA, Gross GA (2013) A randomized controlled trial comparing a multimodal intervention and standard obstetrics care for low back and pelvic pain in pregnancy. American Journal of Obstetric Gynecology. 208(4):295. e1–7.

Geranmayeh M, Rezaei Habibabadi Z, Fallahkish B, Farahani MA, Khakbazan Z, Mehran A (2012) Reducing perineal trauma through perineal massage with vaseline in second stage of labor. Archives of Gynecology and Obstetrics. 285(1):77–81.

Ghaly RG, Fitzpatrick KT, Dundee JW (1987) Antiemetic studies with traditional Chinese acupuncture: a comparison of manual needling with electrical stimulation and commonly used antiemetics. Anaesthesia. 42(10):1108–10.

Ghasemi V, Kheirkhah M, Vahedi M (2015) The effect of herbal tea containing fenugreek seed on the signs of breast milk sufficiency in Iranian girl infants. Iranian Red Crescent Medical Journal. 17(8):e21848.

Ghayur MN, Gilani AH (2005) Ginger lowers blood pressure through blockade of voltage-dependent calcium channels. Journal of Cardiovascular Pharmacology. 45(1):74–80.

Gholami F, Neisani Samani L, Kashanian M, Naseri M, Hosseini AF, Hashemi Nejad SA (2016) Onset of labor in post-term pregnancy by chamomile. Iranian Red Crescent Medical Journal. 18(11):e19871.

Giacosa A, Morazzoni P, Bombardelli E, Riva A, Bianchi Porro G, Rondanelli M (2015) Can nausea and vomiting be treated with ginger extract? European Review for Medical and Pharmacological Sciences. 19(7):1291–6.

Giovannini D, Gismondi A, Basso A, Canuti L et al. (2016) Lavandula angustifolia Mill. essential oil exerts antibacterial and anti-inflammatory effect in macrophage mediated immune response to Staphylococcus aureus. Immunological Investigations. 45(1):11–28.

Gläser D, Hilberg T (2006) The influence of bromelain on platelet count and platelet activity in vitro. Platelets. 17(1):37–41.

Glezerman M (2011) To rescue a vanishing obstetric skill-vaginal breech delivery. Harefuah. 150(2):96–8, 207, 208 (Abstract).

Gnazzo A, Guerriero V, Di Folco S, Zavattini GC, de Campora G (2015) Skin to skin interactions. Does the infant massage improve the couple functioning? Frontiers in Psychology. 6:1468.

Golaszewski T, Frigo P, Mark HE, Rattay F, Schaller A (1995) Treatment of hyperemesis gravidarum by electrostimulation of the vestibular apparatus. Zeitschrift fur Geburtshilfe und Neonatologie. 199(3):107–10.

Golberg D, Szilagyi A, Graves L (2007) Hyperemesis gravidarum and Helicobacter pylori infection: a systematic review. Obstetrics and Gynecology. 110:695–703. and doi: 10.1097/01. AOG.0000278571.93861.26.

Golezar S (2016) Ananas comosus: effect on perineal pain and wound healing after episiotomy: a randomized double-blind placebo-controlled clinical trial. Iranian Red Crescent Medical Journal. 18(3):e21019.

Gomes CS, Pedriali FR, Urbano MR, Moreira EH, Averbeck MA, Almeida SHM (2017) The effects of Pilates method on pelvic floor muscle strength in patients with post-prostatectomy urinary incontinence: a randomized clinical trial. Neurourology and Urodynamics. 2 May. doi: 10.1002/nau.23300.

Gong H, Ni C, Shen X, Wu T, Jiang C (2015) Yoga for prenatal depression: a systematic review and meta-analysis. BMC Psychiatry. 15:14. doi: 10.1186/s12888-015-0393-1.

Goodwin TM (2008) Hyperemesis gravidarum. Obstetrics and Gynecology. Clinics of North America. 35(3):401–17.

Gori L, Gallo E, Mascherini V, Mugelli A, Vannacci A, Firenzuoli F (2012) Can estragole in fennel seed decoctions really be considered a danger for human health? A fennel safety update. Evidence-Based Complementary and Alternative Medicine. 2012:860542.

Granath AB, Hellgren MS, Gunnarsson RK (2006) Water aerobics reduces sick leave due to low back pain during pregnancy. Journal of Obstetric, Gynecologic and Neonatal Nursing. 35(4):465–71.

Gregson S, Tiran D, Absalom J, Older L et al. (2015) Acupressure for inducing labour for nulliparous women with post-dates pregnancy. Complementary Therapies in Clinical Practice. 21:1–5.

Gribel GP, Coca-Velarde LG, Moreira de Sá RA (2011) Electroacupuncture for cervical ripening prior to labor induction: a randomized clinical trial. Archives of Gynecology and Obstetrics. 283(6):1233–8.

Gruber CW, O'Brien M (2011) Uterotonic plants and their bioactive constituents. Planta Medica. 77(3):207–20.

Gryder LK, Young SM, Zava D, Norris W, Cross CL, Benyshek DC (2017) Effects of human maternal placentophagy on maternal postpartum iron status: a randomized, double-blind, placebo-controlled pilot study. Journal of Midwifery and Women's Health. 62(1):68–79.

Guittier MJ, Bonnet J, Jarabo G, Boulvain M, Irion O, Hudelson P (2011) Breech presentation and choice of mode of childbirth: a qualitative study of women's experiences. Midwifery. 27(6):e208–13.

Guittier MJ, Klein TJ, Dong H, Andreoli N, Irion O, Boulvain M (2008) Side-effects of moxibustion for cephalic version of breech presentation. Journal of Alternative and Complementary Medicine. 14(10):1231–3.

Guittier MJ, Pichon M, Dong H, Irion O, Boulvain M (2009) Moxibustion for breech version: a randomized controlled trial. Obstetrics and Gynecology. 114(5):1034–40.

Guittier MJ, Pichon M, Irion O, Guillemin F, Boulvain M (2012) Recourse to alternative medicine during pregnancy: motivations of women and impact of research findings. Journal of Alternative and Complementary Medicine. 18(12):1147–53.

Gunn TR, Wright IM (1996) The use of black and blue cohosh in labour. New Zealand Medical Journal. 109:410–11.

Gunnarsdottir TJ, Jonsdottir H (2010) Healing crisis in reflexology: becoming worse before becoming better. Complementary Therapies in Clinical Practice. 16(4):239–43.

Guthrie K, Taylor DJ, Defriend D (1984) Maternal hypnosis induced by husbands. Journal of Obstetrics and Gynaecology. 5:93–6.

Gutke A, Betten C, Degerskär K, Pousette S, Olsén MF (2015) Treatments for pregnancy-related lumbopelvic pain: a systematic review of physiotherapy modalities. Acta Obstetricia et Gynecologica Scandinavica. 94(11):1156–67.

Gutteridge K (2014) The multisensory approach to birth and aromatherapy. The Practising Midwife. 17(5):26–9.

Haavik H, Murphy BA, Kruger J (2016) Effect of spinal manipulation on pelvic floor functional changes in pregnant and nonpregnant women: a preliminary study. Journal of Manipulative and Physiological Therapeutics. 39(5):339–47.

Hadi N, Hanid AA (2011) Lavender essence for post-cesarean pain. Pakistan Journal of Biological Sciences. 14(11):664–7.

Hagen S, Glazener C, McClurg D, Macarthur C et al. (2017) Pelvic floor muscle training for secondary prevention of pelvic organ prolapse (PREVPROL): a multicentre randomised controlled trial. Lancet. 389(10067):393–402.

Haji Seid Javadi E, Salehi F, Mashrabi O (2013) Comparing the effectiveness of vitamin B6 and ginger in treatment of pregnancy-induced nausea and vomiting. Obstetrics and Gynecology International. 2013:927834.

Hajiamini Z, Masoud SN, Ebadi A, Mahboubh A, Matin AA (2012) Comparing the effects of ice massage and acupressure on labor pain reduction. Complementary Therapies in Clinical Practice. 18(3):169–72.

Hall H, Cramer H, Sundberg T, Ward L *et al.* (2016) The effectiveness of complementary manual therapies for pregnancy-related back and pelvic pain: a systematic review with meta-analysis. Medicine (Baltimore). 95(38):e4723.

Hall H, Jolly K (2014) Women's use of complementary and alternative medicines during pregnancy: a cross-sectional study. Midwifery. 30:499–505.

Hall H, Lauche R, Adams J, Steel A, Broom A, Sibbritt D (2016) Healthcare utilisation of pregnant women who experience sciatica, leg cramps and/or varicose veins: a cross-sectional survey of 1835 pregnant women. Women and Birth. 29(1):35–40.

Hall H, McKenna L, Griffiths D (2012) Complementary and alternative medicine for induction of labour. Women and Birth. 25:142–8.

Hall HG, Griffiths DL, McKenna LG (2011) The use of complementary and alternative medicine by pregnant women: a literature review. Midwifery. 27(6):817–24.

Hall HG, Griffiths DL, McKenna LG (2013) Keeping childbearing safe: midwives' influence on women's use of complementary and alternative medicine. International Journal of Nursing Practice. 19(4):437–43.

Hall HG, Griffiths DL, McKenna LG (2015) Complementary and alternative medicine: interaction and communication between midwives and women. Women and Birth. 28(2):137–42.

Haller H, Lauche R, Cramer H, Rampp T *et al.* (2016) Craniosacral therapy for the treatment of chronic neck pain: a randomized sham-controlled trial. The Clinical Journal of Pain. 32(5):441–9.

Halsband U, Wolf TG (2015) Functional changes in brain activity after hypnosis in patients with dental phobia. Journal of Physiology – Paris. 109(4–6):131–42.

Haltzman S, Foy DiGeronimo T (2008) The Secrets of Happily Married Women. San Francisco, CA: Jossey Bass (Wiley imprint).

Hammer KA, Carson CF, Riley TV (1998) In-vitro activity of essential oils, in particular Melaleuca alternifolia (tea tree) oil and tea tree oil products, against Candida spp. Journal of Antimicrobial Chemotherapy. 42(5):591–5.

Hammer KA, Carson CF, Riley TV (2012) Effects of Melaleuca alternifolia (tea tree) essential oil and the major monoterpene component terpinen-4-ol on the development of single- and multistep antibiotic resistance and antimicrobial susceptibility. Antimicrobial Agents and Chemotherapy. 56(2):909–15.

Hammett, FS (1918) The effect of ingestion of desiccated (dried) placenta on milk production. The Journal of Biological Chemistry, 36. American Society of Biological Chemists, Rockefeller Institute for Medical Research, original press: Harvard University.

Han JH, Kim MJ, Yang HJ, Lee YJ, Sung YH (2014) Effects of therapeutic massage on gait and pain after delayed onset muscle soreness. Journal of Exercise Rehabilitation. 10(2):136–40. doi: 10.12965/jer.140106. eCollection 2014.

Han N, Gu Y, Ye C, Cao Y, Liu Z, Yin J (2012) Antithrombotic activity of fractions and components obtained from raspberry leaves (Rubus chingii). Food Chemistry. 132(1):181–5.

Hansen AH, Kristoffersen AE (2016) The use of CAM providers and psychiatric outpatient services in people with anxiety/depression: a cross-sectional survey. BMC Complementary and Alternative Medicine. 16(1):461.

Hardy ML (2000) Herbs of special interest to women. Journal of the American Pharmaceutical Association (Wash). 40(2):234–42.

Harker N, Montgomery A, Fahey T (2004) Treating nausea and vomiting during pregnancy: case outcome. BMJ. 328(7438):503.

Harlev A, Pariente G, Kessous R, Aricha-Tamir B *et al.* (2013) Can we find the perfect oil to protect the perineum? A randomized-controlled double-blind trial. The Journal of Maternal-Fetal and Neonatal Medicine. 26(13):1328–31.

Harmon TM, Hynan MT, Tyre TE (1990) Improved obstetric outcomes using hypnotic analgesia and skill mastery combined with childbirth education. Journal of Consulting and Clinical Psychology. 58(5):525–30.

Harper TC, Coeytaux RR, Chen W, Campbell K *et al.* (2006) A randomized controlled trial of acupuncture for initiation of labor in nulliparous women. The Journal of Maternal-Fetal and Neonatal Medicine. 19(8):465–70.

Hasan FM, Zagarins SE, Pischke KM, Saiyed S *et al.* (2014) Hypnotherapy is more effective than nicotine replacement therapy for smoking cessation: results of a randomized controlled trial. Complementary Therapies in Medicine. 22(1):1–8.

Hashemi M, Jafarian AA, Tofighi S, Mahluji K, Halabchi F (2016) Studying the effectiveness of one type of Iranian traditional massage on lumbar radiculopathy. Iranian Journal of Medical Sciences. 41(3 Suppl):S11.

Hastings-Tolsma M (2014) Antenatal perineal massage decreases risk of perineal trauma during birth. Evidence-Based Nursing. 17(3):77.

Hastings-Tolsma M, Vincent D, Emeis C, Francisco T (2007) Getting through birth in one piece: protecting the perineum. MCN: The American Journal of Maternal/Child Nursing. 32(3):158–64.

Haugen M, Vikanes A, Brantsaeter AL, Meltzer HM, Grjibovski AM, Magnus P (2011) Diet before pregnancy and the risk of hyperemesis gravidarum. British Journal of Nutrition. 106(4):596–602.

Hayes EH (2016) Consumption of the placenta in the postpartum period. Journal of Obstetric, Gynecologic and Neonatal Nursing. 45(1):78–89.

Heinrichs L (2002) Linking olfaction with nausea and vomiting of pregnancy, recurrent abortion, hyperemesis gravidarum, and migraine headache. American Journal of Obstetric Gynecology. 186(5 Suppl Understanding):S215–19.

Heitmann K, Nordeng H, Holst L (2013) Safety of ginger use in pregnancy: results from a large population-based cohort study. European Journal of Clinical Pharmacology. 69(2):269–77.

Helmreich RJ, Shiao SY, Dune LS (2006) Meta-analysis of acustimulation effects on nausea and vomiting in pregnant women. Explore (NY). 2(5):412–21.

Henry L (2015) Chiropractic management of postpartum pubic symphysis diastasis: a case report. Journal of the Canadian Chiropractic Association. 59(1):30–6.

Hensel KL, Buchanan S, Brown SK, Rodriguez M, Cruser A (2015) Pregnancy research on osteopathic manipulation optimizing treatment effects: the PROMOTE study. American Journal of Obstetric Gynecology. 212(1):108.e1–9.

Hensel KL, Carnes MS, Stoll ST (2016) Pregnancy research on osteopathic manipulation optimizing treatment effects: The PROMOTE Study Protocol. The Journal of the American Osteopathic Association. 116(11):716–24.

Hensel KL, Roane BM, Chaphekar AV, Smith-Barbaro P (2016) PROMOTE Study: safety of osteopathic manipulative treatment during the third trimester by labor and delivery outcomes. Journal of the American Osteopathic Association. 116(11):698–703.

Henson J, Brown C, Chow SC, Muir AJ (2017) Complementary and alternative medicine use in United States adults with liver disease. Journal of Clinical Gastroenterology. 51(6):564–70.

Hesse T, Henkel B, Zygmunt M, Mustea A, Usichenko TI (2016) Acupuncture for pain control after Caesarean section: a prospective observational pilot study. Acupuncture in Medicine. 34(1):14–19.

Ho D, Jagdeo J, Waldorf HA (2016) Is there a role for arnica and bromelain in prevention of post-procedure ecchymosis or edema? A systematic review of the literature. Dermatologic Surgery. 42(4):445–63.

Hofmeyr GJ, Kulier R (2012) Cephalic version by postural management for breech presentation. Cochrane Database of Systematic Reviews. (10):CD000051.

Holst L, Haavik S, Nordeng H (2009) Raspberry leaf: should it be recommended to pregnant women? Complementary Therapies in Clinical Practice. 15(4):204–8.

Holt J, Lord J, Acharya U, White A et al. (2009) The effectiveness of foot reflexology in inducing ovulation: a sham-controlled randomized trial. Fertility and Sterility. 91(6):2514–19.

Howard J (2007) Do Bach flower remedies have a role to play in pain control? A critical analysis investigating therapeutic value beyond the placebo effect, and the potential of Bach flower remedies as a psychological method of pain relief. Complementary Therapies in Clinical Practice. 13(3):174–83.

Howell ER (2012) Pregnancy-related symphysis pubis dysfunction management and postpartum rehabilitation: two case reports. Journal of the Canadian Chiropractic Association. 56(2):102–11.

Howland LC, Jallo N, Connelly CD, Pickler RH (2017) Feasibility of a relaxation guided imagery intervention to reduce maternal stress in the NICU. Journal of Obstetric, Gynecologic and Neonatal Nursing. 17 May. pii: S0884–2175(17)30084-9.

Hrgovic I, Hrgovic Z, Habek D, Oreskovic S, Hofmann J, Münstedt K (2010) Use of complementary and alternative medicine in departments of obstetrics in Croatia and a comparison to Germany. Forschende Komplementmedizin. 17(3):144–6. Abstract viewed online 19/09/2017 at www.ncbi.nlm.nih.gov/pubmed/20616518

Hu L, Wang L, Wei J, Ryszard G, Shen X, Wolfgang S (2015) Heat induces adenosine triphosphate release from mast cells in vitro: a putative mechanism for moxibustion. Journal of Traditional Chinese Medicine. 35(3):323–8.

Hu ML, Rayner CK, Wu KL, Chuah SK et al. (2011) Effect of ginger on gastric motility and symptoms of functional dyspepsia. World Journal of Gastroenterology. 17(1):105–10.

Huang TL, Charyton C (2008) A comprehensive review of the psychological effects of brainwave entrainment. Alternative Therapies. 14(5):38–50.

Humphrey T, Tucker J. (2009) Rising rates of obstetric interventions: exploring the determinants of induction of labour. Journal of Public Health. 31(1):88–94.

Hunt KJ, Coelho HF, Wider B, Perry R et al. (2010) Complementary and alternative medicine use in England: results from a national survey. International Journal of Clinical Practice. 64(11):1496–502.

Hunt R, Dienemann J, Norton HJ, Hartley W et al. (2013) Aromatherapy as treatment for postoperative nausea: a randomized trial. Anesthia and Analgesia. 117(3):597–604.

Hunter J, Marshall J, Corcoran K, Leeder S, Phelps K (2013) A positive concept of health: interviews with patients and practitioners in an integrative medicine clinic. Complementary Therapies in Clinical Practice. 19(4):197–203.

Hunter LA (2014) Vaginal breech birth: can we move beyond the term Breech Trial? Journal of Midwifery and Women's Health. 59(3):320–7.

Hur MH, Lee MS, Seong KY, Lee MK (2012) Aromatherapy massage on the abdomen for alleviating menstrual pain in high school girls: a preliminary controlled clinical study. Evidence-Based Complementary and Alternative Medicine. 2012:187163.

Hutton EK, Kasperink M, Rutten M, Reitsma A, Wainman B (2009) Sterile water injection for labour pain: a systematic review and meta-analysis of randomised controlled trials. BJOG. 116(9):1158–66.

Iannitti T, Morales-Medina JC, Bellavite P, Rottigni V, Palmieri B (2016) Effectiveness and safety of arnica montana in post-surgical setting, pain and inflammation. American Journal of Therapeutics. 23(1):e184–97.

Ikeda H, Takasu S, Murase K (2014) Contribution of anterior cingulate cortex and descending pain inhibitory system to analgesic effect of lemon odor in mice. Molecular Pain. 10:14.

Illingworth J (2015) Clinical human factors group continuous improvement of patient safety: the case for change in the NHS. The Health Foundation. www.health.org.uk/sites/health/files/ContinuousImprovementPatientSafety.pdf

Imura M, Misao H, Ushijima H (2006) The psychological effects of aromatherapy-massage in healthy postpartum mothers. Journal of Midwifery and Women's Health. 51(2):e21–7.

Inamori M, Akiyama T, Akimoto K, Fujita K et al. (2007) Early effects of peppermint oil on gastric emptying: a crossover study using a continuous real-time 13C breath test (BreathID system). Journal of Gastroenterology. 42(7):539–42.

Ingram J, Domagala C, Yates S (2005) The effects of shiatsu on post-term pregnancy. Complementary Therapies in Medicine. 13(1):11–15.

Irikura B, Kennelly E (1999) Blue cohosh: a word of caution. American Health Consultants. Viewed online 19/09/2017 at www.ahcmedia.com/articles/50424-blue-cohosh-a-word-of-caution

Isaksson M, Bruze M (1999) Occupational allergic contact dermatitis from olive oil in a masseur. Journal of the American Academy of Dermatology. 41(2 Pt 2):312–15.

Ismail SI, Emery SJ (2013) Patient awareness and acceptability of antenatal perineal massage. Journal of Obstetrics and Gynaecology. 33(8):839–43.

Iversen ML, Midtgaard J, Ekelin M, Hegaard HK (2017) Danish women's experiences of the rebozo technique during labour: a qualitative explorative study. Sexual and Reproductive Healthcare. 11:79–85.

Izzo AA, Hoon-Kim S, Radhakrishnan R, Williamson EM (2016) A critical approach to evaluating clinical efficacy, adverse events and drug interactions of herbal remedies. Phytotherapy Research. 30(5):691–700.

Jabraeile M, Rasooly AS, Farshi MR, Malakouti J (2016) Effect of olive oil massage on weight gain in preterm infants: a randomized controlled clinical trial. Nigerian Medical Journal. 57(3):160–3.

Jackson JE, Grobman WA, Haney E, Casele H (2007) Mid-trimester dilation and evacuation with laminaria does not increase the risk for severe subsequent pregnancy complications. International Journal of Gynecology and Obstetrics. 96(1):12–15.

Jafari-Dehkordi E, Hashem-Dabaghian F, Aliasl F, Aliasl J et al. (2017) Comparison of quince with vitamin B6 for treatment of nausea and vomiting in pregnancy: a randomised clinical trial. Journal of Obstetrics and Gynaecology. 37(8):1048–52.

Jahdi F, Sheikhan F, Haghani H, Sharifi B et al. (2017) Yoga during pregnancy: the effects on labor pain and delivery outcomes (a randomized controlled trial). Complementary Therapies in Clinical Practice. 27:1–4.

Jalili J, Askeroglu U, Alleyne B, Guyuron B (2013) Herbal products that may contribute to hypertension. Plastic and Reconstructive Surgery. 131(1):168–73.

Jallo N, Salyer J, Ruiz RJ, French E (2015) Perceptions of guided imagery for stress management in pregnant African American women. Archives of Psychiatric Nursing. 29(4):249–54.

James U (2009) Practical uses of clinical hypnosis in enhancing fertility, healthy pregnancy and childbirth. Complementary Therapies in Clinical Practice. 15(4):239–41.

Janssen P, Shroff F, Jaspar P (2012) Massage therapy and labor outcomes: a randomized controlled trial. International Journal of Therapeutic Massage and Bodywork. 5(4):15–20.

Jaruzel CB, Kelechi T (2016) Relief from anxiety using complementary therapies in the perioperative period: a principle based concept analysis. Complementary Therapies in Clinical Practice. 24:1–5.

Jay A (2015) Women's experiences of labour induction: a qualitative study. Doctorate thesis. Viewed online 25/10/2017 at http://researchprofiles.herts.ac.uk/portal/files/10116260/Thesis._Dr_Annabel_Jay_2016.pdf

Jenkins MW, Pritchard MH (1993) Hypnosis: practical applications and theoretical considerations in normal labour. British Journal of Obstetrics and Gynaecology. 100(3):221–6.

Jenkinson B, Josey N, Kruske S (2014) BirthSpace: an evidence-based guide to birth environment design. Queensland Centre for Mothers and Babies. Viewed online 19/09/2017 at https://www.researchgate.net/publication/278328878_BirthSpace_An_evidence-based_guide_to_birth_environment_design

Jenner C, Filshie J (2002) Galactorrhoea following acupuncture. Acupuncture in Medicine. 20(2–3):107–8.

Jensen MP, Adachi T, Hakimian S (2015) Brain oscillations, hypnosis, and hypnotizability. American Journal of Clinical Hypnosis. 57(3):230–53.

Jiang H, White MP, Greicius MD, Waelde LC, Spiegel D (2016) Brain activity and functional connectivity associated with hypnosis. Cerebral Cortex. 27(8):4083–93.

Jiang X, Blair EY, McLachlan AJ (2006) Investigation of the effects of herbal medicines on warfarin response in healthy subjects: a population pharmacokinetic-pharmacodynamic modeling approach. The Journal of Clinical Pharmocology. 46(11):1370–8.

Johnson JD, Cocker K, Chang E (2015) Infantile colic: recognition and treatment. American Family Physician. 92(7):577–82.

Johnson JR, Makaji E, Ho S, Boya Xiong, Crankshaw DJ, Holloway AC (2009) Effect of maternal raspberry leaf consumption in rats on pregnancy outcome and the fertility of the female offspring. Reproductive Sciences. 16(6):605–9.

Johnson PJ, Kozhimannil KB, Jou J, Ghildayal N, Rockwood TH (2016) Complementary and alternative medicine use among women of reproductive age in the United States. Women's Health Issues. 26(1):40–7.

Jonasson A, Larsson B, Lecander I, Astedt B (1989) Placental and decidual u-PA, t-PA, PAI-1, and PAI-2 concentrations, as affected by cervical dilatation with laminaria tents or Hegar dilators. Thrombosis Research. 53(2):91–7.

Jones C, Chan C, Farine D (2011) Sex in pregnancy. Canadian Medical Association Journal. 183(7):815–18.

Jones C, Jomeen J, Ogbuehi O (2013) A preliminary survey of the use of complementary and alternative medicines in childbearing women. Evidence Based Midwifery. 11:128–31.

Jones L, Othman M, Dowswell T, Alfirevic Z et al. (2012) Pain management for women in labour: an overview of systematic reviews. Cochrane Database of Systematic Reviews. (3):CD00923.

Jones TK, Lawson BM (1998) Profound neonatal congestive heart failure caused by maternal consumption of blue cohosh herbal medication. Journal of Pediatrics. 132(3 Pt 1):550–2.

Jorge MP, Santaella DF, Pontes IM, Shiramizu VK et al. (2016) Hatha Yoga practice decreases menopause symptoms and improves quality of life: a randomized controlled trial. Complementary Therapies in Medicine. 26:128–35.

Jou J, Kozhimannil KB, Johnson PJ, Sakala C (2015) Patient-perceived pressure from clinicians for labor induction and Cesarean delivery: a population-based survey of U.S. women. Journal of Medicinal Plants Research. 4(24):2609–14.

Joy D, Joy J, Duane P (2008) Black cohosh: a cause of abnormal postmenopausal liver function tests. Climacteric. 11(1):84–8.

Jung SY, Chae HD, Kang UR, Kwak MA, Kim IH (2017) Effect of acupuncture on postoperative ileus after distal gastrectomy for gastric cancer. Journal of Gastric Cancer. 17(1):11–20.

Kalder M, Knoblauch K, Hrgovic I, Münstedt K (2011) Use of complementary and alternative medicine during pregnancy and delivery. Archives of Gynecology and Obstetrics. 283(3):475–82.

Källén B, Lundberg G, Aberg A (2003) Relationship between vitamin use, smoking, and nausea and vomiting of pregnancy. Acta Obstetricia et Gynecologica Scandinavica. 82(10):916–20.

Kamalifard M, Shahnazi M, Sayyah Melli M, Allahverdizadeh S, Toraby S, Ghahvechi A (2012) The efficacy of massage therapy and breathing techniques on pain intensity and physiological responses to labor pain. Journal of Caring Sciences. 1(2):73–6.

Kamatenesi-Mugisha M, Oryem-Origa H (2007) Medicinal plants used to induce labour during childbirth in western Uganda. Journal of Ethnopharmacology. 109(1):1–9.

Kamen C, Tejani MA, Chandwani K, Janelsins M et al. (2014) Anticipatory nausea and vomiting due to chemotherapy. European Journal of Pharmacology. 722:172–9.

Kanakura Y, Kometani K, Nagata T, Niwa K et al. (2001) Moxibustion treatment of breech presentation. The American Journal of Chinese Medicine. 29(1):37–45.

Kanherkar RR, Stair SE, Bhatia-Dey N, Mills PJ, Chopra D, Csoka AB (2017) Epigenetic mechanisms of integrative medicine. Evidence-Based Complementary and Alternative Medicine. 2017:4365429.

Kanji N (2000) Management of pain through autogenic training. Complementary Therapies in Nursing and Midwifery. 6(3):143–8.

Kara B (2009) Herbal product use in a sample of Turkish patients undergoing haemodialysis. Journal of Clinical Nursing. 18(15):2197–205.

Karaçam Z, Ekmen H, Calişir H (2012) The use of perineal massage in the second stage of labor and follow-up of postpartum perineal outcomes. Health Care for Women International. 33(8):697–718.

Katonis P, Kampouroglou A, Aggelopoulos P, Kakavelakis K et al. (2011) Pregnancy-related low back pain. Hippokratia. 15(3):205–10.

Kaur H, Corscadden K, Lott C, Elbatarny HS, Othman M (2016) Bromelain has paradoxical effects on blood coagulability: a study using thromboelastography. Blood Coagulation and Fibrinolysis. 27(7):745–52.

Kavadar G, Demircioğlu DT, Can H, Emre TY, Civelek E, Senyigit A (2016) The clinical factors associated with benefit finding of complementary medicine use in patients with back pain: a cross-sectional study with cluster analysis. Journal of Back and Musculoskeletal Rehabilitation. 30(2):271–7.

Kavanagh J, Kelly AJ, Thomas J (2001) Sexual intercourse for cervical ripening and induction of labour. Cochrane Database of Systematic Reviews. (2):CD003093.

Kaviani M, Maghbool S, Azima S, Tabaei MH (2014) Comparison of the effect of aromatherapy with Jasminum officinale and Salvia officinale on pain severity and labor outcome in nulliparous women. Iranian Journal of Nursing Midwifery Research. 19(6):666–72.

Kavurt S, Bas AY, Aydemir O, Yucel H, Isikoglu S, Demirel N (2013) The effect of galactagogue herbal tea on oxidant and anti-oxidant status of human milk. The Journal of Maternal-Fetal and Neonatal Medicine. 26(10):1048–51.

Kawakita K, Okada K (2014) Acupuncture therapy: mechanism of action, efficacy, and safety: a potential intervention for psychogenic disorders? BioPsychoSocial Medicine. 8:4.

Kawanishi Y, Saijo Y, Yoshioka E, Nakagi Y et al. (2016) The association between prenatal yoga and the administration of ritodrine hydrochloride during pregnancy: an adjunct study of the Japan environment and children's study. PLoS One. 11(6):e0158155.

Kayman-Kose S, Arioz DT, Toktas H, Koken G *et al.* (2014) Transcutaneous electrical nerve stimulation (TENS) for pain control after vaginal delivery and Cesarean section. The Journal of Maternal-Fetal and Neonatal Medicine. 27(15):1572–5.

Kazzi GM, Bottoms SF, Rosen MG (1982) Efficacy and safety of Laminaria digitata for preinduction ripening of the cervix. Obstetrics and Gynecology. 60(4):440–3.

Kennedy DA, Lupattelli A, Koren G, Nordeng H (2013) Herbal medicine use in pregnancy: results of a multinational study. BMC Complementary and Alternative Medicine. 13:355.

Kenyon C (2013) Clinical hypnosis for labour and birth: a consideration. The Practising Midwife. 16(5):10–13.

Keskin EA, Onur O, Keskin HL, Gumus II, Kafali H, Turhan N (2012) Transcutaneous electrical nerve stimulation improves low back pain during pregnancy. Gynecologic and Obstetric Investigation. 74(1):76–83.

Khambalia AZ, Roberts CL, Nguyen M, Algert S, Nicholl NC, Morris J (2013) Predicting date of birth and examining the best time to date a pregnancy. International Journal of Gynecology and Obstetrics. 123(2):105–9.

Khianman B, Pattanittum P, Thinkhamrop J, Lumbiganon P (2012) Relaxation therapy for preventing and treating preterm labour. Cochrane Database of Systematic Reviews. (8):CD007426.

Khorsand A, Tadayonfar MA, Badiee S, Aghaee MA, Azizi H, Baghani S (2015) Evaluation of the effect of reflexology on pain control and analgesic consumption after appendectomy. Journal of Alternative and Complementary Medicine. 21(12):774–80.

Khosravan S, Mohammadzadeh-Moghadam H, Mohammadzadeh F, Fadafen SA, Gholami M (2017) The effect of hollyhock (Althaea officinalis L) leaf compresses combined with warm and cold compress on breast engorgement in lactating women: a randomized clinical trial. Journal of Evidence-Based Complementary and Alternative Medicine. 22(1):25–30 (Abstract).

Kianpour M, Mansouri A, Mehrabi T, Asghari G (2016) Effect of lavender scent inhalation on prevention of stress, anxiety and depression in the postpartum period. Iranian Journal of Nursing and Midwifery Research. 21(2):197–201.

Kiba T, Abe T, Kanbara K, Kato F *et al.* (2017) The relationship between salivary amylase and the physical and psychological changes elicited by continuation of autogenic training in patients with functional somatic syndrome. BioPsychoSocial Medicine. 11:17.

Kiechl-Kohlendorfer U, Berger C, Inzinger R (2008) The effect of daily treatment with an olive oil/lanolin emollient on skin integrity in preterm infants: a randomized controlled trial. Pediatric Dermatology. 25(2):174–8.

Kim JI, Choi JY, Lee H, Lee MS, Ernst E (2010) Moxibustion for hypertension: a systematic review. BMC Cardiovascular Disorders. 10:33.

Kim JT, Wajda M, Cuff G, Serota D *et al.* (2006) Evaluation of aromatherapy in treating postoperative pain: pilot study. Pain Practice. 6(4):273–7.

Kim SH, Chang YH, Kim WK, Kim YK *et al.* (2003) Two cases of anaphylaxis after laminaria insertion. Journal of Korean Medical Science. 18(6):886–8.

Kimber L, McNabb M, McCourt C, Haines A, Brocklehurst P (2008) Massage or music for pain relief in labour: a pilot randomised placebo controlled trial. European Journal of Pain. 12(8):961–9.

King's Fund (2009) Safe Births: Everybody's Business. An independent inquiry into the safety of maternity services in England. Viewed online 19/09/2017 at www.kingsfund.org.uk/sites/files/kf/Safe%20Births.pdf

Kinser P, Masho S (2015) "Yoga was my saving grace": the experience of women who practice prenatal yoga. Journal of the American Psychiatric Nurses Association. 21(5):319–26.

Kinser PA, Pauli J, Jallo N, Shall M *et al.* (2017) Physical activity and yoga-based approaches for pregnancy-related low back and pelvic pain. Journal of Obstetric, Gynecologic and Neonatal Nursing. 13 Mar. pii: S0884-2175(17)30012-6.

Klier CM, Schmid-Siegel B, Schäfer MR, Lenz G *et al.* (2006) St. John's wort (Hypericum perforatum) and breastfeeding: plasma and breast milk concentrations of hyperforin for 5 mothers and 2 infants. Journal of Clinical Psychiatry. 67(2):305–9.

Knowles SR, Djordjevic K, Binkley K, Weber EA (2002) Allergic anaphylaxis to Laminaria. Allergy. 57(4):370.

Ko YL, Lee HJ (2014) Randomised controlled trial of the effectiveness of using back massage to improve sleep quality among Taiwanese insomnia postpartum women. Midwifery. 30(1):60–4.

Ko YL, Yang CL, Fang CL, Lee MY, Lin PC (2013) Community-based postpartum exercise program. Journal of Clinical Nursing. 22(15–16):2122–31.

Kobayashi K (1988) Organic components of moxa. American Journal of Chinese Medicine. 16(3–4):179–85.

Kordi M, Meybodi FA, Tara F, Nemati M, Shakeri MT (2014) The effect of late pregnancy consumption of date fruit on cervical ripening in nulliparous women. Journal of Midwifery and Reproductive Health. 2(3):150–6.

Korman SH, Cohen E, Preminger A (2001) Pseudo-maple syrup urine disease due to maternal prenatal ingestion of fenugreek. Journal of Paediatrics and Child Health. 37(4):403–4.

Korukcu O, Kukulu K (2017) The effect of the mindfulness-based transition to motherhood program in pregnant women with preterm premature rupture of membranes. Health Care for Women International. 38(7):765–85.

Koto R, Imamura M, Watanabe C, Obayashi S *et al.* (2006) Linalyl acetate as a major ingredient of lavender essential oil relaxes the rabbit vascular smooth muscle through dephosphorylation of myosin light chain. Journal of Cardiovascular Pharmacology. 48(1):850–6.

Kozhimannil KB, Johnson PJ, Attanasio LB, Gjerdingen DK, McGovern PM (2013) Use of non-medical methods of labor induction and pain management among U.S. women. Birth. 40(4):227–36.

Kramer J, Bowen A, Stewart N, Muhajarine N (2013) Nausea and vomiting of pregnancy: prevalence, severity and relation to psychosocial health. MCN: The American Journal of Maternal/Child Nursing. 38(1):21–7.

Kumar S, Rampp T, Kessler C, Jeitler M *et al.* (2016) Effectiveness of Ayurvedic massage (Sahacharadi Taila) in patients with chronic low back pain: a randomized controlled trial. Journal of Alternative and Complementary Medicine. 5 Oct.

Kumarappah A, Senderovich H (2016) Therapeutic touch in the management of responsive behavior in patients with dementia. Advances in Mind-Body Medicine. 30(4):8–13.

Kuo SY, Tsai SH, Chen SL, Tzeng YL (2016) Auricular acupressure relieves anxiety and fatigue, and reduces cortisol levels in post-caesarean section women: a single-blind, randomised controlled study. International Journal of Nursing Studies. 53:17–26.

Kurebayashi LF, Turrini RN, Souza TP, Takiguchi RS, Kuba G, Nagumo MT (2016) Massage and Reiki used to reduce stress and anxiety: randomized clinical trial. Revista Latino-Americana de Enfermagem. 28(24):e2834.

Kuriyan R, Kumar DR, R R, Kurpad AV (2010) An evaluation of the hypolipidemic effect of an extract of Hibiscus Sabdariffa leaves in hyperlipidemic Indians: a double blind, placebo controlled trial. BMC Complementary and Alternative Medicine. 10:27.

Kusaka M, Matsuzaki M, Shiraishi M, Haruna M (2016) Immediate stress reduction effects of yoga during pregnancy: one group pre-post test. Women and Birth. 29(5):e82–e88. doi: 10.1016/j.wombi.2016.04.003.

Kvist LJ, Hall-Lord ML, Rydhstroem H, Larsson BW (2007) A randomised-controlled trial in Sweden of acupuncture and care interventions for the relief of inflammatory symptoms of the breast during lactation. Midwifery. 23(2):184–95.

Kwon OS, Cho SJ, Choi KH, Yeon SH *et al.* (2017) Safety recommendations for moxa use based on the concentration of noxious substances produced during commercial indirect moxibustion. Acupuncture in Medicine. 35(2):93–9. Abstract viewed online 19/09/2017 at www.ncbi. nlm.nih.gov/pubmed/27515415

Labrecque M, Nouwen A, Bergeron M, Rancourt JF (1999) A randomized controlled trial of nonpharmacologic approaches for relief of low back pain during labor. The Journal of Family Practice. 48(4):259–63.

Lacasse A, Rey E, Ferreira E, Morin C, Bérard A (2009) Epidemiology of nausea and vomiting of pregnancy: prevalence, severity, determinants, and the importance of race/ethnicity. BMC Pregnancy and Childbirth. 9:26.

Lacroix R, Eason E, Melzack R (2000) Nausea and vomiting during pregnancy: a prospective study of its frequency, intensity, and patterns of change. American Journal of Obstetric Gynecology. 182(4):931–7.

Lai MM, D'Acunto G, Guzzetta A, Boyd RN *et al.* (2016) PREMM: preterm early massage by the mother: protocol of a randomised controlled trial of massage therapy in very preterm infants. BMC Pediatrics. 16(1):146.

Laivuori H, Hovatta O, Viinikka L, Yikoala O (1993) Dietary supplementation with primrose oil or fish oil does not change urinary excretion of prostacyclin and thromboxane metabolites in pre-eclamptic women. PLEFA. 49(3):691–4.

Landgren K, Hallström I (2017) Effect of minimal acupuncture for infantile colic: a multicentre, three-armed, single-blind, randomised controlled trial (ACU-COL). Acupuncture in Medicine. 16 Jan. pii: acupmed-2016-011208.

Landolt AS, Milling LS (2011) The efficacy of hypnosis as an intervention for labor and delivery pain: a comprehensive methodological review. Clinical Psychology Review. 31(6):1022–31.

Lane B, Cannella K, Bowen C, Copelan D *et al.* (2012) Examination of the effectiveness of peppermint aromatherapy on nausea in women post C-section. Journal of Holistic Nursing. 30(2):90–104.

Langhammer AJ, Nilsen OG (2014) In vitro inhibition of human CYP1A2, CYP2D6, and CYP3A4 by six herbs commonly used in pregnancy. Phytotherapy Research. 28(4):603–10.

Laopaiboon M, Lumbiganon P, Martis R, Vatanasapt P, Somjaivong B (2009) Music during caesarean section under regional anaesthesia for improving maternal and infant outcomes. Cochrane Database of Systematic Reviews. (2):CD006914.

Larden CN, Palmer ML, Janssen P (2004) Efficacy of therapeutic touch in treating pregnant inpatients who have a chemical dependency. Journal of Holistic Nursing. 22(4):320–32.

Laursen M, Johansen C, Hedegaard M (2009) Fear of childbirth and risk for birth complications in nulliparous women in the Danish National Birth Cohort. BJOG. 116(10):1350–5.

Lavelle JM (2012) Osteopathic manipulative treatment in pregnant women. The Journal of the American Osteopathic Association. 112(6):343–6.

Lee A (2010) The effectiveness of cabbage leaf application (treatment) on breast engorgement in breastfeeding women. JBI Library of Systematic Reviews. 8(34):1–21.

Lee A, Chan SKC, Fan LTY (2015) Stimulation of the wrist acupuncture point PC6 for preventing postoperative nausea and vomiting. Cochrane Database of Systematic Reviews. (11):CD003281.

Lee HJ, Ko YL (2015) Back massage intervention for relieving lower back pain in puerperal women: a randomized control trial study. International Journal of Nursing Practice. 21 Suppl 2:32–7.

Lee KB, Cho E, Kang YS (2014) Changes in 5-hydroxytryptamine and cortisol plasma levels in menopausal women after inhalation of clary sage oil. Phytotherapy Research. 28(11):1599–605.

Lee NM, Saha S (2011) Nausea and vomiting of pregnancy. Gastroenterology Clinics of North America. 40(2):309–34.

Leeners B, Sauer I, Rath W (2000) Nausea and vomiting in early pregnancy/hyperemesis gravidarum: current status of psychosomatic factors. Zeitschrift fur Geburtshilfe und Neonatologie. 204(4):128–34.

Leite PM, Martins MA, Castilho RO (2016) Review on mechanisms and interactions in concomitant use of herbs and warfarin therapy. Biomedicine and Pharmacotherapy. 83:14–21.

Lete I, Allué J (2016) The effectiveness of ginger in the prevention of nausea and vomiting during pregnancy and chemotherapy. Integrative Medicine Insights. 11:11–17.

Levett KM, Smith CA, Bensoussan A, Dahlen HG (2016a) The Complementary Therapies for Labour and Birth Study making sense of labour and birth: experiences of women, partners and midwives of a complementary medicine antenatal education course. Midwifery. 40:124–31.

Levett KM, Smith CA, Bensoussan A, Dahlen HG (2016b) Complementary Therapies for Labour and Birth Study: a randomised controlled trial of antenatal integrative medicine for pain management in labour. Viewed online 19/09/2017 at http://bmjopen.bmj.com/content/6/7/e010691.full

Levitas E, Parmet A, Lunenfeld E, Bentov Y et al. (2006) Impact of hypnosis during embryo transfer on the outcome of in vitro fertilization-embryo transfer: a case-control study. Fertility and Sterility. 85(5):1404–8.

Li CY, Chen SC, Li CY, Gau ML, Huang CM (2011) Randomised controlled trial of the effectiveness of using foot reflexology to improve quality of sleep amongst Taiwanese postpartum women. Midwifery. 27(2):181–6.

Li H, Liu S (2008) 2 cases of moxibustion allergy. Journal of Emergency in Traditional Chinese Medicine. 17(6):859–60.

Li X, Hu J, Wang X, Zhang H, Liu J (2009) Moxibustion and other acupuncture point stimulation methods to treat breech presentation: a systematic review of clinical trials. Chinese Medicine. 4:4.

Licciardone JC, Gatchel RJ, Aryal S (2016) Recovery from chronic low back pain after osteopathic manipulative treatment: a randomized controlled trial. The Journal of the American Osteopathic Association. 116(3):144–55.

Lichtenberg ES (2004) Complications of osmotic dilators. Obstetrical and Gynecological Survey. 59(7):528–36.

Liddle SD, Pennick V (2015) Interventions for preventing and treating low-back and pelvic pain during pregnancy. Cochrane Database of Systematic Reviews. (8):CD001139.

Lim S, Lee SH (2017) Clinical effectiveness of acupuncture on Parkinson disease: a PRISMA-compliant systematic review and meta-analysis. Medicine (Baltimore). 96(3):e5836.

Lim CE, Ng RW, Xu K (2013) Non-hormonal methods for induction of labour. Current Opinion in Obstetrics and Gynecology. 25(6):441–7.

Lim CE, Wilkinson JM, Wong WS, Cheng NC (2009) Effect of acupuncture on induction of labor. Journal of Alternative and Complementary Medicine. 15(11):1209–14.

Lin SY, Cheng WF, Su YN, Chen CA, Lee CN (2006) Septic shock after intracervical laminaria insertion. Taiwanese Journal of Obstetrics and Gynecology. 45(1):76–8.

Lindblad AJ, Koppula S (2016) Ginger for nausea and vomiting of pregnancy. Canadian Family Physician. 62(2):145.

Linde K, Berner MM, Kriston L (2008) St John's wort for major depression. Cochrane Database of Systematic Reviews. (4):CD000448.

Linde K, Knüppel L (2005) Large-scale observational studies of hypericum extracts in patients with depressive disorders – a systematic review. Phytomedicine. 12(1–2):148–57.

Lindholm A, Hildingsson I (2015) Women's preferences and received pain relief in childbirth: a prospective longitudinal study in a northern region of Sweden. Sexual and Reproductive Healthcare. 6(2):74–81.

Littel M, Kenemans JL, Baas JMP, Logemann HNA et al. (2017) The effects of β-adrenergic blockade on the degrading effects of eye movements on negative autobiographical memories. Biological Psychiatry. pii: S0006-3223(17)31369-0.

Liu J, Han Y, Zhang N, Wang B et al. (2008) The safety of electroacupuncture at Hegu (LI 4) plus oxytocin for hastening uterine contraction of puerperants: a randomized controlled clinical observation. Journal of Traditional Chinese Medicine. 28(3):163–7.

Liu Y, Xu M, Che X, He J et al. (2015) Effect of direct current pulse stimulating acupoints of JiaJi (T10–13) and Ciliao (BL 32) with Han's acupoint nerve stimulator on labour pain in women: a randomized controlled clinical study. Journal of Traditional Chinese Medicine. 35(6):620–5.

Liu YH, Chang MY, Chen CH (2010) Effects of music therapy on labour pain and anxiety in Taiwanese first-time mothers. Journal of Clinical Nursing. 19(7–8):1065–72.

Liu Z, Meng R, Zhao X, Shi C et al. (2016) Inhibition effect of tea tree oil on Listeria monocytogenes growth and exotoxin proteins listeriolysin O and p60 secretion. Letters in Applied Microbiology. 63(6):450–7.

Löffler A, Trojan J, Zieglgänsberger W, Diers M (2017) Visually induced analgesia during massage treatment in chronic back pain patients. European Journal of Pain. doi: 10.1002/ejp.1066 (Abstract).

Lontos S, Jones RM, Angus PW, Gow PJ (2003) Acute liver failure associated with the use of herbal preparations containing black cohosh. Medical Journal of Australia. 178(8):411–12.

López-Garrido B, García-Gonzalo J, Patrón-Rodriguez C, Marlasca-Gutiérrez MJ et al. (2015) Influence of acupuncture on the third stage of labor: a randomized controlled trial. Journal of Midwifery and Women's Health. 60(2):199–205.

Lu CY, Kang SY, Liu SH, Mai CW, Tseng CH (2016) Controlling indoor air pollution from moxibustion. International Journal of Environmental Research and Public Health. 13(6). pii: E612.

Lu QB, Wang ZP, Gao LJ, Gong R et al. (2015) Nausea and vomiting in early pregnancy and the risk of neural tube defects: a case-control study. Scientific Reports. 5:7674.

Luff D, Thomas JK (2000) "Getting somewhere", feeling cared for: patients' perspectives on complementary therapies in the NHS. Complementary Therapies in Medicine. 8(4): 253–9.

Lund I, Lundeberg T, Lönnberg L, Svensson E (2006) Decrease of pregnant women's pelvic pain after acupuncture: a randomized controlled single-blind study. Acta Obstetricia et Gynecologica Scandinavica. 85(1):12–19.

Lundberg GD (2008) Sterile water is better than acupuncture in relieving the pain of labor. The Medscape Journal of Medicine. 10(6):151.

Lunny CA, Fraser SN (2010) The use of complementary and alternative medicines among a sample of Canadian menopausal-aged women. Journal of Midwifery and Women's Health. 55(4):335–43.

Lytle J, Mwatha C, Davis KK (2014) Effect of lavender aromatherapy on vital signs and perceived quality of sleep in the intermediate care unit: a pilot study. American Journal of Critical Care. 23(1):24–9.

Macdonald S (ed.) (2011) Mayes' Midwifery: A Textbook for Midwives, 14th edition. Edinburgh: Bailliere Tindall.

Macharey G, Gissler M, Rahkonen L, Ulander VM *et al.* (2017) Breech presentation at term and associated obstetric risks factors: a nationwide population based cohort study. Archives of Gynecology and Obstetrics. 295(4):833–8.

MacPherson H, Thomas K, Walters S, Fitter M (2001) The York acupuncture safety study: prospective survey of 34 000 treatments by traditional acupuncturists. BMJ. 323:486.

Madden K, Middleton P, Cyna AM, Matthewson M, Jones L (2016) Hypnosis for pain management during labour and childbirth. Cochrane Database of Systematic Reviews. (5):CD009356.

Madgula VL, Ali Z, Smillie T, Khan IA, Walker LA, Khan SI (2009) Alkaloids and saponins as cytochrome P450 inhibitors from blue cohosh (Caulophyllum thalictroides) in an in vitro assay. Planta Medica. 75(4):329–32.

Madrid A, Giovannoli R, Wolfe M (2011) Treating persistent nausea of pregnancy with hypnosis: four cases. American Journal of Clinical Hypnosis. 54(2):107–15.

Mafetoni RR, Shimo AK (2015) Effects of acupressure on progress of labor and cesarean section rate: randomized clinical trial. Revista de Saude Publica. 49:9.

Mahady GB, Low Dog T, Barrett ML, Chavez ML *et al.* (2008) United States Pharmacopeia Review of the black cohosh case reports of hepatotoxicity. Menopause. 15(4 Pt 1):628–38.

Makaji E, Ho SH, Holloway AC, Crankshaw DJ (2011) Effects in rats of maternal exposure to raspberry leaf and its constituents on the activity of cytochrome p450 enzymes in the offspring. International Journal of Toxicology. 30(2):216–24.

Maliwichi-Nyirenda CP, Maliwichi LL (2010) Medicinal plants used to induce labour and traditional techniques used in determination of onset of labour in pregnant women in Malawi: a case study of Mulanje District. Journal of Medicinal Plants Research. 4(24):2609–14.

Malmqvist S, Kjaermann I, Andersen K, Økland I, Brønnick K, Larsen JP (2012) Prevalence of low back and pelvic pain during pregnancy in a Norwegian population. Journal of Manipulative and Physiological Therapeutics. 35(4):272–8.

Mangesi L, Zakarija-Grkovic I (2016) Treatments for breast engorgement during lactation. Cochrane Database of Systematic Reviews. (6):CD006946.

Manik RK, Mahapatra AK, Gartia R, Bansal S, Patnaik A (2017) Effect of selected yogic practices on pain and disability in patients with lumbar spondylitis. International Journal of Yoga. 10(2):81–7.

Manyande A, Grabowska C (2009) Factors affecting the success of moxibustion in the management of a breech presentation as a preliminary treatment to external cephalic version. Midwifery. 25(6):774–80.

Marc I, Toureche N, Ernst E, Hodnett ED *et al.* (2011) Mind-body interventions during pregnancy for preventing or treating women's anxiety. Cochrane Database of Systematic Reviews. (7):CD007559.

Marchioni Beery RM, Birk JW (2015) Wheat-related disorders reviewed: making a grain of sense. Expert Review of Gastroenterology and Hepatology. 9(6):851–64.

Marra C, Pozzi I, Ceppi L, Sicuri M, Veneziano F, Regalia AL (2011) Wrist-ankle acupuncture as perineal pain relief after mediolateral episiotomy: a pilot study. Journal of Alternative and Complementary Medicine. 17(3):239–41.

Mårtensson L, Stener-Victorin E, Wallin G (2008) Acupuncture versus subcutaneous injections of sterile water as treatment for labour pain. Acta Obstetricia et Gynecologica Scandinavica. 87(2):171–7.

Martin AA, Schauble PG, Rai SH, Curry RW Jr. (2001) The effects of hypnosis on the labor processes and birth outcomes of pregnant adolescents. The Journal of Family Practice. 50(5):441–3.

Martinez GJ (2008) Traditional practices, beliefs and uses of medicinal plants in relation to maternal-baby health of Criollo woman in central Argentina. Midwifery. 24:490–502.

Martingano D (2016) Management of cesarean deliveries and cesarean scars with osteopathic manipulative treatment: a brief report. The Journal of the American Osteopathic Association. 116(7):e22–30.

Martins RF, Pinto e Silva JL (2014) Treatment of pregnancy-related lumbar and pelvic girdle pain by the yoga method: a randomized controlled study. Journal of Alternative and Complementary Medicine. 20(1):24–31.

Marx M, McKavanagh D, McCarthy AL, Bird R *et al.* (2015) The effect of ginger (Zingiber officinale) on platelet aggregation: a systematic literature review. PLoS One. 10(10): e0141119. Viewed online 19/09/2017 at www.ncbi.nlm.nih.gov/pmc/articles/PMC4619316

Marzouk T, Barakat R, Ragab A, Badria F, Badawy A (2015) Lavender-thymol as a new topical aromatherapy preparation for episiotomy: a randomised clinical trial. Journal of Obstetrics and Gynaecology. 35(5):472–5.

Masoumi SZ, Asl HR, Poorolajal J, Panah MH, Oliaei SR (2016) Evaluation of mint efficacy regarding dysmenorrhea in comparison with mefenamic acid: a double blinded randomized crossover study. Iranian Journal of Nursing and Midwifery Research. 21(4):363–7.

Mathie JG, Dawson BH (1959) Effect of castor oil, soap enema, and hot bath on the pregnant human uterus near term: a tocographic study. BMJ. 1(5130):1162–5.

Matos LC, Santos SC, Anderson JG, Machado J, Greten HJ, Monteiro FJ (2017) Instrumental measurements of water and the surrounding space during a randomized blinded controlled trial of focused intention. Journal of Evidence-Based Complementary and Alternative Medicine. 2156587217707117.

Mayberry L, Daniel J (2016) "Birthgasm": a literary review of orgasm as an alternative mode of pain relief in childbirth. Journal of Holistic Nursing. 34(4):331–42.

Mayo L (2001) A sound remedy? A new treatment for "morning sickness". The Practising Midwife. 4(20):16–17.

Mazzarino M, Kerr D, Wajswelner H, Morris ME (2015) Pilates method for women's health: systematic review of randomized controlled trials. Archives of Physical Medicine and Rehabilitation. 96(12):2231–42.

McAllister S, Coxon K, Murrells T, Sandall J (2017) Healthcare professionals' attitudes, knowledge and self-efficacy levels regarding the use of self-hypnosis in childbirth: a prospective questionnaire survey. Midwifery. 47:8–14.

McCauley M, Stewart C, Kebede B (2017) A survey of healthcare providers' knowledge and attitudes regarding pain relief in labor for women in Ethiopia. BMC Pregnancy and Childbirth. 17(1):56.

McCormack D (2010) Hypnosis for hyperemesis gravidarum. Journal of Obstetrics and Gynaecology. 30(7):647–53.

McCulloch M, Nachat A, Schwartz J, Casella-Gordon V, Cook J (2015) Acupuncture safety in patients receiving anticoagulants: a systematic review. The Permanente Journal. 19(1):68–73.

McEwen BJ (2015) The influence of herbal medicine on platelet function and coagulation: a narrative review. Seminars in Thrombosis and Hemostasis. 41(3):300–14.

McFarlin BL, Gibson MH, O'Rear J, Harman P (1999) A national survey of herbal preparation use by nurse-midwives for labor stimulation: review of the literature and recommendations for practice. Journal of Nurse-Midwifery. 44:205–16.

McGlone F, Cerritelli F, Walker S, Esteves J (2016) The role of gentle touch in perinatal osteopathic manual therapy. Neuroscience and Biobehavioral Reviews. 72:1–9.

McNabb MT, Kimber L, Haines A, McCourt C (2006) Does regular massage from late pregnancy to birth decrease maternal pain perception during labour and birth? A feasibility study to investigate a programme of massage, controlled breathing and visualization, from 36 weeks of pregnancy until birth. Complementary Therapies in Clinical Practice. 12(3):222–31.

McNeile, LG (1918) Enhancement of opioid-mediated analgesia: a solution to the enigma of placentophagia. The American Journal of Obstetrics and Diseases of Women and Children, 77. W.A. Townsend & Adams, original press: University of Michigan.

Meamarbashi A, Rajabi A (2013) The effects of peppermint on exercise performance. Journal of the International Society of Sports Nutrition. 10(1):15.

Mehl LE (1994) Hypnosis and conversion of the breech to the vertex presentation. Archives of Family Medicine. 3(10):881–7.

Mehl-Madrona LE (2004) Hypnosis to facilitate uncomplicated birth. American Journal of Clinical Hypnosis. 46(4):299–312.

Mei-dan E, Walfisch A, Raz I, Levy A, Hallak M (2008) Perineal massage during pregnancy: a prospective controlled trial. The Israel Medicine Association Journal. 10(7):499–502.

Mello LF, Nóbrega LF, Lemos A (2011) Transcutaneous electrical stimulation for pain relief during labor: a systematic review and meta-analysis. Revista Brasileira de Fisioterapia. 15(3):175–84.

Melzack R, Wall PW (1965) Pain mechanisms: a new theory. Science. 150(3699):971–9.

Meng S, Deng Q, Feng C, Pan Y, Chang Q (2015) Effects of massage treatment combined with topical cactus and aloe on puerperal milk stasis. Breast Disease. 35(3):173–8.

Mens JM, Damen L, Snijders CJ, Stam HJ (2006) The mechanical effect of a pelvic belt in patients with pregnancy-related pelvic pain. Clinical Biomechanics (Bristol, Avon). 21(2):122–7.

Mevissen L, Didden R, Korzilius H, de Jongh A (2017) Eye movement desensitisation and reprocessing therapy for posttraumatic stress disorder in a child and an adolescent with mild to borderline intellectual disability: a multiple baseline across subjects study. Journal of Applied Research in Intellectual Disability. 1–8. Doi: 10.1111/jar.12335.

Meyerson J, Uziel N (2014) Application of hypno-dissociative strategies during dental treatment of patients with severe dental phobia. International Journal of Clinical and Experimental Hypnosis. 62(2):179–87.

Michel JL, Caceres A, Mahady GB (2016) Ethnomedical research and review of Q'eqchi Maya women's reproductive health in the Lake Izabal region of Guatemala: past, present and future prospects. Journal of Ethnopharmacology. 178:307–22.

Midilli TS, Eser I (2015) Effects of Reiki on post-cesarean delivery pain, anxiety, and hemodynamic parameters: a randomized, controlled clinical trial. Pain Management Nursing. 16(3):388–99.

Miller J, Beharie MC, Taylor AM, Simmenes EB, Way S (2016) Parent reports of exclusive breastfeeding after attending a combined midwifery and chiropractic feeding clinic in the United Kingdom: a cross-sectional service evaluation. Journal of Evidence-Based Complementary and Alternative Medicine. 21(2):85–91.

Miller JE, Newell D, Bolton JE (2012) Efficacy of chiropractic manual therapy on infant colic: a pragmatic single-blind, randomized controlled trial. Journal of Manipulative and Physiological Therapeutics. 35(8):600–7.

Miller JE, Phillips HL (2009) Long-term effects of infant colic: a survey comparison of chiropractic treatment and nontreatment groups. Journal of Manipulative and Physiological Therapeutics. 32(8):635–8.

Miquelutti MA, Cecatti JG, Makuch MY (2013) Antenatal education and the birthing experience of Brazilian women: a qualitative study. BMC Pregnancy and Childbirth. 13:171.

Mitchell M, Allen K (2008) An exploratory study of women's experiences and key stakeholders views of moxibustion for cephalic version in breech presentation. Complementary Therapies in Clinical Practice. 14(4):264–72.

Mitri F, Hofmeyr GJ, van Gelderen CJ (1987) Meconium during labour: self-medication and other associations. South African Medical Journal. 71(7):431–3.

Modlock J, Nielsen BB, Uldbjerg N (2010) Acupuncture for the induction of labour: a double-blind randomised controlled study. BJOG. 117(10):1255–61.

Moghimi-Hanjani S, Mehdizadeh-Tourzani Z, Shoghi M (2015) The effect of foot reflexology on anxiety, pain, and outcomes of the labor in primigravida women. Acta Medica Iranica. 53(8):507–11.

Mogren IM (2005) Previous physical activity decreases the risk of low back pain and pelvic pain during pregnancy. Scandinavian Journal of Public Health. 33(4):300–6.

Mogren IM, Pohjanen AI (2005) Low back pain and pelvic pain during pregnancy: prevalence and risk factors. Spine (Philadelphia Pa 1976). 30(8):983–91.

Mohammadi A, Mohammad-Alizadeh-Charandabi S, Mirghafourvand M, Javadzadeh Y et al. (2014) Effects of cinnamon on perineal pain and healing of episiotomy: a randomized placebo-controlled trial. Journal of Integrative Medicine. 12(4):359–66.

Mohammed OJ, McAlpine R, Chiewhatpong P, Latif ML, Pratten MK (2016) Assessment of developmental cardiotoxic effects of some commonly used phytochemicals in mouse embryonic D3 stem cell differentiation and chick embryonic cardiomyocyte micromass culture models. Reproductive Toxicology. 64:86–97.

Mollart L (2003) Single-blind trial addressing the differential effects of two reflexology techniques versus rest, on ankle and foot oedema in late pregnancy. Complementary Therapies in Nursing and Midwifery. 9(4):203–8.

Mollart L, Adam J, Foureur M (2015) Impact of acupressure on onset of labour and labour duration: a systematic review. Women and Birth. 28(3):199–206.

Mollart L, Skinner V, Adams J, Foureur M (2017) Midwives' personal use of complementary and alternative medicine (CAM) influences their recommendations to women experiencing a post-date pregnancy. Women and Birth. 11 Jul. pii: S1871–5192(17)30048-3.

Monji F, Adaikan PG, Lau LC, Bin Said B et al. (2016) Investigation of uterotonic properties of Ananas comosus extracts. Journal of Ethnopharmacology. 193:21–9.

Montross-Thomas LP, Meier EA, Reynolds-Norolahi K, Raskin EE et al. (2017) Inpatients' preferences, beliefs, and stated willingness to pay for complementary and alternative medicine treatments. Journal of Alternative and Complementary Medicine. 23(4):259–63.

Moon RJ, Harvey NC, Cooper C (2015) Endocrinology in pregnancy: influence of maternal vitamin D status on obstetric outcomes and the fetal skeleton. European Journal of Endocrinology. 173(2):R69–83.

Moore CB, Hickey AH (2017) Increasing access to auricular acupuncture for postoperative nausea and vomiting. Journal of PeriAnesthesia Nursing. 32(2):96–105.

Moreno-Alcázar A, Radua J, Landín-Romero R, Blanco L et al. (2017) Eye movement desensitization and reprocessing therapy versus supportive therapy in affective relapse prevention in bipolar patients with a history of trauma: study protocol for a randomized controlled trial. Trials. 18(1):160.

Moretti ME, Maxson A, Hanna F, Koren G (2009) Evaluating the safety of St. John's Wort in human pregnancy. Reproductive Toxicology. 28(1):96–9. doi: 10.1016/j.reprotox.2009.02.003.

Mori HM, Kawanami H, Kawahata H, Aoki M (2016) Wound healing potential of lavender oil by acceleration of granulation and wound contraction through induction of TGF-β in a rat model. BMC Complementary and Alternative Medicine. 16:144.

Morimoto C, Satoh Y, Hara M, Inoue S, Tsujita T, Okuda H (2005) Anti-obese action of raspberry ketone. Life Sciences. 77(2):194–204.

Mørkved S, Salvesen KA, Schei B, Lydersen S, Bø K (2007) Does group training during pregnancy prevent lumbopelvic pain? A randomized clinical trial. Acta Obstetricia et Gynecologica Scandinavica. 86(3):276–82.

Mortel M, Mehta SD (2013) Systematic review of the efficacy of herbal galactogogues. Journal of Human Lactation. 29(2):154–62.

Mozaffari-Khosravi H, Talaei B, Jalali BA, Najarzadeh A, Mozayan MR (2014) The effect of ginger powder supplementation on insulin resistance and glycemic indices in patients with type 2 diabetes: a randomized, double-blind, placebo-controlled trial. Complementary Therapies in Medicine. 22(1):9–16.

Mozurkewich EL, Chilimigras JL, Berman DR, Perni UC et al. (2011) Methods of induction of labour: a systematic review. BMC Pregnancy and Childbirth. 11:84.

Mu Y, Zhang J, Zhang S, Zhou HH et al. (2006) Traditional Chinese medicines Wu Wei Zi (Schisandra chinensis Baill) and Gan Cao (Glycyrrhizauralensis Fisch) activate pregnane X receptor and increase warfarin clearance in rats. The Journal of Pharmacology and Experimental Therapeutics. 316(3):1369–77.

Mucuk S, Baser M (2014) Effects of noninvasive electroacupuncture on labour pain and duration. Journal of Clinical Nursing. 23(11–12):1603–10.

Mucuk S, Baser M, Ozkan T (2013) Effects of noninvasive electroacupuncture on labor pain, adrenocorticotropic hormone, and cortisol. Alternative Therapies in Health and Medicine. 19(3):26–30.

Münstedt K, Brenken A, Kalder M (2009) Clinical indications and perceived effectiveness of complementary and alternative medicine in departments of obstetrics in Germany: a questionnaire study. European Journal of Obstetrics & Gynecology and Reproductive Biology. 146(1):50–4.

Murphy DR, Hurwitz EL, McGovern EE (2009) Outcome of pregnancy-related lumbopelvic pain treated according to a diagnosis-based decision rule: a prospective observational cohort study. Journal of Manipulative and Physiological Therapeutics. 32(8):616–24.

Murphy PA, Kern SE, Stanczyk FZ, Westhoff CL (2005) Interaction of St. John's Wort with oral contraceptives: effects on the pharmacokinetics of norethindrone and ethinyl estradiol, ovarian activity and breakthrough bleeding. Contraception. 71(6):402–8.

Murtagh M, Folan M (2014) Women's experiences of induction of labour for post-date pregnancy. British Journal of Midwifery. 22(2):105–10.

Muzik M, Hamilton SE, Lisa Rosenblum K, Waxler E, Hadi Z (2012) Mindfulness yoga during pregnancy for psychiatrically at-risk women: preliminary results from a pilot feasibility study. Complementary Therapies in Clinical Practice. 18(4):235–40.

Nagai K, Niijima A, Horii Y, Shen J, Tanida M (2014) Olfactory stimulatory with grapefruit and lavender oils change autonomic nerve activity and physiological function. Autonomic Neuroscience. 185:29–35.

Nahidi F, Gazerani N, Yousefi P, Abadi AR (2017) The comparison of the effects of massaging and rocking on infantile colic. Iranian Journal of Nursing and Midwifery Research. 22(1):67–71.

Nakakita Kenyon M (2015) Randomized controlled trial on the relaxation effects of back massages for puerperants on the first post-partum day. Japan Journal of Nursing Science. 12(2):87–98.

Nanthakomon T, Pongrojpaw D (2006) The efficacy of ginger in prevention of postoperative nausea and vomiting after major gynecologic surgery. Journal of the Medical Association of Thailand. 89 Suppl 4:S130–6.

Naser B, Bodinet C, Tegtmeier M, Lindequist U (2005) Thuja occidentalis (Arbor vitae): a review of its pharmaceutical, pharmacological and clinical properties. Evidence-Based Complementary and Alternative Medicine. 2(1):69–78.

Naser B, Schnitker J, Minkin MJ, de Arriba SG, Nolte KU, Osmers R (2011) Suspected black cohosh hepatotoxicity: no evidence by meta-analysis of randomized controlled clinical trials for isopropanolic black cohosh extract. Menopause. 18(4):366–75.

Nazari F, Soheili M, Hosseini S, Shaygannejad V (2016) A comparison of the effects of reflexology and relaxation on pain in women with multiple sclerosis. Journal of Complementary and Integrative Medicine. 13(1):65–71.

Neri I, Airola G, Contu G, Allais G, Facchinetti F, Benedetto C (2004) Acupuncture plus moxibustion to resolve breech presentation: a randomized controlled study. The Journal of Maternal-Fetal and Neonatal Medicine. 15(4):247–52.

Neri I, Allais G, Vaccaro V, Minniti S *et al.* (2011) Acupuncture treatment as breastfeeding support: preliminary data. Journal of Alternative and Complementary Medicine. 17(2):133–7.

Neri I, Dante G, Pignatti L, Salvioli C, Facchinetti F (2017) Castor oil for induction of labour: a retrospective study. The Journal of Maternal-Fetal and Neonatal Medicine. 15:1–4.

Neri I, De Pace V, Venturini P, Facchinetti F (2007) Effects of three different stimulations (acupuncture, moxibustion, acupuncture plus moxibustion) of BL.67 acupoint at small toe on fetal behavior of breech presentation. The American Journal of Chinese Medicine. 35(1):27–33.

Neri I, Fazzio M, Menghini S, Volpe A, Facchinetti F (2002) Non-stress test changes during acupuncture plus moxibustion on BL67 point in breech presentation. Journal of the Society for Gynecologic Investigation. 9(3):158–62.

Neri I, Monari F, Midwife CS, Facchinetti F (2014) Acupuncture in post-date pregnancy: a pilot study. The Journal of Maternal-Fetal and Neonatal Medicine. 27(9):874–8.

Nettis E, Napoli G, Ferrannini A, Tursi A (2001) IgE-mediated allergy to bromelain. Allergy. 56(3):257–8.

Newburn, M, Singh D (2003) Creating a Better Birth Environment. Women's Views about the Design and Facilities in Maternity Units: A National Survey. London: National Childbirth Trust. Viewed online 20/09/2017 at www.arquitecturadematernidades.com/sites/default/files/nct2003_bbe_report.pdf

Ng SS, Leung WW, Mak TW, Hon SS *et al.* (2013) Electroacupuncture reduces duration of postoperative ileus after laparoscopic surgery for colorectal cancer. Gastroenterology. 144(2):307–313.e1.

NHS Choices (2017) Complementary and alternative medicine. Viewed online 20/09/2017 at www.nhs.uk/Livewell/complementary-alternative-medicine/Pages/complementary-alternative-medicines.aspx

NHS Digital (2015) Maternity statistics 2013–2014. Viewed online 25/10/2017 at http://content.digital.nhs.uk/catalogue/PUB16725

NHS England (2016) Better births: improving outcomes of maternity services in England. A five year forward view for maternity care. Viewed online 20/09/2017 at www.england.nhs.uk/wp-content/uploads/2016/02/national-maternity-review-report.pdf

NHS Institute for Innovation and Improvement (2009) High impact actions for nursing and midwifery. Viewed online 25/10/2017 at https://www.qualitasconsortium.com/index.cfm/reference-material/innovation/high-impact-actions-for-nursing-midwifery

NICE (2008) Inducing labour (CG70) Viewed online 22/11/2017 at www.nice.org.uk/guidance/cg70/resources/inducing-labour-pdf-975621704389

NICE (2017a) Antenatal care for uncomplicated pregnancies (CG62). Viewed online 20/09/2017 at www.nice.org.uk/guidance/cg62

NICE (2017b) Intrapartum care for healthy women and babies (CG190). Viewed online 20/09/2017 at www.nice.org.uk/guidance/cg190

Nikodem VC, Danziger D, Gebka N, Gulmezoglu AM, Hofmeyr GJ (1993) Do cabbage leaves prevent breast engorgement? A randomized, controlled study. Birth. 20(2):61–4.

Nimma VL, Talla HV, Bairi JK, Gopaldas M, Bathula H, Vangdoth S (2017) Holistic healing through herbs: effectiveness of aloe vera on post extraction socket healing. Journal of Clinical and Diagnostic Research. 11(3):ZC83–ZC86.

Nlooto M, Naidoo P (2016) Traditional, complementary and alternative medicine use by HIV patients a decade after public sector antiretroviral therapy roll out in South Africa: a cross sectional study. BMC Complementary and Alternative Medicine. 16:128.

NMC (2009) Standards for pre-registration midwifery education. Viewed online 20/09/2017 at www.nmc.org.uk/globalassets/sitedocuments/standards/nmc-standards-for-preregistration-midwifery-education.pdf

NMC (2010) Standards for medicines management. Viewed online 20/09/2017 at www.nmc.org.uk/globalassets/sitedocuments/standards/nmc-standards-for-medicines-management.pdf

NMC (2015) The Code: professional standards of practice and behaviour for nurses and midwives. Viewed online 20/09/2017 at www.nmc.org.uk/globalassets/sitedocuments/nmc-publications/nmc-code.pdf

Noori S, Hassan ZM, Salehian O (2013) Sclareol reduces CD4+ CD25+ FoxP3+ Treg cells in a breast cancer model in vivo. Iranian Journal of Immunology. 10(1):10–21.

Nordeng H, Bayne K, Havnen GC, Paulsen BS (2011) Use of herbal drugs during pregnancy among 600 Norwegian women in relation to concurrent use of conventional drugs and pregnancy outcome. Complementary Therapies in Clinical Practice. 17(3):147–51.

Nordeng H, Saboni M, Samuelsen AB (2014) Assessment report on Rubus idaeus L., folium. European Medicines Agency, Committee on Herbal Medicinal Products. Viewed online 20/09/2017 at www.ema.europa.eu/docs/en_GB/document_library/Herbal_-_HMPC_assessment_report/2014/03/WC500163552.pdf

Norén L, Ostgaard S, Johansson G, Ostgaard HC (2002) Lumbar back and posterior pelvic pain during pregnancy: a 3-year follow-up. European Spine Journal. 11(3):267–71.

Norman JA, Pickford CJ, Sanders TW, Waller M (1988) Human intake of arsenic and iodine from seaweed-based food supplements and health foods available in the UK. Food Additives and Contaminants. 5(1):103–9.

Nutter E, Meyer S, Shaw-Battista J, Marowitz A (2014) Waterbirth: an integrative analysis of peer-reviewed literature. Journal of Midwifery and Women's Health. 59(3):286–319.

Nyeko R, Tumwesigye NM, Halage AA (2016) Prevalence and factors associated with use of herbal medicines during pregnancy among women attending postnatal clinics in Gulu district, Northern Uganda. BMC Pregnancy and Childbirth. 16(1):296.

Oakley S, Evans E (2014) The role of yoga: breathing, meditation and optimal fetal positioning. The Practising Midwife. 17(5):30–2.

O'Connor NA, Graham DM, McCaffrey J, Carney DN (2011) The use of complementary and alternative medicine (CAM) by Irish patients with cancer. Journal of Clinical Oncology. 29(15suppl):e19618.

Oderinde O, Noronha C, Oremosu A, Kusemiju T, Okanlawon OA (2002) Abortifacient properties of aqueous extract of Carica papaya (Linn) seeds on female Sprague-Dawley rats. Nigerian Postgraduate Medical Journal. 9(2):95–8.

Oh JY, Park MA, Kim YC (2014) Peppermint oil promotes hair growth without toxic signs. Toxicology Research. 30(4):297–304.

Olapour A, Behaeen K, Akhondzadeh R, Soltani F, Al Sadat Razavi F, Bekhradi R (2013) The effect of inhalation of aromatherapy blend containing lavender essential oil on cesarean postoperative pain. Anesthesiology and Pain Medicine. 3(1):203–7.

Omar NS, Tan PC, Sabir N, Yusop ES, Omar SZ (2013) Coitus to expedite the onset of labour: a randomised trial. BJOG. 120(3):338–45.

O'Mathúna DP (2016) Therapeutic touch for healing acute wounds. Cochrane Database of Systematic Reviews. (8):CD002766.

Onozawa K, Glover V, Adams D, Modi N, Kumar RC (2001) Infant massage improves mother-infant interaction for mothers with postnatal depression. Journal of Affective Disorders. 63(1–3):201–7.

Orhan N, Berkkan A, Deliorman Orhan D, Aslan M, Ergun F (2011) Effects of Juniperus oxycedrus ssp. oxycedrus on tissue lipid peroxidation, trace elements (Cu, Zn, Fe) and blood glucose levels in experimental diabetes. Journal of Ethnopharmacology. 133(2):759–64.

Ormsby SM, Smith CA, Dahlen HG, Hay PJ, Lind JM (2016) Evaluation of an antenatal acupuncture intervention as an adjunct therapy for antenatal depression (AcuAnteDep): study protocol for a pragmatic randomised controlled trial. Trials. 17(1):1–14.

Ososki AL, Lohr P, Reiff M, Balick MJ et al. (2002) Ethnobotanical literature survey of medicinal plants in the Dominican Republic used for women's health conditions. Journal of Ethnopharmacology. 79:285–98.

Oswald C, Higgins CC, Assimakopoulos D (2013) Optimizing pain relief during pregnancy using manual therapy. Canadian Family Physician. 59(8):841–2.

Ou MC, Hsu TF, Lai AC, Lin YT, Lin CC (2012) Pain relief assessment by aromatic essential oil massage on outpatients with primary dysmenorrhea: a randomized, double-blind clinical trial. Journal of Obstetrics and Gynaecological Research. 38(5):817–22.

Ouzir M, El Bairi K, Amzazi S (2016) Toxicological properties of fenugreek (Trigonella foenum graecum). Food and Chemical Toxicology. 96:145–54.

Oyedemi SO, Yakubu MT, Afolayan AJ (2010) Effect of aqueous extract of Leonotis leonurus (L.) R. Br. leaves in male Wistar rats. Human and Experimental Toxicology. 29(5):377–84.

Ozgoli G, Goli M, Simbar M (2009) Effects of ginger capsules on pregnancy, nausea, and vomiting. Journal of Alternative and Complementary Medicine. 15(3):243–6.

Ozgoli G, Sedigh Mobarakabadi S, Heshmat R, Alavi Majd H, Sheikhan Z (2016) Effect of LI4 and BL32 acupressure on labor pain and delivery outcome in the first stage of labor in primiparous women: a randomized controlled trial. Complementary Therapies in Medicine. 29:175–80.

Pach D, Brinkhaus B, Willich SN (2009) Moxa sticks: thermal properties and possible implications for clinical trials. Complementary Therapies in Medicine. 17(4):243–6.

Padua L, Padua R, Bondì R, Ceccarelli E et al. (2002) Patient-oriented assessment of back pain in pregnancy. European Spine Journal. 11(3):272–5.

Palaniappan K, Holley RA (2010) Use of natural antimicrobials to increase antibiotic susceptibility of drug resistant bacteria. International Journal of Food Microbiology. 140(2–3):164–8.

Pallivalappila AR, Stewart D, Shetty A, Pande B, McLay J (2013) Complementary and alternative medicines use during pregnancy: a systematic review of pregnant women and healthcare professional views and experiences. Evidence-Based Complementary and Alternative Medicine. 2013:205639. Viewed online 20/09/2017 at www.hindawi.com/journals/ecam/2013/205639

Panahi Y, Saadat A, Sahebkar A, Hashemian F, Taghikhani M, Abolhasani E (2012) Effect of ginger on acute and delayed chemotherapy-induced nausea and vomiting: a pilot, randomized, open-label clinical trial. Integrative Cancer Therapies. 11(3):204–11.

Paris A, Gonnet N, Chaussard C, Belon P *et al.* (2008) Effect of homeopathy on analgesic intake following knee ligament reconstruction: a phase III monocentre randomized placebo controlled study. British Journal of Clinical Pharmocology. 65(2):180–7.

Park JE, Lee SS, Lee MS, Choi SM, Ernst E (2010) Adverse events of moxibustion: a systematic review. Complementary Therapies in Medicine. 18(5):215–23.

Parsons M, Simpson M, Ponton T (1999) Raspberry leaf and its effect on labour: safety and efficacy. Australian College of Midwives Incorporated Journal. 12:20–5.

Pasha H, Behmanesh F, Mohsenzadeh F, Hajahmadi M, Moghadamnia AA (2012) Study of the effect of mint oil on nausea and vomiting during pregnancy. Iranian Red Crescent Medical Journal. 14(11):727–30.

Pauley T, Percival R (2014) Reducing post-dates induction numbers with complementary post dates clinics. British Journal of Midwifery. 22(9):630–3.

Paulsen E, Andersen KE (2012) Patch testing with constituents of Compositae mixes. Contact Dermatitis. 66(5):241–6.

Paulsen E, Chistensen LP, Andersen KE (2008) Cosmetics and herbal remedies with Compositae plant extracts: are they tolerated by Compositae-allergic patients? Contact Dermatitis. 58(1):15–23.

Pavan R, Jain S, Shraddha S, Kumar V (2012) Properties and therapeutic application of bromelain: a review. Biotechnology Research International. 2012:976203. Viewed online 20/09/2017 at www.hindawi.com/journals/btri/2012/976203

Peirce C, Murphy C, Fitzpatrick M, Cassidy M *et al.* (2013) Randomised controlled trial comparing early home biofeedback physiotherapy with pelvic floor exercises for the treatment of third-degree tears (EBAPT Trial). BJOG. 120(10):1240–7.

Pennell CE, Henderson JJ, O'Neill MJ, McCleery S, Doherty DA, Dickinson JE (2009) Induction of labour in nulliparous women with an unfavourable cervix: a randomised controlled trial comparing double and single balloon catheters and PGE2gel. BJOG. 116(11):1443–52.

Pennick V, Liddle SD (2013) Interventions for preventing and treating pelvic and back pain in pregnancy. Cochrane Database of Systematic Reviews. (8):CD001139.

Pennick VE, Young G (2007) Interventions for preventing and treating pelvic and back pain in pregnancy. Cochrane Database of Systematic Reviews. (8):CD001139.

Perez-Blasco J, Viguer P, Rodrigo MF (2013) Effects of a mindfulness-based intervention on psychological distress, well-being, and maternal self-efficacy in breast-feeding mothers: results of a pilot study. Archives of Women's Mental Health. 16(3):227–36.

Pérol D, Provençal J, Hardy-Bessard AC, Coeffic D *et al.* (2012) Can treatment with Cocculine improve the control of chemotherapy-induced emesis in early breast cancer patients? A randomized, multi-centered, double-blind, placebo-controlled Phase III trial. BMC Cancer. 12:603.

Perry R, Hunt K, Ernst E (2011) Nutritional supplements and other complementary medicines for infantile colic: a systematic review. Pediatrics. 127(4):720–33.

Perry R, Terry R, Watson LK, Ernst E (2012) Is lavender an anxiolytic drug? A systematic review of randomised clinical trials. Phytomedicine. 19(8–9):825–35.

Peters NA, Schlaff RA (2016) Examining the energy cost and intensity level of prenatal yoga. International Journal of Yoga. 9(1):77–80.

Petersen I, McCrea RL, Lupattelli A, Nordeng H (2015) Women's perception of risks of adverse fetal pregnancy outcomes: a large-scale multinational survey. BMJ Open. 5(6):e007390.

Peterson CD, Haas M, Gregory WT (2012) A pilot randomized controlled trial comparing the efficacy of exercise, spinal manipulation, and neuro emotional technique for the treatment of pregnancy-related low back pain. Chiropractic and Manual Therapies. 20(1):18.

Peterson CK, Mühlemann D, Humphreys BK (2014) Outcomes of pregnant patients with low back pain undergoing chiropractic treatment: a prospective cohort study with short term, medium term and 1 year follow-up. Chiropractic and Manual Therapies. 22(1):15.

Pintov S, Hochman M, Livne A, Heyman E, Lahat E (2005) Bach flower remedies used for attention deficit hyperactivity disorder in children: a prospective double blind controlled study. European Journal of Paediatric Neurology. 9(6):395–8.

Pistolese RA (2002) The Webster Technique: chiropractic technique with obstetric implications. Journal of Manipulative and Physiological Therapeutics. 25(6):E1–9.

Pitangui AC, Araújo RC, Bezerra MJ, Ribeiro CO, Nakano AM (2014) Low and high-frequency TENS in post-episiotomy pain relief: a randomized, double-blind clinical trial. Brazilian Journal of Physical Therapy. 18(1):72–8.

Plakornkul V, Vannabhum M, Viravud Y, Roongruangchai J *et al.* (2016) The effects of the court-type Thai traditional massage on anatomical relations, blood flow, and skin temperature of the neck, shoulder, and arm. BMC Complementary and Alternative Medicine. 16:363.

Polis RL, Gussman D, Kuo YH (2015) Yoga in pregnancy: an examination of maternal and fetal responses to 26 yoga postures. Obstetrics and Gynecology. 126(6):1237–41.

Pongrojpaw D, Somprasit C, Chanthasenanont A (2007) A randomized comparison of ginger and dimenhydrinate in the treatment of nausea and vomiting in pregnancy. Journal of the Medical Association of Thailand. 90(9):1703–9.

Poole H, Glenn S, Murphy P (2007) A randomised controlled study of reflexology for the management of chronic low back pain. European Journal of Pain. 11(8):878–87.

Portela GS, Azoubel R, Batigália, F (2007) Effects of aspartame on maternal-fetal and placental weights, length of umbilical cord and fetal liver: a kariometric experimental study. International Journal of Morphology. 25(3):549–54.

Prairie BA, Lauria MR, Kapp N, Mackenzie T, Baker ER, George KE (2007) Mifepristone versus laminaria: a randomized controlled trial of cervical ripening in midtrimester termination. Contraception. 76(5):383–8.

Pregnancy Sickness Support (2013) Women's experiences of NVP and HG: results from an online survey of 975 women. Unpublished. London: PSS. Cited in Dean C, Marsden J (2017) Satisfaction for treatment of hyperemesis gravidarum in day case settings compared to hospital admissions. MIDIRS Midwifery Digest. 27(1):11–20.

Price DD, Finniss DG, Benedetti F (2008) A comprehensive review of the placebo effect: recent advances and current thought. Annual Review of Psychology. 59:565–90.

Pumpa KL, Fallon KE, Bensoussan A, Papalia S (2014) The effects of topical Arnica on performance, pain and muscle damage after intense eccentric exercise. European Journal of Sport Science. 14(3):294–300.

Purepong N, Channak S, Boonyong S, Thaveeratitham P, Janwantanakul P (2015) The effect of an acupressure backrest on pain and disability in office workers with chronic low back pain: a randomized, controlled study and patients' preferences. Complementary Therapies in Medicine. 23(3):347–55.

Puri BK (2007) The safety of evening primrose oil in epilepsy. Pakistan Journal of Pharmaceutical Sciences. 22(4):355–9.

Pye KG, Kelsey SM, House IM, Newland AC (1992) Severe dyserythropoiesis and autoimmune thrombocytopenia associated with ingestion of kelp supplements. Lancet. 339(8808):1540.

Qayyum R, Qamar HM, Khan S, Salma U, Khan T, Shah AJ (2016) Mechanisms underlying the antihypertensive properties of Urtica dioica. Journal of Translational Medicine. 14:254.

Qin GF, Tang HJ (1989) Cases of abnormal fetal position corrected by auricular plaster therapy. Journal of Traditional Chinese Medicine. 9(4):235–7.

Quinn VF, Colagiuri B (2016) Sources of placebo-induced relief from nausea: the role of instruction and conditioning. Psychosomatic Medicine. 78(3):365–72.

Quraishy K (2016) Feeding in the NICU: a perspective from a craniosacral therapist. Neonatal Network. 35(2):105–7.

Rabl M, Ahner R, Bitschnau M, Zeisler H, Husslein P (2001) Acupuncture for cervical ripening and induction of labor at term: a randomized controlled trial. Wiener Klinische Wochenschrift. 113(23–24):942–6.

Rahimi R, Nikfar S, Abdollahi M (2009) Efficacy and tolerability of Hypericum perforatum in major depressive disorder in comparison with selective serotonin reuptake inhibitors: a meta-analysis. Progress in Neuropsychopharmacology and Biological Psychiatry. 33(1):118–27.

Rahmawati R, Bajorek BV (2017) Self-medication among people living with hypertension: a review. Family Practice. 34(2):147–53.

Räikkönen K, Seckl JR, Heinonen K, Pyhälä R et al. (2010) Maternal prenatal licorice consumption alters hypothalamic-pituitary-adrenocortical axis function in children. Psychoneuroendocrinology. 35(10):1587–93.

Raith W, Marschik PB, Sommer C, Maurer-Fellbaum U et al. (2016) General movements in preterm infants undergoing craniosacral therapy: a randomised controlled pilot-trial. BMC Complementary and Alternative Medicine. 16:12.

Raith W, Urlesberger B, Schmölzer GM (2013) Efficacy and safety of acupuncture in preterm and term infants. Evidence-Based Complementary and Alternative Medicine. 2013:739414.

Rao RB, Hoffman RS (2002) Nicotinic toxicity from tincture of blue cohosh (Caulophyllum thalictroides) used as an abortifacient. Veterinary and Human Toxicology. 44(4):221–2.

Rashidi-Fakari F, Tabatabaeichehr M, Kamali H, Rashidi Fakari F, Naseri M (2015) Effect of inhalation of aroma of geranium essence on anxiety and physiological parameters during first stage of labor in nulliparous women: a randomized clinical trial. Journal of Caring Sciences. 4(2):135–41.

Rashidi-Fakari F, Tabatabaeichehr M, Mortazavi H (2015) The effect of aromatherapy by essential oil of orange on anxiety during labor: a randomized clinical trial. Iranian Journal of Nursing and Midwifery Research. 20(6):661–4.

Razali N, Mohd Nahwari SH, Sulaiman S, Hassan J (2017) Date fruit consumption at term: effect on length of gestation, labour and delivery. Journal of Obstetrics and Gynaecology. 37(5):595–600.

RCOG (2016) The Management of Nausea and Vomiting in Pregnancy and Hyperemesis Gravidarum. Green-top guideline no. 69. Viewed online 20/09/2017 at www.rcog.org.uk/globalassets/documents/guidelines/green-top-guidelines/gtg69-hyperemesis.pdf

RCOG (2017) Management of Breech Presentation. Green-top guideline no. 20b. Viewed online 20/09/2017 at http://onlinelibrary.wiley.com/doi/10.1111/1471-0528.14465/epdf

Reddy S, Mishra P, Qureshi S, Nair S, Straker T (2016) Hepatotoxicity due to red bush tea consumption: a case report. Journal of Clinical Anesthesia. 35:96–8.

Reeder C, Legrand A, O'Connor-Von SK (2013) The effect of fenugreek on milk production and prolactin levels in mothers of preterm infants. Clinical Lactation. 4(4):159–65.

Reinhard J, Heinrich TM, Reitter A, Herrmann E, Smart W, Louwen F (2012) Clinical hypnosis before external cephalic version. American Journal of Clinical Hypnosis. 55(2):184–92.

Reinhard J, Peiffer S, Sanger N, Herrmann E, Yuan J, Louwen F (2012) The effects of clinical hypnosis versus neurolinguistic programming (NLP) before external cephalic version (ECV): a prospective off-centre randomised, double-blind, controlled trial. Evidence-Based Complementary and Alternative Medicine. Article ID 626740. doi:10.1155/2012/626740.

Relton C, Cooper K, Viksveen P, Fibert P, Thomas K (2017) Prevalence of homeopathy use by the general population worldwide: a systematic review. Homeopathy. 106(2):69–78.

Resende MM, Costa FE, Gardona RG, Araújo RG, Mundim FG, Costa MJ (2014) Preventive use of Bach flower Rescue Remedy in the control of risk factors for cardiovascular disease in rats. Complementary Therapies in Medicine. 22(4):719–23.

Rhodes VA, McDaniel RW (1999) The Index of Nausea, Vomiting, and Retching: a new format of the Index of Nausea and Vomiting. Oncology Nursing Forum. 26(5):889–94.

Riaz A, Khan RA, Ahmed SP (2009) Assessment of anticoagulant effect of evening primrose oil. Pakistan Journal of Pharmaceutical Sciences. 22(4):355–9.

Richards E, van Kessel G, Virgara R, Harris P (2012) Does antenatal physical therapy for pregnant women with low back pain or pelvic pain improve functional outcomes? A systematic review. Acta Obstetricia et Gynecologica Scandinavica. 91(9):1038–45.

Richardson J (2004) What patients expect from complementary therapy: a qualitative study. American Journal of Public Health. 94(6):1049–53.

Rivas-Suárez SR, Águila-Vázquez J, Suárez-Rodríguez B, Vázquez-León L et al. (2015) Exploring the effectiveness of external use of Bach flower remedies on carpal tunnel syndrome: a pilot study. Journal of Evidence-Based Complementary and Alternative Medicine. pii: 2156587215610705.

Rivera D, Verde A, Obón C, Alcaraz F et al. (2017) Is there nothing new under the sun? The influence of herbals and pharmacopoeias on ethnobotanical traditions in Albacete (Spain). Journal of Ethnopharmacology. 195:96–117.

Roberts KL, Reiter M, Schuster D (1995) A comparison of chilled and room temperature cabbage leaves in treating breast engorgement. Journal of Human Lactation. 11(3):191–4.

Robertson A, Suryanarayanan R, Banerjee A (2007) Homeopathic Arnica montana for post-tonsillectomy analgesia: a randomised placebo control trial. Homeopathy. 96(1):17–21.

Robertson E, Johansson SE (2010) Use of complementary, non-pharmacological pain reduction methods during childbirth among foreign-born and Swedish-born women. Midwifery. 26(4):442–9.

Rock NL, Shipley TE, Campbell C (1969) Hypnosis with untrained, nonvolunteer patients in labor. International Journal of Clinical and Experimental Hypnosis. 17(1):25–36.

Rodriguez-Blanque R, Sánchez-García JC, Sánchez-López AM, Mur-Villar N, Aguilar-Cordero MJ (2017) The influence of physical activity in water on sleep quality in pregnant women: a randomised trial. Women and Birth. pii: S1871–5192(16)30267-0.

Roecker CB (2013) Breech repositioning unresponsive to Webster technique: coexistence of oligohydramnios. Journal of Chiropractic Medicine. 12(2):74–8.

Rojas-Vera J, Patel AV, Dacke CG (2002) Relaxant activity of raspberry (Rubus idaeus) leaf extract in guinea-pig ileum in vitro. Phytotherapy Research. 16(7):665–8.

Romei V, Bauer M, Brooks JL, Economides M et al. (2016) Causal evidence that intrinsic beta-frequency is relevant for enhanced signal propagation in the motor system as shown through rhythmic TMS. Neuroimage. 126:120–30.

Ross A, Touchton-Leonard K, Yang L, Wallen G (2016) A national survey of yoga instructors and their delivery of yoga therapy. International Journal of Yoga Therapy. 26(1):83–91.

Rosti L, Nardini A, Bettinelli ME, Rosti D (1994) Toxic effects of a herbal tea mixture in two newborns. Acta Paediatrica. 83(6):683.

Rothberg S, Friedman BW (2016) Complementary therapies in addition to medication for patients with nonchronic, nonradicular low back pain: a systematic review. American Journal of Emergency Medicine. 35(1):55–61. pii: S0735–6757(16)30690-8

Roy Malis F, Meyer T, Gross MM (2017) Effects of an antenatal mindfulness-based childbirth and parenting programme on the postpartum experiences of mothers: a qualitative interview study. BMC Pregnancy and Childbirth. 17(1):57.

Ruffini N, D'Alessandro G, Cardinali L, Frondaroli F, Cerritelli F (2016) Osteopathic manipulative treatment in gynecology and obstetrics: a systematic review. Complementary Therapies in Medicine. 26:72–8.

Russell K, Walsh D, Scott I, McIntosh T (2014) Effecting change in midwives' waterbirth practice behaviours on labour ward: an action research study. Midwifery. 30(3):e96–e101.

Ryan JL, Heckler CE, Roscoe JA, Dakhil SR et al. (2012) Ginger (Zingiber officinale) reduces acute chemotherapy-induced nausea: a URCC CCOP study of 576 patients. Supportive Care in Cancer. 20(7):1479–89.

Ryu KH, Shin HS, Yang EY (2015) Effects of laughter therapy on immune responses in postpartum women. Journal of Alternative and Complementary Medicine. 21(12):781–8.

Saatsaz S, Rezaei R, Alipour A, Beheshti Z (2016) Massage as adjuvant therapy in the management of post-cesarean pain and anxiety: a randomized clinical trial. Complementary Therapies in Clinical Practice. 24:92–8.

Saberi F, Sadat Z, Abedzadeh-Kalahroudi M, Taebi M (2013) Acupressure and ginger to relieve nausea and vomiting in pregnancy: a randomized study. Iranian Red Crescent Medical Journal. 15:854–61.

Sado M, Ota E, Stickley A, Mori R (2012) Hypnosis during pregnancy, childbirth, and the postnatal period for preventing postnatal depression. Cochrane Database of Systematic Reviews. (6):CD009062.

Sadr S, Pourkiani-Allah-Abad N, Stuber K (2012) The treatment experience of patients with low back pain during pregnancy and their chiropractors: a qualitative study. Chiropractic and Manual Therapies. 20(1):32.

Sagkal Midilli T, Ciray Gunduzoglu N (2016) Effects of reiki on pain and vital signs when applied to the incision area of the body after Cesarean section surgery: a single-blinded, randomized, double-controlled study. Holistic Nursing Practice. 30(6):368–78.

Saini P, Saini R (2014) Cabbage leaves and breast engorgement. Indian Journal of Public Health. 58(4):291–2.

Salehi M, Karegar-Borzi H, Karimi M, Rahimi R (2016) Medicinal plants for management of gastroesophageal reflux disease: a review of animal and human studies. Journal of Alternative and Complementary Medicine. 23(2):82–95.

Salim R, Zafran N, Nachum Z, Garmi G, Kraiem N, Shalev E (2011) Single-balloon compared with double-balloon catheters for induction of labor: a randomized controlled trial. Obstetrics and Gynecology. 118(1):79–86.

Sananes N, Roth GE, Aissi GA, Meyer N et al. (2016) Acupuncture version of breech presentation: a randomized sham-controlled single-blinded trial. European Journal of Obstetrics & Gynecology and Reproductive Biology. 204:24–30.

Santana LS, Gallo RB, Ferreira CH, Duarte G, Quintana SM, Marcolin AC (2016) Transcutaneous electrical nerve stimulation (TENS) reduces pain and postpones the need for pharmacological analgesia during labour: a randomised trial. Journal of Physiotherapy. 62(1):29–34.

Sarris J, Robins Wahlin TB, Goncalves DC, Byrne GJ (2010) Comparative use of complementary medicine, allied health, and manual therapies by middle-aged and older Australian women. Journal of Women and Aging. 22(4):273–82.

Savino F, Cresi F, Castagno E, Silvestro L, Oggero R (2005) A randomized double-blind placebo-controlled trial of a standardized extract of Matricariae recutita, Foeniculum vulgare and Melissa officinalis (ColiMil) in the treatment of breastfed colicky infants. Phytotherapy Research. 19(4):335–40.

Sayorwan W, Siripornpanich V, Piriyapunyaporn T, Hongratanaworakit T, Kotchabhakdi N, Ruangrungsi N (2012) The effects of lavender oil inhalation on emotional states, autonomic nervous system, and brain electrical activity. Journal of the Medical Association of Thailand. 95(4):598–606.

Sayyah Melli M, Rashidi MR, Delazar A, Madarek E *et al.* (2007) Effect of peppermint water on prevention of nipple cracks in lactating primiparous women: a randomized controlled trial. International Breastfeeding Journal. 2:7.

Schachtman TR, Klakotskaia D, Walker JM, Hill AJ (2016) Psychological factors in food aversions, nausea, and vomiting during pregnancy. Journal of Food and Nutrition Research. 4(10):677–89.

Schäfer I, Chuey-Ferrer L, Hofmann A, Lieberman P, Mainusch G, Lotzin A (2017) Effectiveness of EMDR in patients with substance use disorder and comorbid PTSD: study protocol for a randomized controlled trial. BMC Psychiatry. 17(1):95.

Schaffir J, Czapla C (2012) Survey of lactation instructors on folk traditions in breastfeeding. Breastfeed Medicine. 7:230–3.

Schuette SA, Brown KM, Cuthbert DA, Coyle CW *et al.* (2017) Perspectives from patients and healthcare providers on the practice of maternal placentophagy. Journal of Alternative and Complementary Medicine. 23(1):60–7.

Schüle C, Baghai T, Ferrera A, Laakmann G (2001) Neuroendocrine effects of Hypericum extract WS 5570 in 12 healthy male volunteers. Pharmacopsychiatry. 34 Suppl 1:S127–33.

Schweimer JV, Mallet N, Sharp T, Ungless MA (2011) Spike-timing relationship of neurochemically-identified dorsal raphe neurons during cortical slow oscillations. Neuroscience. 196:115–23.

Schwerla F, Rother K, Rother D, Ruetz M, Resch KL (2015) Osteopathic manipulative therapy in women with postpartum low back pain and disability: a pragmatic randomized controlled trial. The Journal of the American Osteopathic Association. 115(7):416–25.

Sebastian MK (2014) Effect of acupressure on labour pain during first stage of labour among Primi mothers in a selected hospital of Delhi. The Nursing Journal of India. 105(3):136–9.

Seehusen DA, Raleigh M (2014) Antenatal perineal massage to prevent birth trauma. American Family Physician. 89(5):335–6.

Seely D, Dugoua JJ, Perri D, Mills E, Koren G (2008) Safety and efficacy of panax ginseng during pregnancy and lactation. The Canadian Journal of Clinical Pharmacology. 15(1):e87–94.

Sejari N, Kamaruddin K, Ramasamy K, Lim SM, Neoh CF, Ming LC (2016) The immediate effect of traditional Malay massage on substance P, inflammatory mediators, pain scale and functional outcome among patients with low back pain: study protocol of a randomised controlled trial. BMC Complementary and Alternative Medicine. 16:16.

Selander J, Cantor A, Young SM, Benyshek DC (2013) Human maternal placentophagy: a survey of self-reported motivations and experiences associated with placenta consumption. Ecology of Food and Nutrition. 52(2):93–115.

Select Committee on Science and Technology (2000) Sixth report of the Committee on Science and Technology: Complementary and Alternative Medicine. Viewed online 19/09/2017 at www.publications.parliament.uk/pa/ld199900/ldselect/ldsctech/123/12302.htm

Selmer-Olsen T, Lydersen S, Mørkved S (2007) Does acupuncture used in nulliparous women reduce time from prelabour rupture of membranes at term to active phase of labour? A randomised controlled trial. Acta Obstetricia et Gynecologica Scandinavica. 86(12):1447–52.

Seol GH, Lee YH, Kang P, You JH, Park M, Min SS (2013) Randomized controlled trial for Salvia sclarea or Lavandula angustifolia: differential effects on blood pressure in female patients with urinary incontinence undergoing urodynamic examination. Journal of Alternative and Complementary Medicine. 19(7):664–70.

Seol GH, Shim HS, Kim PJ, Moon HK *et al.* (2010) Antidepressant-like effect of Salvia sclarea is explained by modulation of dopamine activities in rats. Journal of Ethnopharmacology. 130(1):187–90.

Sewell AC, Mosandl A, Böhles H (1999) False diagnosis of maple syrup urine disease owing to ingestion of herbal tea. The New England Journal of Medicine. 341(10):769.

Seyyedrasooli A, Valizadeh L, Hosseini MB, Asgari Jafarabadi M, Mohammadzad M (2014) Effect of vimala massage on physiological jaundice in infants: a randomized controlled trial. Journal of Caring Sciences. 3(3):165–73.

Shalansky S, Lynd L, Richardson K, Ingaszewski A, Kerr C (2007) Risk of warfarin-related bleeding events and supratherapeutic international normalized ratios associated with complementary and alternative medicine: a longitudinal analysis. Pharmacotherapy. 27(9):1237–47 (Abstract).

Sharifzadeh F, Kashanian M, Koohpayehzadeh J, Rezaian F, Sheikhansari N, Eshraghi N (2017) A comparison between the effects of ginger, pyridoxine (vitamin B6) and placebo for the treatment of the first trimester nausea and vomiting of pregnancy (NVP). The Journal of Maternal-Fetal and Neonatal Medicine. doi: 10.1080/14767058.2017.1344965.

Shawahna R, Taha A (2017) Which potential harms and benefits of using ginger in the management of nausea and vomiting of pregnancy should be addressed? A consensual study among pregnant women and gynaecologists. BMC Complementary and Alternative Medicine. 17:204.

Sheidaei A, Abadi A, Zayeri F, Nahidi F, Gazerani N, Mansouri A (2016) The effectiveness of massage therapy in the treatment of infantile colic symptoms: a randomized controlled trial. Medical Journal of the Islamic Republic of Iran. 30:351.

Sheikhan F, Jahdi F, Khoei EM, Shamsalizadeh N, Sheikhan M, Haghani H (2012) Episiotomy pain relief: use of lavender oil essence in primiparous Iranian women. Complementary Therapies in Clinical Practice. 18(1):66–70.

Shin HS, Song YA, Seo S (2007) Effect of Nei-Guan point (P6) acupressure on ketonuria levels, nausea and vomiting in women with hyperemesis gravidarum. Journal of Advanced Nursing. 59(5):510–19.

Shirazi M, Mohebitabar S, Bioos S, Yekaninejad MS *et al.* (2016) The effect of topical Rosa damascena (rose) oil on pregnancy-related low back pain: a randomized controlled clinical trial. Journal of Evidence-Based Complementary and Alternative Medicine. 22(1):121–6. pii: 2156587216654601.

Shuster J (1996) Black cohosh root? Chasteberry tree? Seizures! Hospital Pharmacy. 31:1553–4.

Sibbritt D, Catling CJ, Adams J, Shaw AJ, Homer CS (2014) The self-prescribed use of aromatherapy oils by pregnant women. Women and Birth. 27(1):41–5.

Sibbritt D, Ladanyi S, Adams J (2016) Healthcare practitioner utilisation for back pain, neck pain and/or pelvic pain during pregnancy: an analysis of 1835 pregnant women in Australia. International Journal of Clinical Practice. 70(10):825–31.

Sienkiewicz M, Głowacka A, Kowalczyk E, Wiktorowska-Owczarek A, Jóźwiak-Bębenista M, Łysakowska M (2014) The biological activities of cinnamon, geranium and lavender essential oils. Molecules. 19(12):20929–40.

Sigurjónsdóttir HA, Franzson L, Manhem K, Ragnarsson J, Sigurdsson G, Wallerstedt S (2001) Liquorice-induced rise in blood pressure: a linear dose-response relationship. Journal of Human Hypertension. 15(8):549–52.

Silva F, Brito RS, Carvalho JB, Lopes TR (2016) Using acupressure to minimize discomforts during pregnancy. Revista Gaucha de Enfermagem. Viewed online 21/09/2017 at www.scielo.br/scielo.php?pid=S1983-14472016000200412&script=sci_arttext&tlng=en

Silva F, Dias F, Costa G, da Graça Campos M (2017) Chamomile reveals to be a potent galactogogue: the unexpected effect. The Journal of Maternal-Fetal and Neonatal Medicine. Apr, 101–3. doi: 10.1080/14767058.2016.1274300.

Sim TF, Sherriff J, Hattingh HL, Parsons R, Tee LB (2013) The use of herbal medicines during breastfeeding: a population-based survey in Western Australia. BMC Complementary and Alternative Medicine. 13:317.

Simavli S, Gumus I, Kaygusuz I, Yildirim M, Usluogullari B, Kafali H (2014) Effect of music on labor pain relief, anxiety level and postpartum analgesic requirement: a randomized controlled clinical trial. Gynecologic and Obstetric Investigation. 78(4):244–50.

Simon EP, Schwartz J (1999) Medical hypnosis for hyperemesis gravidarum. Birth. 26(4):248–54.

Simsek G, Sari E, Kilic R, Bayar Muluk N (2016) Topical application of arnica and mucopolysaccharide polysulfate attenuates periorbital edema and ecchymosis in open rhinoplasty: a randomized controlled clinical study. Plastic and Reconstructive Surgery. 137(3):530e–535e.

Singh N, Tripathi R, Manikya Mala Y, Yedla N (2014) Breast stimulation in low-risk primigravidas at term: does it aid in spontaneous onset of labour and vaginal delivery? A pilot study. BioMed Research International. Article ID 695037. http://dx.doi.org/10.1155/2014/695037

Singh SK, Barreto GE, Aliev G, Echeverria V (2016) Ginkgo biloba as an alternative medicine in the treatment of anxiety in dementia and other psychiatric disorders. Current Drug Metabolism. 18(2):112–19.

Sinha A, Paech MJ, Thew ME, Rhodes M, Luscombe K, Nathan E (2011) A randomised, double-blinded, placebo-controlled study of acupressure wristbands for the prevention of nausea and vomiting during labour and delivery. International Journal of Obstetric Anesthesia. 20(2):110–17.

Sites DS, Johnson NT, Miller JA, Torbush PH *et al.* (2014) Controlled breathing with or without peppermint aromatherapy for postoperative nausea and/or vomiting symptom relief: a randomized controlled trial. Journal of Perianesthesia Nursing. 29(1):12–19.

Skjeie H, Skonnord T, Fetveit A, Brekke M (2013) Acupuncture for infantile colic: a blinding-validated, randomized controlled multicentre trial in general practice. Scandinavian Journal of Primary Health Care. 31(4):190–6.

Sklempe Kokic I, Ivanisevic M, Uremovic M, Kokic T, Pisot R, Simunic B (2017) Effect of therapeutic exercises on pregnancy-related low back pain and pelvic girdle pain: secondary analysis of a randomized controlled trial. Journal of Rehabilitation Medicine. 49(3):251–7.

Slater PM (2015) Post-traumatic stress disorder managed successfully with hypnosis and the rewind technique: two cases in obstetric patients. International Journal of Obstetric Anesthesia. 24(3):272–5.

Smith CA (2010) Homeopathy for induction of labour. Cochrane Pregnancy and Childbirth Group. doi: 10.1002/14651858.CD003399

Smith CA, Betts D (2014) The practice of acupuncture and moxibustion to promote cephalic version for women with a breech presentation: implications for clinical practice and research. Complementary Therapies in Medicine. 22(1):75–80.

Smith CA, Collins CT, Crowther CA (2011a) Aromatherapy for pain management in labour. Cochrane Database of Systematic Reviews. (7):CD009215.

Smith CA, Collins CT, Crowther CA, Levett KM (2011b) Acupuncture or acupressure for pain management in labour. Cochrane Database of Systematic Reviews. (7):CD009232.

Smith CA, Crowther CA, Grant SJ (2013) Acupuncture for induction of labour. Cochrane Database of Systematic Reviews. (8):CD002962.

Sobrinho LG (2003) Prolactin, psychological stress and environment in humans: adaptation and maladaptation. Pituitary. 6(1):35–9.

Sobrinho LG, Simões M, Barbosa L, Raposo JF *et al.* (2003) Cortisol, prolactin, growth hormone and neurovegetative responses to emotions elicited during an hypnoidal state. Psychoneuroendocrinology. 28(1):1–17.

Soh KS, Kang KA, Ryu YH (2013) 50 years of bong-han theory and 10 years of primo vascular system. Evidence-Based Complementary and Alternative Medicine. 2013:587827. Viewed online 21/09/2017 at www.ncbi.nlm.nih.gov/pmc/articles/PMC3747427

Solcà M, Mottaz A, Guggisberg AG (2016) Binaural beats increase interhemispheric alpha-band coherence between auditory cortices. Hearing Research. 332:233–7.

Soliday E, Hapke P (2014) Patient expectations of acupuncture in pregnancy. Global Advances in Health and Medicine. 3(4):14–19.

Sorrentino L, Piraneo S, Riggio E, Basilicò S *et al.* (2017) Is there a role for homeopathy in breast cancer surgery? A first randomized clinical trial on treatment with Arnica montana to reduce post-operative seroma and bleeding in patients undergoing total mastectomy. Journal of Intercultural Ethnopharmacology. 6(1):1–8.

Spinella M (2001) Herbal medicines and epilepsy: the potential for benefit and adverse effects. Prostaglandins, Leukotrienes and Essential Fatty Acids. 77(2):101–3.

Spolarich AE, Andrews L (2007) An examination of the bleeding complications associated with herbal supplements, antiplatelet and anticoagulant medications. Journal of Dental Hygiene. 81(3):67.

Sridharan S, Archer N, Manning N (2009) Premature constriction of the fetal ductus arteriosus following the maternal consumption of camomile herbal tea. Ultrasound in Obstetrics and Gynecology. 34(3):358–9.

Sripramote M, Lekhyananda N (2003) A randomized comparison of ginger and vitamin B6 in the treatment of nausea and vomiting of pregnancy. Journal of the Medical Association of Thailand. 86(9):846–53.

Stapleton DB, MacLennan AH, Kristiansson P (2002) The prevalence of recalled low back pain during and after pregnancy: a South Australian population survey. Australian and New Zealand Journal of Obstetrics and Gynaecology. 42(5):482–5.

Steel A, Frawley J, Sibbritt D, Broom A, Adams J (2016) The characteristics of women who use hypnotherapy for intrapartum pain management: preliminary insights from a nationally-representative sample of Australian women. Complementary Therapies in Medicine. 25:67–70.

Steingrub JS, Lopez T, Teres D, Steingart R (1988) Amniotic fluid embolism associated with castor oil ingestion. Critical Care Medicine. 16(6):642–3.

Stenglin M, Foureur M (2013) Designing out the fear cascade to increase the likelihood of normal birth. Midwifery. 29(8):819–25.

Stickel F, Seitz HK (2000) The efficacy and safety of comfrey. Public Health Nutrition. 3(4A):501–8.

Strandberg TE, Andersson S, Järvenpää AL, McKeigue PM (2002) Preterm birth and licorice consumption during pregnancy. American Journal of Epidemiology. 156(9):803–5.

Strandberg TE, Järvenpää AL, Vanhanen H, McKeigue PM (2001) Birth outcome in relation to licorice consumption during pregnancy. American Journal of Epidemiology. 153(11):1085–8.

Streibert LA, Reinhard J, Yuan J, Schiermeier S, Louwen F (2015) Clinical study: change in outlook towards birth after a midwife led antenatal education programme versus hypnoreflexogenous self-hypnosis training for childbirth. Geburtshilfe und Frauenheilkunde. 75(11):1161–6.

Stub T, Alraek T, Salamonsen A (2012) The red flag! Risk assessment among medical homeopaths in Norway: a qualitative study. BMC Complementary and Alternative Medicine. 12:150.

Suranyi S, Nagy T (1957) Energetic dehydration as a simple and harmless measure for induction of labor. Zeitschrift für Geburtshilfe und Gynäkologie. 148(2):137–49.

Sutar R, Yadav S, Desai G (2016) Yoga intervention and functional pain syndromes: a selective review. International Review of Psychiatry. 28(3):316–22.

Suzuki M, Isonishi S, Morimoto O, Ogawa M, Ochiai K (2012) Effect of sophrology on perinatal stress monitored by biopyrrin. Open Journal of Obstetrics and Gynaecology. 2(2):176–81.

Taavoni S, Abdolahian S, Haghani H (2013) Effect of sacrum-perineum heat therapy on active phase labor pain and client satisfaction: a randomized, controlled trial study. Pain Medicine. 14(9):1301–6.

Tabatabaee A, Tafreshi MZ, Rassouli M, Aledavood SA, AlaviMajd H, Farahmand SK (2016) Effect of therapeutic touch in patients with cancer: a literature review. Medical Archives. 70(2):142–7.

Tafazoli M, Saeedi R, Gholami Robatsangi M, Mazloom R (2010) Aloe vera gel vs. lanolin ointment in the treatment of nipple sore: arandomized clinical trial. Tehran University Medical Journal. 67:699–704 (Abstract).

Taghinejad H, Delpisheh A, Suhrabi Z (2010) Comparison between massage and music therapies to relieve the severity of labor pain. Women's Health (London). 6(3):377–81.

Tam TW, Liu R, Saleem A, Arnason JT et al. (2014) The effect of Cree traditional medicinal teas on the activity of human cytochrome P450-mediated metabolism. Journal of Ethnopharmacology. 155(1):841–6.

Tamer S, Öz M, Ülger Ö (2016) Effects of sacroiliac joint mobilization on hamstring muscle flexibility and quadriceps muscle strength. Orthopaedic Journal of Sports Medicine. 2(3 Suppl):2325967114S00174.

Tan PC, Andi N, Azmi A, Noraihan MN (2006) Effect of coitus at term on length of gestation, induction of labor, and mode of delivery. Obstetrics and Gynecology. 108(1):134–40.

Taavoni S, Sheikhan F, Abdolahian S, Ghavi F (2016) Birth ball or heat therapy? A randomized controlled trial to compare the effectiveness of birth ball usage with sacrum-perineal heat therapy in labor pain management. Complementary Therapies in Clinical Practice. 24:99–102.

Takayama S, Seki T, Watanabe M, Takashima S et al. (2011) Changes of blood flow volume in the superior mesenteric artery and brachial artery with abdominal thermal stimulation. Evidence-Based Complementary and Alternative Medicine. 2011:214089.

Tanchoco N, Aguilar AS (2015) Cervical priming prior to operative hysteroscopy: a randomized controlled study comparing the efficacy of laminaria versus evening primrose oil (EPO). Journal of Minimally Invasive Gynecology. 22(6S):S45.

Taussig SJ, Batkin S (1988) Bromelain, the enzyme complex of pineapple (Ananas comosus) and its clinical application: an update. Journal of Ethnopharmacology. 22(2):191–203.

Teng L, Shaw D, Barnes J (2015) Characteristics and practices of Traditional Chinese Medicine retail shops in London, UK: a cross-sectional study using an observational approach. Journal of Ethnopharmacology. 173:318–29.

Teoh CS, Aizul MHI, Wan Fatimah Suriyani WM, Ang SH et al. (2013) Herbal ingestion during pregnancy and post-partum period is a cause for concern. Medical Journal of Malaysia. 68(2):157–60.

Thaler K, Kaminski A, Chapman A, Langley T, Gartlehner G (2009) Bach Flower Remedies for psychological problems and pain: a systematic review. BMC Complementary and Alternative Medicine. 9:16.

Thomson M, Corbin R, Leung L (2014) Effects of ginger for nausea and vomiting in early pregnancy: a meta-analysis. Journal of the American Board of Family Medicine. 27(1):115–22.

Thomson P, Jones J, Browne M, Leslie SJ (2014) Why people seek complementary and alternative medicine before conventional medical treatment: a population based study. Complementary Therapies in Clinical Practice. 20:339–46.

Thring TS, Hili P, Naughton D (2011) Antioxidant and potential anti-inflammatory activity of extracts and formulations of white tea, rose, and witch hazel on primary human dermal fibroblast cells. Journal of Inflammation (London, England). 8:27.

Ticktin T, Dalle SP (2005) Medicinal plant use in the practice of midwifery in rural Honduras. Journal of Ethnopharmacology. 96:233–48.

Tiran D (2000) Clinical Aromatherapy for Pregnancy and Childbirth, 2nd edition. Edinburgh: Churchill Livingstone.

Tiran D (2004) Nausea and Vomiting in Pregnancy: An Integrated Approach to Care. Edinburgh: Churchill Livingstone.

Tiran D (2010a) Avoiding the Chinese whispers effect in maternity complementary therapies: educational issues for midwives. MIDIRS Midwifery Digest. 20(1):15–19.

Tiran D (2010b) Reflexology in Pregnancy and Childbirth. Edinburgh: Elsevier.

Tiran D (2011) The need to include the subject of natural remedies in midwifery education. Complementary Therapies in Clinical Practice. 17(4):187–8.

Tiran D (2012) Ginger to reduce nausea and vomiting during pregnancy: evidence of effectiveness is not the same as proof of safety. Complementary Therapies in Clinical Practice. 18(1):22–5.

Tiran D (2014a) Aromatherapy in Midwifery Practice: Draft Clinical Guidelines for NHS Trusts. London: Expectancy.

Tiran D (2014b) Maternity Complementary Therapies: Professional Code of Practice. London: Expectancy.

Tiran D (2016a) Aromatherapy in Midwifery Practice. London: Singing Dragon.

Tiran D (2016b) Hot topic: aromatherapy in midwifery, a cause for concern? MIDIRS. Viewed online 21/09/2017 at www.midirs.org/aromatherapy-in-midwifery-cause-for-concern

Tiran D (2017) Baillière's Midwives' Dictionary, 13th edition. Edinburgh: Baillière Tindall.

Tiran D, Mack S (2000) Complementary Therapies for Pregnancy and Birth, 2nd edition. Edinburgh: Baillière Tindall.

Tiran D, Mackereth P (2010) Clinical Reflexology: A Guide for Integrated Practice. Edinburgh: Churchill Livingstone.

Tisserand R (2010) Is clary sage oil estrogenic? Viewed online 25/10/2017 at http://roberttisserand.com/2010/04/is-clary-sage-oil-estrogenic

Tito A, Bimonte M, Carola A, De Lucia A et al. (2015) An oil-soluble extract of Rubus idaeus cells enhances hydration and water homeostasis in skin cells. International Journal of Cosmetic Science. 37(6):588–94.

Todd AJ, Carroll MT, Robinson A, Mitchell EK (2015) Adverse events due to chiropractic and other manual therapies for infants and children: a review of the literature. Journal of Manipulative and Physiological Therapeutics. 38(9):699–712.

Torkzahrani S, Ghobadi K, Heshmat R, Shakeri N, Jalali Aria K (2015) Effect of acupressure on cervical ripening. Iranian Red Crescent Medical Journal. 17(8):e28691. doi:10.5812/ircmj.28691.

Torkzahrani S, Mahmoudikohani F, Saatchi K, Sefidkar R, Banaei M (2017) The effect of acupressure on the initiation of labor: a randomized controlled trial. Women and Birth. 30(1):46–50.

Tovey P (2002) A single-blind trial of reflexology for irritable bowel syndrome. British Journal of General Practice. 52(474):19–23.

Tozer J (2009) Midwife struck off after her error led to pregnant patient drinking aromatherapy oils. Daily Mail, 7 August 2009. Viewed online 21/09/2017 at www.dailymail.co.uk/news/article-1205011/Midwife-struck-giving-pregnant-woman-cup-aromatherapy-oils-DRINK-headache-cure.html

Trabace L, Tucci P, Ciuffreda L, Matteo M, Fortunato F, Campolongo P, Trezza V, Cuomo V (2015) "Natural" relief of pregnancy-related symptoms and neonatal outcomes: above all do no harm. Journal of Ethnopharmacology 174:396–402.

Tuchin PJ (1998) The effect of chiropractic spinal manipulative therapy on salivary cortisol levels. Australasian Chiropractic and Osteopathy. 7(2):86–92.

Tunaru S, Althoff TF, Nüsing RM, Diener M, Offermanns S (2012) Castor oil induces laxation and uterus contraction via ricinoleic acid activating prostaglandin EP3 receptors. Proceedings of the National Academy of Sciences (USA). 109(23):9179–84.

Turan N, Aşt TA (2016) The effect of abdominal massage on constipation and quality of life. Gastroenterology Nursing. 39(1):48–59.

Turkyılmaz C, Onal E, Hirfanoglu IM, Turan O et al. (2011) The effect of galactagogue herbal tea on breast milk production and short-term catch-up of birth weight in the first week of life. Journal of Alternative and Complementary Medicine. 17(2):139–42.

Tuuli MG, Keegan MB, Odibo AO, Roehl K, Macones GA, Cahill AG (2013) Progress of labor in women induced with misoprostol versus the Foley catheter. American Journal of Obstetric Gynecology. 209(3):237.e1–7.

Ty-Torredes KA (2006) The effect of oral evening primrose oil on Bishop score and cervical length amongst term gravidas. American Journal of Obstetric Gynecology. 195(6 Suppl 1):S30.

Uebelacker LA, Battle CL, Sutton KA, Magee SR, Miller IW (2016) A pilot randomized controlled trial comparing prenatal yoga to perinatal health education for antenatal depression. Archives of Women's Mental Health. 19(3):543–7.

Ulbricht C, Armstrong J, Basch E, Basch S et al. (2007) An evidence-based systematic review of Aloe vera by the natural standard research collaboration. Journal of Herbal Pharmacotherapy. 7(3–4):279–323.

Unger M, Frank A (2004) Simultaneous determination of the inhibitory potency of herbal extracts on the activity of six major cytochrome P450 enzymes using liquid chromatography/mass spectrometry and automated online extraction. Rapid Communications in Mass Spectrometry. 18(19):2273–81 (Abstract).

Uppal E, Manley J, Schofield A (2016) Pilates for pregnancy and beyond: a study. The Practising Midwife. 19(5):25–7.

Usman MI, Abubakar MK, Muhammad S, Rabiu A, Garba I (2017) Low back pain in pregnant women attending antenatal clinic: the Aminu Kano teaching hospital experience. Annals of African Medicine. 16(3):136–40.

Uvnäs-Moberg K (1998) Oxytocin may mediate the benefits of positive social interaction and emotions. Psychoneuroendocrinology. 23(8):819–35.

Vacillotto G, Favretto D, Seraglia R, Pagiotti R, Traldi P, Mattoli L (2013) A rapid and highly specific method to evaluate the presence of pyrrolizidine alkaloids in Boragoofficinalis seed oil. Journal of Mass Spectrometry. 48(10):1078–82.

Vakilian K, Atarha M, Bekhradi R, Chaman R (2011) Healing advantages of lavender essential oil during episiotomy recovery: a clinical trial. Complementary Therapies in Clinical Practice. 17(1):50–3.

Vakilian K, Keramat A (2013) The effect of the breathing technique with and without aromatherapy on the length of the active phase and second stage of labor. Nursing and Midwifery Studies. 2(1):115–19.

Valiani M, Shiran E, Kianpour M, Hasanpour M (2010) Reviewing the effect of reflexology on the pain and certain features and outcomes of the labor on the primiparous women. Iranian Journal of Nursing and Midwifery Research. 15(Suppl 1):302–10.

Valizadeh L, Seyyedrasooli A, Zamanazadeh V, Nasiri K (2015) Comparing the effects of reflexology and footbath on sleep quality in the elderly: a controlled clinical trial. Iranian Red Crescent Medical Journal. 17(11):e20111.

Vallim AL, Osis MJ, Cecatti JG, Baciuk ÉP, Silveira C, Cavalcante SR (2011) Water exercises and quality of life during pregnancy. Reproductive Health. 8:14.

van den Berg I, Bosch JL, Jacobs B, Bouman I, Duvekot JJ, Hunink MG (2008) Effectiveness of acupuncture-type interventions versus expectant management to correct breech presentation: a systematic review. Complementary Therapies in Medicine. 16(2):92–100.

van den Berg I, Kaandorp GC, Bosch JL, Duvekot JJ, Arends LR, Hunink MG (2010) Cost-effectiveness of breech version by acupuncture-type interventions on BL 67, including moxibustion, for women with a breech foetus at 33 weeks gestation: a modelling approach. Complementary Therapies in Medicine. 18(2):67–77.

van den Heuvel E, Goossens M, Vanderhaegen H, Sun HX, Buntinx F (2016) Effect of acustimulation on nausea and vomiting and on hyperemesis in pregnancy: a systematic review of Western and Chinese literature. BMC Complementary and Alternative Medicine. 16:13.

van der Kooi R, Theobald S (2006) Traditional medicine in late pregnancy and labour: perceptions of kgaba remedies amongst the Tswana in South Africa. African Journal of Traditional, Complementary and Alternative Medicines. 3(1):11–22.

van Exsel DC, Pool SM, van Uchelen JH, Edens MA, van der Lei B, Melenhorst WB (2016) Arnica ointment 10% does not improve upper blepharoplasty outcome: a randomized, placebo-controlled trial. Plastic and Reconstructive Surgery. 138(1):66–73.

van Kampen M, Devoogdt N, De Groef A, Gielen A, Geraerts I (2015) The efficacy of physiotherapy for the prevention and treatment of prenatal symptoms: a systematic review. International Urogynecological Journal. 26(11):1575–86.

Vanderperren B, Rizzo M, Angenot L, Haufroid V, Jadoul M, Hantson P (2005) Acute liver failure with renal impairment related to the abuse of senna anthraquinone glycosides. Annals of Pharmacotherapy. 39(7–8):1353–7.

Vandervaart S, Berger H, Tam C, Goh YI et al. (2011) The effect of distant reiki on pain in women after elective Caesarean section: a double-blinded randomised controlled trial. BMJ Open. 1(1):e000021.

Varshney JP, Naresh R (2005) Comparative efficacy of homeopathic and allopathic systems of medicine in the management of clinical mastitis of Indian dairy cows. Homeopathy. 94(2):81–5.

Vas J, Aranda JM, Nishishinya B, Mendez C et al. (2009) Correction of nonvertex presentation with moxibustion: a systematic review and metaanalysis. American Journal of Obstetric Gynecology. 201(3):241–59.

Vas J, Aranda-Regules JM, Modesto M, Ramos-Monserrat M et al. (2013) Using moxibustion in primary healthcare to correct non-vertex presentation: a multicentre randomised controlled trial. Acupuncture in Medicine. 31(1):31–8.

Venkatramani DV, Goel S, Ratra V, Gandhi RA (2013) Toxic optic neuropathy following ingestion of homeopathic medication Arnica-30. Cutaneous and Ocular Toxicology. 32(1):95–7.

Vidas M, Folnegović-Smalc V, Catipović M, Kisić M (2011) The application of autogenic training in counseling center for mother and child in order to promote breastfeeding. Collegium Antropologicum. 35(3):723–31. Abstract viewed online 21/09/2017 at www.ncbi.nlm.nih.gov/pubmed/22053548

Viljoen E, Visser J, Koen N, Musekiwa A (2014) A systematic review and meta-analysis of the effect and safety of ginger in the treatment of pregnancy-associated nausea and vomiting. Nutrition Journal. 13:20.

Villani V, Prosperini L, Palombini F, Orzi F, Sette G (2017) Single-blind, randomized, pilot study combining shiatsu and amitriptyline in refractory primary headaches. Neurological Sciences. 38(6):999–1007.

Visconti L, Capra G, Carta G, Forni C, Janin D (2015) Effect of massage on DOMS in ultramarathon runners: a pilot study. Journal of Bodywork and Movement Therapies. 19(3):458–63.

Vitetta L, Thomsen M, Sali A (2003) Black cohosh and other herbal remedies associated with acute hepatitis. Medical Journal of Australia. 148(8):411–2.

Vithoulkas G (2017) Serious mistakes in meta-analysis of homeopathic research. Journal of Medicine and Life. 10(1):47–9.

Vixner L, Mårtensson LB, Schytt E (2015) Acupuncture with manual and electrical stimulation for labour pain: a two month follow up of recollection of pain and birth experience. BMC Complementary and Alternative Medicine. 15:180.

Vixner L, Schytt E, Stener-Victorin E, Waldenström U, Pettersson H, Mårtensson LB (2014) Acupuncture with manual and electrical stimulation for labour pain: a longitudinal randomised controlled trial. BMC Complementary and Alternative Medicine. 14:187.

von Rühle G (1995) Pilot study of Bach flower essences administered to first-time mothers in prolonged pregnancy. Erfahrungsheilkunde. 44(12):854–60 (Abstract).

Walach H, Rilling C, Engelke U (2001) Efficacy of Bach-flower remedies in test anxiety: a double-blind, placebo-controlled, randomized trial with partial crossover. Journal of Anxiety Disorders. 15(4):359–66.

Waller B, Lambeck J, Daly D (2009) Therapeutic aquatic exercise in the treatment of low back pain: a systematic review. Clinical Rehabilitation. 23(1):3–14.

Wang JY, Chen R, Chen SP, Gao YH et al. (2016) Electroacupuncture reduces the effects of acute noxious stimulation on the electrical activity of pain-related neurons in the hippocampus of control and neuropathic pain rats. Neural Plasticity. 2016:6521026. Viewed online 21/09/2017 at www.hindawi.com/journals/np/2016/6521026

Wang LL, Nankorn W, Fukui K (2003) Food and medicinal plants used for childbirth among Yunanese Chinese in Northern Thailand. Journal of Ethnobiology. 23:209–26.

Wang WB, Yang LF, He QS, Li T et al. (2016) Mechanisms of electroacupuncture effects on acute cerebral ischemia/reperfusion injury: possible association with upregulation of transforming growth factor beta 1. Neural Regeneration Research. 11(7):1099–101.

Wanyua S, Kaneko S, Karama M, Makokha A et al. (2014) Roles of traditional birth attendants and perceptions of the policy discouraging home delivery in coastal Kenya. East African Medical Journal. 91(3):83–93.

Warriner S, Bryan K, Brown AM (2014) Women's attitude towards the use of complementary and alternative medicines (CAM) in pregnancy. Midwifery. 30:138–43.

Waterfield J, Bartlam B, Bishop A, Holden MA, Barlas P, Foster NE (2015) Physical therapists' views and experiences of pregnancy-related low back pain and the role of acupuncture: qualitative exploration. Physical Therapy. 95(9):1234–43.

Wedig KE, Whitsett JA (2008) Down the primrose path: petechiae in a neonate exposed to herbal remedy for parturition. International Journal of Cancer. 85(5):643–8.

Wei L, Wang H, Han Y, Li C (2008) Clinical observation on the effects of electroacupuncture at Shaoze (SI 1) in 46 cases of postpartum insufficient lactation. Journal of Traditional Chinese Medicine. 28(3):168–72.

Weis CA, Nash J, Triano JJ, Barrett J (2017) Ultrasound assessment of abdominal muscle thickness in women with and without low back pain during pregnancy. Journal of Manipulative and Physiological Therapeutics. 40(4):230–5.

Weis CA, Triano JJ, Barrett J, Campbell MD, Croy M, Roeder J (2015) Ultrasound assessment of abdominal muscle thickness in postpartum vs nulliparous women. Journal of Manipulative and Physiological Therapeutics. 38(5):352–7.

Weizman Z, Alkrinawi S, Goldfarb D, Bitran C (1993) Efficacy of herbal tea preparation in infantile colic. Journal of Pediatrics. 122(4):650–2.

Wells C, Kolt GS, Marshall P, Hill B, Bialocerkowski A (2014) The effectiveness of Pilates exercise in people with chronic low back pain: a systematic review. Viewed online 21/09/2017 at http://journals.plos.org/plosone/article?id=10.1371/journal.pone.0100402

Werner A, Uldbjerg N, Zachariae R, Rosen G, Nohr EA (2013) Self-hypnosis for coping with labour pain: a randomised control trial. BJOG. 120(3):346–53.

Weston M, Grabowska C (2013) Complementary therapy for induction of labour. The Practising Midwife. 16(8):S16–18.

White A (2004) A cumulative review of the range and incidence of significant adverse events associated with acupuncture. Acupuncture in Medicine. 22(3):122–33.

White A, Hayhoe S, Hart A, Ernst E (2001) Adverse events following acupuncture: prospective survey of 32,000 consultations with doctors and physiotherapists. BMJ. 323:485.

Whiting PW, Clouston A, Kerlin P (2003) Black cohosh and other herbal remedies associated with acute hepatitis. Maturitas. 44(Suppl 1):S67–77.

Wiberg KR, Wiberg JM (2010) Retrospective study of chiropractic treatment of 276 Danish infants with infantile colic. Journal of Manipulative and Physiological Therapeutics. 33(7):536–41A.

Wibowo N, Purwosunu Y, Sekizawa A, Farina A, Tambunan V, Bardosono S (2012) Vitamin B6 supplementation in pregnant women with nausea and vomiting. International Journal of Gynecology and Obstetrics. 116(3):206–10.

Williamson M, Gregory C (2015) Hypnotherapy: the salutogenic solution to dealing with phobias. The Practising Midwife. 18(5):35–7.

Wilson PM, Greiner MV, Duma EM (2012) Posterior rib fractures in a young infant who received chiropractic care. Pediatrics. 130(5):e1359–62.

Witt CM, Pach D, Brinkhaus B, Wruck K et al. (2009) Safety of acupuncture: results of a prospective observational study with 229,230 patients and introduction of a medical information and consent form. Forschende Komplementärmedizin. 16(2):91–7.

Wolf TG, Wolf D, Below D, d'Hoedt B, Willershausen B, Daubländer M (2016) Effectiveness of self-hypnosis on the relief of experimental dental pain: a randomized trial. International Journal of Clinical and Experimental Hypnosis. 64(2):187–99.

Wolff M, Rogers K, Erdal B, Chalmers JP, Sundquist K, Midlöv P (2016) Impact of a short home-based yoga programme on blood pressure in patients with hypertension: a randomized controlled trial in primary care. Journal of Human Hypertension. 30(10):599–605.

Wood S, Cooper S, Ross S (2014) Does induction of labour increase the risk of caesarean section? A systematic review and meta-analysis of trials in women with intact membranes. BJOG. 121:674–85.

Wu M, Hu Y, Ali Z, Khan IA, Verlangeiri AJ, Dasmahapatra AK (2010) Teratogenic effects of blue cohosh (Caulophyllum thalictroides) in Japanese medaka (Oryzias latipes) are probably mediated through GATA2/EDN1 signaling pathway. Chemical Research in Toxicology. 23(8):1405–16.

Wuttke W, Seidlova-Wuttke D, Gorkow C (2003) The Cimicifuga preparation BNO 1055 vs. conjugated estrogens in a double-blind placebo-controlled study: effects on menopause symptoms and bone markers. Medical Journal of Australia. 179(7):390–1.

Wye L, Shaw L, Sharp D (2013) Same difference? Complementary therapy consultations delivered in NHS and private settings – a qualitative study. European Journal of Integrative Medicine. 5(4):339–46.

Xu J, Deng H, Shen X (2014) Safety of moxibustion: a systematic review of case reports. Evidence-Based Complementary and Alternative Medicine. Viewed online 21/09/2017 at www.hindawi.com/journals/ecam/2014/783704

Yamahara J, Miki K, Chisaka T, Sawada T et al. (1985) Cholagogic effect of ginger and its active constituents. Journal of Ethnopharmacology. 13(2):217–25.

Yamamoto S, Kagawa K, Hori N, Akezaki Y, Mori K, Nomura T (2016) Preliminary validation of an exercise program suitable for pregnant women with abnormal glucose metabolism: inhibitory effects of Tai Chi Yuttari-exercise on plasma glucose elevation. Journal of Physical Therapy Science. 28(12):3411–15.

Yang M, Chen X, Bo L, Lao L et al. (2017) Moxibustion for pain relief in patients with primary dysmenorrhea: a randomized controlled trial. PLoS One. 12(2):e0170952.

Yang X, Xiong X, Yang G, Wang J (2014) Effectiveness of stimulation of acupoint ki 1 by artemisia vulgaris (moxa) for the treatment of essential hypertension: a systematic review of randomized controlled trials. Evidence-Based Complementary and Alternative Medicine. Viewed online 21/09/2017 at www.hindawi.com/journals/ecam/2014/187484

Yao M, Ritchie HE, Brown-Woodman PD (2006) A reproductive screening test of feverfew: is a full reproductive study warranted? Reproductive Toxicology. 22(4):688–93.

Yardley L, Dennison L, Coker R, Webley F et al. (2010) Patients' views of receiving lessons in the Alexander technique and an exercise prescription for managing back pain in the ATEAM trial. Family Practice. 27(2):198–204.

Yasue H, Itoh T, Mizuno Y, Harada E (2007) Severe hypokalemia, rhabdomyolysis, muscle paralysis, and respiratory impairment in a hypertensive patient taking herbal medicines containing licorice. Internal Medicine. 46(9):575–8.

Yavari Kia P, Safajou F, Shahnazi M, Nazemiyeh H (2014) The effect of lemon inhalation aromatherapy on nausea and vomiting of pregnancy: a double-blinded, randomized, controlled clinical trial. Iranian Red Crescent Medical Journal. 16(3):e1436.

Yemele MD, Telefo PB, Lienou LL, Tagne SR et al. (2015) Ethnobotanical survey of medicinal plants used for pregnant women's health conditions in Menoua division-West Cameroon. Journal of Ethnopharmacology. 3(160):14–31.

Yip YB, Tse SH (2006) An experimental study on the effectiveness of acupressure with aromatic lavender essential oil for sub-acute, non-specific neck pain in Hong Kong. Complementary Therapies in Clinical Practice. 12(1):18–26.

Yoshida S, Takayama Y (2003) Licorice-induced hypokalemia as a treatable cause of dropped head syndrome. Clinical Neurology and Neurosurgery. 105(4):286–7.

Young E (2008) Maternal expectations: do they match experience? Community Practitioner. 81(10):27–30.

Young HY, Liao JC, Chang YS, Luo YL, Lu MC, Peng WH (2006) Synergistic effect of ginger and nifedipine on human platelet aggregation: a study in hypertensive patients and normal volunteers. American Journal of Chinese Medicine. 34(4):545–51.

Young SM, Benyshek DC (2010) In search of human placentophagy: a cross-cultural survey of human placenta consumption, disposal practices, and cultural beliefs. Ecology of Food and Nutrition. 49(6):467–84.

Yousuf Azeemi ST, Mohsin Raza S (2005) A critical analysis of chromotherapy and its scientific evolution. Evidence-Based Complementary and Alternative Medicine. 2(4):481–8.

Yu SH, Seol GH (2017) Lavandula angustifolia Mill. oil and its active constituent linalyl acetate alleviate pain and urinary residual sense after colorectal cancer surgery: a randomised controlled trial. Evidence-Based Complementary and Alternative Medicine. Viewed online 22/09/2017 at www.hindawi.com/journals/ecam/2017/3954181

Zafar S, Najam Y, Arif Z, Hafeez A (2016) A randomized controlled trial comparing Pentazocine and Chamomilla recutita for labor pain relief. Homeopathy. 105(1):66–70.

Zahra A, Leila MS (2013) Lavender aromatherapy massages in reducing labor pain and reduction of labor: a randomized controlled trial. African Journal of Pharmacy and Pharmacology. 7:426–30.

Zangeneh FZ, Minaee M, Amirzargar A, Ahangarpour A, Mousavizadeh K (2010) Effects of Chamomile extract on biochemical and clinical parameters in a rat model of polycystic ovary syndrome. Journal of Reproduction and Infertility. 11(3):169–74.

Zeng Y, Zhou Y, Chen P, Luo T, Huang M (2014) Use of complementary and alternative medicine across the childbirth spectrum in China. Complementary Therapies in Medicine. 22(6):1047–52.

Zhao BX, Chen HY, Shen XY, Lao L (2014) Can moxibustion, an ancient treatment modality, be evaluated in a double-blind randomized controlled trial? A narrative review. Journal of Integrative Medicine. 12(3):131–4.

Zheng J, Pistilli MJ, Holloway AC, Crankshaw DJ (2010) The effects of commercial preparations of red raspberry leaf on the contractility of the rat's uterus in vitro. Reproductive Sciences. 17(5):494–501 (Abstract).

Zhou HY, Li L, Li D, Li X et al. (2009) Clinical observation on the treatment of post-cesarean hypogalactia by auricular point sticking-pressing. Chinese Journal of Integrative Medicine. 15(2):117–20.

Zhou J, Fang L, Wu WY, He F et al. (2017) The effect of acupuncture on chemotherapy-associated gastrointestinal symptoms in gastric cancer. Current Oncology. 24(1):e1–e5.

Zhu LL, Zhou JY, Luo L, Wang X et al. (2017) Comparison of the efficacy between conventional moxibustion and smoke-free moxibustion on knee osteoarthritis: study protocol of a randomized controlled trial. Trials. 18(1):188.

Ziółkowska-Klinkosz M, Kedzia A, Meissner HO, Kedzia AW (2016) Evaluation of the tea tree oil activity to anaerobic bacteria: in vitro study. Acta Poloniae Pharmaceutica. 73(2):389–94.

Zuppa AA, Sindico P, Orchi C, Carducci C, Cardiello V, Romagnoli C (2010) Safety and efficacy of galactogogues: substances that induce, maintain and increase breast milk production. Journal of Pharmacy and Pharmaceutical Sciences. 13(2):162–74.

Subject Index

Author Index

CPI Antony Rowe
Eastbourne, UK
October 04, 2022